Series editor
Daniel Horton-Szar
BSc (Hons)
United Medical and Dental
Schools of Guy's and
St Thomas's Hospitals
(UMDS),
London

Faculty advisors
Susan Whitten
MA, PhD
Lecturer in Medical
Science,
School of Biological
and Medical Sciences,
University of St
Andrews,
Fife

Ian Campbell
MBChB, FRCP
(Edin & Glasg),
Consultant Physician,
Victoria Hospital,
Kilcaldy,
Fife

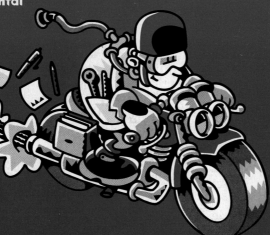

Endocrine and Reproductive Systems

Madeleine Debuse
BSc (Hons)
United Medical and Dental
Schools of Guy's and
St Thomas's Hospitals
(UMDS),
London

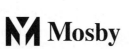

Mosby

London • Philadelphia
St Louis • Sydney • Tokyo

Publisher	Dianne Zack
Managing Editor	Louise Crowe
Development Editors	Filipa Maia
	Marion Jowett
Project Manager	Jane Tozer
Designer	Greg Smith
Layout	Rob Curran
Illustration Management	Danny Pyne
Illustrators	Evi Antoniou
	Kevin Faerber
	Deborah Maizels
	Jenni Miller
	Danny Pyne
	Mike Saiz
	Elisabeth Smith
	Annette Whalley
Cover Design	Greg Smith
Production	Gudrun Hughes
Index	Liza Weinkove

ISBN 0 7234 2996 0

Copyright © Mosby International Ltd, 1998.

Published by Mosby, an imprint of Mosby International Ltd, Lynton House, 7–12 Tavistock Square, London WC1H 9LB, UK.

Printed in Barcelona, Spain, by Grafos S.A. Arte sobre papel, 1998.
Text set in Crash Course–VAG Light; captions in Crash Course–VAG Thin.

Cataloguing in Publication Data
Catalogue records for this book are available from the British Library.

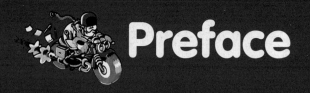

Preface

Professor Harold Ellis and Sir Roy Calne wrote in their textbook of General Surgery: 'The ideal medical student at the end of his clinical course will have written his own textbook—a digest of the lectures and tutorials he has assiduously attended and of the textbooks he had meticulously read.' I am not sure if they ever intended that students should actually publish their own textbooks, but a number of us at St Thomas's and Guy's Medical School have done just that!

This book aims to provide a complete overview of the endocrine and reproduction systems in a format that the majority of medical schools are now teaching—it integrates the relevant anatomy, biochemistry, physiology, pathology, and pharmacology, and gives an introduction to their clinical applications. As well as being packed with information, this text is rich in diagrams and tables to help you understand and remember the essential material. Hints and Tips boxes highlight important concepts and Comprehension Check boxes highlight the facts that the student should know from each section. Practising exam questions are always a useful way to revise and the self-assessment section, with its model answers, should be most helpful.

Good luck in your forthcoming exams—this text is designed to help you through your endocrinology and reproduction exams, but I also hope it encourages you to look further into this fascinating area of medicine.

Maddy Debuse

Medical education is in the process of dramatic change. The British General Medical Council has recommended that subject boundaries should be broken down and clinical applications introduced from the beginning of medical training. Integrated courses now illuminate basic science by emphasising clinical applications. We believe that the Crash Course series is an excellent example of this concept put into practice.

We know that medical students are educational experts! They are exposed to a vast range of teaching and learning experiences throughout their training. The extension of the traditional apprenticeship training in medicine to the creation of rapid review texts written by medical students for medical students seems an excellent idea. The undergraduate who has written this volume has created a lively, concise review based on her own recent learning experience. The text is integrated and user friendly, with a wealth of summary diagrams and helpful tables. It has pulled together the basic scientific concepts of endocrinology and reproduction and clearly linked them with clinical applications.

As Faculty Advisors for this title, we have reviewed the balance and accuracy of the text. We are delighted with this comprehensive overview of an increasingly important field and congratulate the young author for her effort in producing this book in the throes of medical studies!

Susie Whiten
Ian Campbell
Faculty Advisors

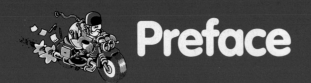

Preface

OK, no-one ever said medicine was going to be easy, but the thing is, there are very few parts of this enormous subject that are actually difficult to understand. The problem for most of us is the sheer volume of information that must be absorbed before each round of exams. It's not fun when time is getting short and you realize that: a) you really should have done a bit more work by now; and b) there are large gaps in your lecture notes that you meant to copy up but never quite got round to.

This series has been designed and written by senior medical students and doctors with recent experience of basic medical science exams. We've brought together all the information you need into compact, manageable volumes that integrate basic science with clinical skills. There is a consistent structure and layout across the series, and every title is checked for accuracy by senior faculty members from medical schools across the UK.

I hope this book makes things a little easier!

Danny Horton-Szar
Series Editor (Basic Medical Sciences)

Contents

Contents

Acknowledgements

I would like to thank all my lecturers at Durham University and St Thomas's and Guy's Hospitals for their stimulating teaching over the years. Thanks also to Anja Halfyard and Danny Horton-Szar for their contributions, to Dr Susie Whiten and Professor Ian Campbell for their direction, and to all those at Mosby who were involved with the book—dealing with novice authors can't have been easy! Finally I would like to acknowledge the support of my parents to whom this book is dedicated.

Figure Credits

Figures 3.1 and 10.16, adapted from *Human Histology 2e*, by A Stevens & J Lowe, Mosby, 1997.

Figure 10.5 adapted from *Clinical Examination* by GD Perkin and O Epstein, Mosby, 1997.

Figure 10.15 from *Integrated Pharmacology* by C Page, M Curtis, M Sutter, M Walker, and B Hoffman, Mosby, 1997.

Figures 11.7, 14.4, 14.8, 14.10, 14.11, 14.14, 14.15, 17.3, and 17.4 courtesy of *Fundamentals of Obstetrics and Gynaecolgy 6e*, by D Llewellyn-Jones, Mosby, 1994.

Figures 14.6, 14.7, 14.12, 14.13, 14.17, 14.18, 14.19, 14.20, and 14.21 from *Atlas of Endocrine Imaging* by M Besser and M Thorner, Mosby Europe Ltd, 1993.

Figure 14.9 from *A Colour Atlas of The Eye and Systemic Disease,* by EE Kritzinger and BE Wright, Wolfe Medical Publications Ltd, 1994.

Figure 14.16 from *A Colour Atlas of Endocrinology 2e,* by R Hall and D Evered, Wolfe Medical Publications Ltd, 1990.

To my parents

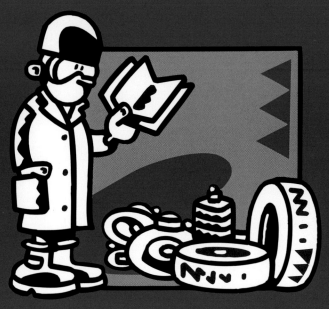

DEVELOPMENT, STRUCTURE, AND FUNCTION

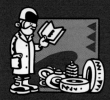

1. Overview of the Endocrine System

The role of the endocrine system

The endocrine and nervous systems regulate the body's internal environment, keeping it in a state of homoeostasis (Greek for 'staying the same'), and allow it to alter appropriately when the internal and external environments demand.

Both the endocrine and the nervous systems act by the release of chemical messengers that allow cells in different parts of the body to coordinate their activities.

- The nervous system releases neurotransmitters (e.g. acetylcholine, noradrenaline) from its nerve endings within the targeted tissues.
- The endocrine system releases hormones into the bloodstream from specialized ductless glands and tissues which may be a distance from the targeted tissues.

Endocrine glands and organs that contain endocrine tissue but have other primary functions are distributed throughout the body (Fig. 1.1).

The organization of the endocrine system

The endocrine system is coordinated by the hypothalamus and the anterior pituitary gland (see Chapter 2):

- The hypothalamic hormones control the secretion of the anterior pituitary hormones.
- The anterior pituitary hormones control the secretion of hormones from the peripheral endocrine organs.

Many peripheral tissues secrete hormones, but only the thyroid gland, parathyroid glands, and adrenal glands are primarily endocrine in function. Other glands and organs that have important endocrine roles, but are not primarily endocrine in function are shown in Fig. 1.1, e.g. the kidney secretes the hormones renin and erythropoietin, and activates the hormone vitamin D, but its primary functions are excretion and metabolism.

Furthermore, there are many other tissues and cells that also have an endocrine function, e.g. the skin is involved in the synthesis of the hormone vitamin D.

[NB Cells of the immune system secrete numerous chemical messengers called cytokines (e.g. interleukins, interferons, tumour necrosis factor) that regulate defence responses; however, these are not classified as true hormones and are covered in the *Crash Course! Immune, Blood, and Lymphatics*.

The following criteria are required to establish that an organ has an endocrine function:

- An endocrine organ contains specialized secretory cells that synthesize and release hormones *directly* into the bloodstream. The secretory cells can be distributed diffusely within an organ (e.g. gastrointestinal tract), form islets of cells embedded in an organ (e.g. endocrine pancreas), or constitute a discrete endocrine gland (e.g. thyroid gland).
- The function of the secretory cells is controlled by nervous, hormonal, or biochemical stimuli.
- The hormone released has specific actions on specific target cells.
- Pathology of the endocrine tissue causes physical or biochemical disorders, e.g. autoimmune damage to the pancreas causes diabetes mellitus; hyperplasia of the pituitary gland can cause enlargement of certain organs and facial changes (acromegaly).

- **What is the role of the endocrine system?**
- **Outline the organization of the endocrine system.**
- **List the criteria required to establish that an organ has an endocrine function.**

MECHANISMS OF HORMONE ACTIVITY

Role of hormones

The term 'hormone', first coined by Bayliss and Starling

in 1905, is derived from the Greek word *hormaein*, meaning 'to arouse' (although hormonal effects can be both stimulatory and inhibitory).

A hormone is a chemical substance that is secreted by specialized epithelial cells, without the benefit of a duct, into the extracellular space (and from here into the bloodstream), and which can act at long or short range, often slowly, on specific organs and tissues.

Hormones possibly control the function of every cell in the body—they act as chemical messengers, allowing cells in different parts of the body to coordinate their activities.

Hormones act alongside the nervous system to regulate a wide range of body functions, as shown in Fig. 1.2.

Mode of delivery of hormones

Hormones were classically described as being secreted into the bloodstream by ductless glands; however, it is now realized that hormones reach their target cells by a variety of methods (Fig. 1.3):

- **Autocrine delivery**—chemical message released acts on the cells that synthesized it, e.g. the cytokine prostaglandin E_2 stimulates the myometrial cells that produced it [NB Most 'true'

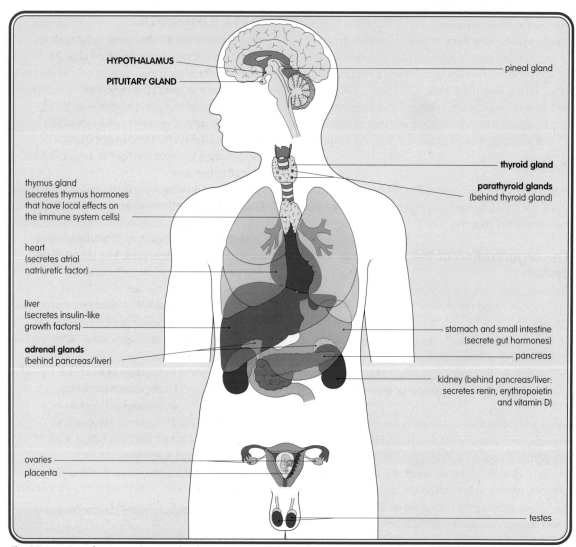

Fig. 1.1 Location of many endocrine glands, organs containing endocrine tissue, and their surrounding structures. The hypothalmus and the pituitary gland are the main controllers of the endocrine system. The glands shown in bold have a primarily endocrine function. The other glands and organs shown here have important endocrine roles but have other primary functions.

hormones do not classically have an autocrine action.]

- **Paracrine delivery**—chemical message or hormone released into the extracellular space acts on neighbouring or distant cells, e.g. *insulin* secreted in the pancreas acts on neighbouring cells to inhibit the secretion of the hormone glucagon; *histamine* released by mast cells affects nearby blood vessels to cause a local inflammatory reaction.
- **Endocrine delivery**—hormone released into the extracellular space circulates in the bloodstream or lymphatics and acts on cells at distant sites, e.g. *insulin* secreted by the pancreas has its effect throughout the body; *pituitary hormones* act on distant endocrine organs.
- **Neuroendocrine delivery**—chemical message or

hormone released into the extracellular space by nerve cells reaches the target cells in a paracrine or endocrine fashion, e.g. *gonadotrophin-releasing hormone* (GnRH), synthesized by nerves in the hypothalamus, is released into the portal blood system and acts on the anterior pituitary gland; the neurotransmitter *acetylcholine* is released by nerve end terminals and acts on neighbouring cells.
- **Pheromonal delivery**—volatile hormones (classified as pheromones) released into the environment act on olfactory cells in another individual (pheromones, although only found in other species, may be important in controlling human sexual behaviour).

Hormone classification

Hormones are classified into four major groups depending on their biochemical structure and method of synthesis:

Peptides and proteins
- Form the great majority of all hormones.
- Range in size from very small peptides with only three amino acids (e.g. thyrotrophin-releasing hormone—TRH) to small proteins with over 200 amino acids (e.g. luteinizing hormone—LH; thyroid-stimulating hormone—TSH).
- Include all of the hormones of the hypothalamus, pituitary gland, parathyroid glands, gastrointestinal tract, and pancreas.
- Synthesized by transciption and translation from nuclear DNA (i.e. gene expression) and stored in secretory granules (in active or inactive form).
- Hormone release is regulated at the level of secretion, not by the rate of synthesis.

Amino acid derivatives
- Small water-soluble compounds derived from amino acids (e.g. tyrosine).
- Hormones derived from tyrosine include the thyroid hormones (T_3 and T_4), the catecholamines (adrenaline and noradrenaline), and dopamine.
- Melatonin is derived from the amino acid tryptophan.
- Synthesized in the cytoplasm and stored in secretory granules prior to their release.
- Hormone release is regulated at the level of secretion, although the rate of synthesis is limited at the initial conversion of tyrosine to dopa.

Steroids
- Fat-soluble lipids that can pass through plasma membranes but need to circulate bound to plasma proteins because they are water insoluble.
- Derived from cholesterol.

Physiological effects of hormones on body functions	
Body function	**Effects of hormones**
metabolism	regulate metabolic processes, i.e. the rate of synthesis and degradation of carbohydrates, proteins, and lipids
reproduction	control reproductive processes, including the development of the sex organs, secondary sexual characteristics, gametogenesis, and the menstrual cycle
digestion	control digestive processes, including gut motility and the secretion of digestive enzymes, bile, gastric acid, and bicarbonate
blood circulation	regulate blood pressure by altering cardiac output, vascular constriction, and blood volume via the control of water excretion by the kidneys
transport of substrates to tissues (blood composition)	regulate blood plasma concentrations of glucose, minerals (e.g. sodium, potassium, calcium), gases (oxygen, carbon dioxide), blood cells, water, and hydrogen ions (pH regulation)
defence against pathogens	regulate immune system responses, including leucocyte activation, inflammation, antibody production, and fever
growth	control cell division and differentiation
stress response	regulate the body's response to stress
behaviour	control sexual and social behaviour

Fig. 1.2 Physiological effects of hormones on body functions.

- Include hormones of the adrenal cortex, gonads (ovary and testes), and placenta.
- Synthesized in mitochondria and smooth endoplasmic reticulum and are not stored pre-made in the cell.
- Hormone release is dependent on the rate of cholesterol ester hydrolysis (hence, rate of secretion = rate of synthesis).

Eicosanoids

- Derived from arachidonic acid.
- Act primarily as local (paracrine) hormones but also as intracellular messengers.
- Produced by all cells of the body except red blood cells.

- Prostaglandins and leukotrienes are the two major types.
- Synthesized in the cell membrane and are not stored in the cell.

The synthetic pathways of the four groups are shown in Fig. 1.4.

The steroid hormones

All steroid hormones are composed of a 4-carbon-ring structure (Fig. 1.5) possessing many hydroxyl and keto groups and have between 18 and 21 carbon molecules .

As previously mentioned, all steroid hormones are synthesized from cholesterol. Cholesterol is acquired from the diet or is synthesized in the steroid-hormone-

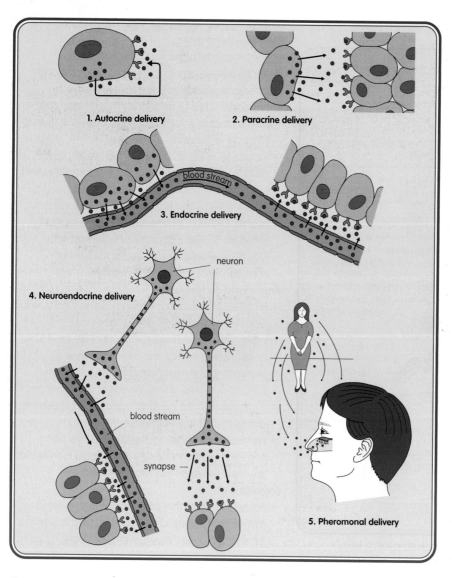

Fig. 1.3 Mode of delivery of hormones to their target cells.

1. Autocrine delivery

2. Paracrine delivery

3. Endocrine delivery

4. Neuroendocrine delivery

neuron

blood stream

synapse

5. Pheromonal delivery

secreting cells, and is stored in fat droplets in the cytoplasm.

Stimuli that promote steroid hormone secretion induce the release of cholesterol from its stores and its transport into the mitochondria. The mitochondria convert cholesterol into pregnenolone—this is the rate-limiting step in steroidogenesis.

Pregnenolone undergoes further modifications (catalysed by enzymes), to make active steroid hormones in the mitochondria and/or the smooth endoplasmic reticulum.

Fig. 1.6 shows the basic pathway of steroidogenesis. This pathway does not represent steroid synthesis in any one cell because not all the enzymes are always present, hence the different cell types synthesize different end product e.g.:

- Cells of the adrenal cortex secrete mineralocorticoids, glucocorticoids or androgens.
- Cells of the testes secrete testosterone.
- Cells of the ovary and placenta secrete oestrogens or progesterone.

Cholesterol, pregnenolone, and dehydroepiandrosterone (DHEA) do not have the 3oxy Δ 4 structure in the A ring that is found in the active steroid hormones, instead they have a Δ 5 structure in the B ring.

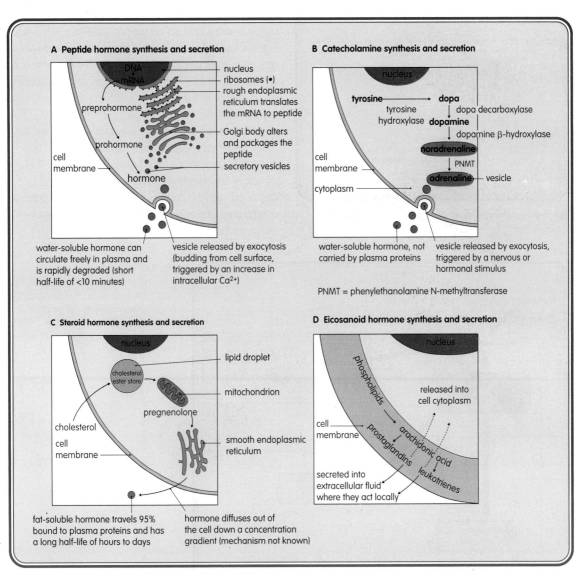

Fig. 1.4 Synthetic pathways of the four main types of hormone.

Overview of the Endocrine System

The δ 5 pathway involves the reactions that modify pregnenolone or its derivatives but preserve the double bond in position 5 of the B ring.

The δ 4 pathway involves the reactions that modify pregnenolone or its derivatives causing or retaining the double bond at position 4 of the A ring.

Some intermediate molecules in the synthetic pathway themselves have weak biological activities, e.g.:

- Deoxycorticosterone (an intermediate in the synthesis of aldosterone) is a weak mineralocorticoid.
- DHEA (an intermediate in the synthesis of the

androgens) is weakly active even though it has the A ring double bond at position 5.

Inherited defects or deficiencies of the enzymes that catalyse steroidogenesis can cause hormone imbalance. For example, deficiency of 21-hydroxylase causes cortisol and aldosterone deficiency, resulting in the accumulation of progesterone as the cells fail to convert it any further (aldosterone deficiency and progesterone excess cause salt loss and virilism)—95% of cases of steroidogenic enzyme deficiencies are caused by 21-hydroxylase deficiency.

Hormone receptors

Hormones are secreted into the blood in very low concentrations and act on specific cell types, e.g. TSH acts exclusively on the thyroid gland, whereas insulin acts on numerous different cell types. The capacity of a cell to respond to a hormone depends on the presence of receptor proteins that are specific for that hormone, e.g. thyroid follicular cells possess TSH receptors.

Cells that exhibit hormone receptor proteins are called target cells. Each target cell has between 2000 and 100 000 receptors for a particular hormone. These receptors are constantly being synthesized and degraded, and the number of receptors per cell can be upregulated or downregulated (increased or decreased) to increase or decrease the hormone's effect.

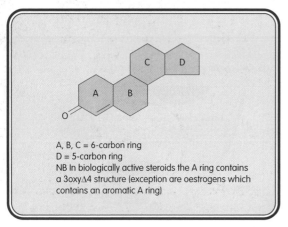

A, B, C = 6-carbon ring
D = 5-carbon ring
NB In biologically active steroids the A ring contains a 3oxyΔ4 structure (exception are oestrogens which contains an aromatic A ring)

Fig. 1.5 Basic 4-carbon-ring structure of the active steroid hormones.

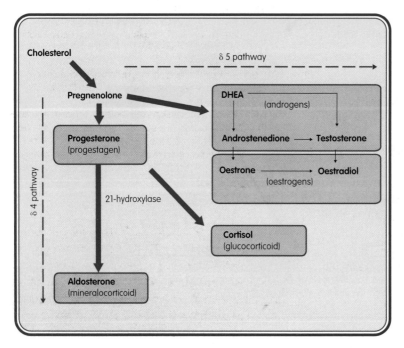

Fig. 1.6 The pathways of steroidogenesis—enzyme-catalysed reactions involved in the conversion of pregnenolone into active steroid hormones. (NB Intermediate molecules in the synthetic pathway are not shown.)

Hormone receptor proteins can be:

- Extracellular (on the cell membrane)—water-soluble molecules (e.g. peptide hormones) bind to these receptors.
- Intracellular (in the cell cytoplasm or nucleus)—fat-soluble molecules (e.g. steroid hormones) diffuse into the cell and bind to these receptors.

Binding of the hormone to the receptor causes a conformational change in the receptor protein which can stimulate protein synthesis directly (intracellular receptors) or trigger a cascade of cytoplasmic responses (extracellular receptors).

The action of the hormone at a specific target cell is determined by the genetic programming of the particular cell, therefore the same hormone may have different actions on different tissues, e.g. insulin stimulates gluconeogenesis in liver cells but promotes lipogenesis in adipose tissue.

There are three types of hormone receptor proteins—G-protein-coupled receptors, tyrosine kinase receptors and steroid receptors:

G-protein-coupled receptors

These receptors mediate the cytoplasmic responses by 'second messenger' systems. Molecules that act as intracellular second messengers include cyclic adenosine monophosphate (cAMP), inositol triphosphate (IP_3), diacylglycerol (DAG) and calcium ions (Ca^{2+}).

The sequence of events at G-protein-coupled receptors using cAMP as the second messenger is shown in Fig. 1.7.

Second-messenger pathways amplify the effect of the hormone binding to the receptor—for every hormone–receptor complex formed, 100 000 000 substrate molecules are acted on.

Specificity of the response comes from the specific receptors and protein kinases involved in the pathway, e.g. target cells for adrenaline have β, α_1, and/or α_2 receptors on their surface, therefore the response can be stimulatory (via β receptors) or inhibitory (via α_2 receptors), depending on which receptor the hormone binds to.

The sequence of events at G-protein-coupled receptors using IP_3, DAG, and Ca^{2+} as the second messengers is shown in Fig. 1.8.

Tyrosine kinase receptors

Hormones that bind to this type of receptor include insulin

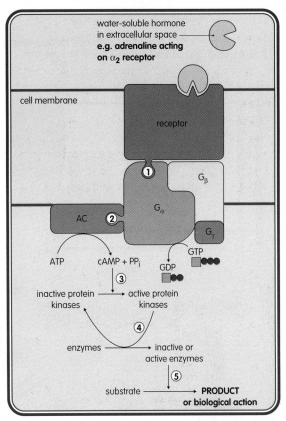

Fig. 1.7 G-protein-coupled receptor with cAMP as the second messenger.

1. The action of hormone binding to the receptor causes a conformational change in about 100 G-protein molecules ($G_\alpha, G_\beta, G_\gamma$), which enables GTP to bind to and activate the G_α subunits.
2. The activated G_α subunits in turn activate the enzyme adenylate cyclase (AC), and each activated AC breaks down about 1000 molecules of ATP into cAMP and pyrophosphate (PPi).
3. cAMP, acting as the second messenger, activates a protein kinase enzyme (the type of protein kinase activated varies with different target cells).
4. Each activated protein kinase initiates a series of reactions that alter the activity of a specific set of enzymes—it does this by donating a phosphate molecule to the enzyme.
5. One thousand enzyme molecules are either activated or inactivated by the action of each protein kinase, so the amount of product made is altered.

and epidermal growth factor (EGF). The insulin receptor molecule is shown in Fig. 1.9. No second messenger associated with this receptor has yet been identified. When hormone binds to the receptor, the tyrosine kinase causes an intracellular cascade of phosphorylation and dephosphorylation reactions that activate or deactivate specific enzyme proteins.

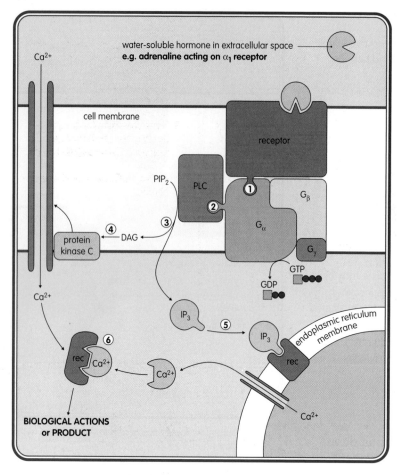

Fig. 1.8 G-protein-coupled receptor with IP_3 and DAG, and Ca^{2+} as second messengers.
1. Hormone–receptor complex activates G_α subunits.
2. Activated G_α subunits trigger the membrane enzyme phospholipase C (PLC).
3. PLC catalyses the hydrolysis of phosphoinositol (PIP_2) to produce IP_3 and DAG.
4. DAG activates the membrane enzyme protein kinase C, which opens the membrane Ca^{2+} channels to cause extracellular Ca^{2+} to influx into the cell.
5. IP_3 binds to receptors on the endoplasmic reticulum, which causes Ca^{2+} channels to open and reticular Ca^{2+} to influx into the cell.
6. Ca^{2+} ions bind to a cytoplasmic receptor (composed of calmodulin and enzyme) and this complex causes the cellular response.

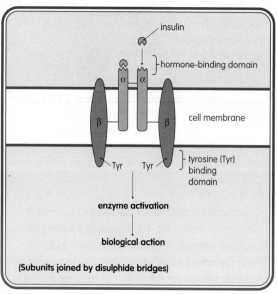

Fig. 1.9 Tyrosine kinase receptors.

Peptide hormones exert a faster cellular response than steroid hormones. This is because peptide hormones activate pre-existing protein enzymes, whereas steroid hormones activate the synthesis of new proteins (it takes longer to make a protein from scratch than merely to activate it).

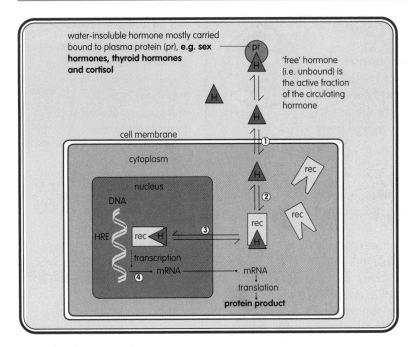

Fig. 1.10 Steroid (intracellular) receptor.
1. Unbound hormone (H) passes easily through the cell membrane.
2. Hormone binds to receptor protein (REC) in the cytoplasm or nucleus.
3. Hormone–receptor complex binds to specific hormone response elements (HRE) on the DNA.
4. mRNA and protein synthesis are altered.

Steroid receptors

The sequence of events at steroid receptors is shown in Fig. 1.10.

Hormone antagonists

An agonist is a hormone or analogue that binds to a receptor and elicits the normal biological response.

An antagonist is a molecule that prevents the normal response, either by binding to the hormone receptor and blocking the hormone from binding, or by blocking the signal transduction.

A partial agonist is a molecule that binds to a hormone receptor but is less biologically active than the hormone. Hence in the absence of hormone it acts as an agonist, but when hormone is present it competes with the hormone for binding and the resultant biological effect is less (i.e. antagonizes the hormonal response). Methods of hormone antagonism are shown in Fig. 1.11 and include:

1. **Direct receptor block**—the antagonist binds to the same site as the hormone, preventing the hormone from binding, e.g. the drug curare irreversibly blocks the acetylcholine receptor binding site, causing muscle paralysis as nerves fail to convey impulses.
2. **Indirect (allosteric) receptor block**—the antagonist binds to another (allosteric) site on the receptor protein, causing a change in its conformation so that the hormone can no longer bind at its usual site.

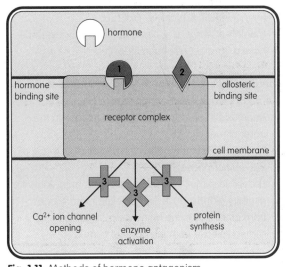

Fig. 1.11 Methods of hormone antagonism.
1. Direct receptor block.
2. Indirect (allosteric receptor block).
3. Direct signal block.

3. **Direct signal block**—the antagonist blocks the signal after it has been generated by the normal hormone–receptor interaction, e.g. phenytoin blocks the Ca^{2+} channels that the hormone-receptor complex has activated; tamoxifen blocks specific transcriptional activation sites on the DNA, so that when the oestrogen–receptor complex binds to the HRE site there is no transcription.

Binding of the antagonist to the receptor is usually, but not always, reversible.
- Reversible binding means the antagonist is in direct competition with the hormone, therefore the relative amounts of each determine the extent of the response.
- Irreversible binding means the hormone will not elicit a response until new receptor molecules have been synthesized.

Control of hormone secretion

Hormone secretion is regulated so that the concentrations in the blood are appropriate to elicit the required response, e.g. in children, growth hormone (GH) coordinates growth processes—oversecretion results in gigantism, undersecretion in dwarfism.

Basal secretion of hormones may be continuous (e.g. prolactin), in short bursts (e.g. insulin), or episodic (e.g. luteinizing hormone—LH and follicle-stimulating hormone—FSH).

Hormone release often has rhythmic patterns:
- Day–night (circadian) rhythms, e.g. adrenocorticotrophic hormone (ACTH), prolactin, GH, TSH.
- Monthly rhythms, e.g. oestrogen and progesterone have a 28-day cycle (menstrual cycle).

Specific stimuli received by the endocrine cells cause them to increase their hormone secretion, e.g.:
- Nervous stimuli induce adrenaline release in the adrenal medulla.
- Biochemical stimuli induce the secretion of many of the gut hormones.
- Endocrine stimuli (releasing factors) from the anterior pituitary gland induce the secretion of hormones from other endocrine glands, e.g. ACTH induces cortisol release from the adrenal cortex.

Often there are multiple stimuli operating, e.g. insulin is released in response to parasympathetic nerve stimulation, glucose, and glucose-dependent insulinotrophic peptide GIP (a gut hormone).

Some stimuli decrease hormone secretion, e.g. somatostatin (GHIH) released by the hypothalamus decreases the amount of GH released by the anterior pituitary gland.

The concentration of the secreted hormone in the blood, and/or the effects produced by the hormone, control subsequent secretion of the hormone, i.e. hormone secretion is controlled by a feedback loop system (Figs 1.12 and 1.13).

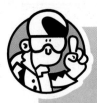
Hormone antagonism plays a large part in the treatment of many endocrine disorders, e.g. tamoxifen (partial agonist) is an antioestrogen drug sometimes used in the treatment of breast cancer. NB Some drugs increase the hormone response, e.g. caffeine potentiates the action of adrenaline by inhibiting the breakdown of its second messenger, cAMP.

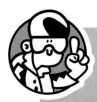
The hypothalamus and the anterior pituitary gland control the secretion of many hormones.

The secretion of hormones is usually controlled by complex feedback loop systems involving a number of regulatory mechanisms.

Integration of the endocrine and nervous systems

The nervous system and the endocrine system are integrated. The mechanisms by which one effects the function of the other are shown in Fig. 1.14 (and described below).

Comparison between the nervous and endocrine systems

Both systems are composed of cells that secrete chemical messengers which act on target cells.

Some chemical messengers are common to both systems, e.g. somatostatin is secreted by neurons in the central nervous system as a neurotransmitter, by neurons in the hypothalamus as a neural hormone, and by gut endocrine cells as a hormone.

Endocrine responses tend to be slow but prolonged, whereas neural responses tend to be fast but short-lasting.

There is some overlap between the two systems, e.g. the posterior pituitary gland and the hypothalamus are composed of nervous tissue but they secrete hormones; the adrenal medulla is composed of modified sympathetic nerve cells that secrete the hormones adrenaline and noradrenaline.

Neural control of endocrine function

The hypothalamus is part of the brain but it controls the release of pituitary hormones (via its hormones) and is the main coordinator of the endocrine system.

The nervous system regulates the secretion of:

- Hormones from the *posterior pituitary gland* and the *hypothalamus,* via afferent neural pathways from the central nervous system.
- *Melatonin,* via postganglionic sympathetic nerves, initially from the retina.

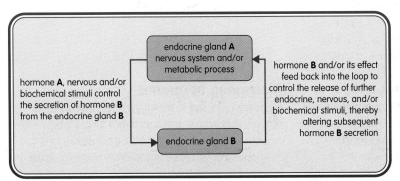

Fig. 1.12 Theory behind endocrine feedback systems.

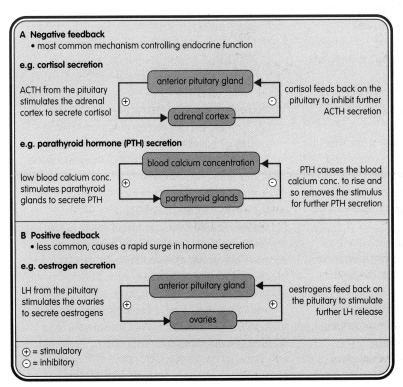

Fig. 1.13 Examples of negative and positive feedback loop systems involved in hormone secretion.

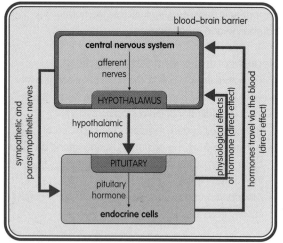

Fig. 1.14 Integration of the nervous and endocrine control systems.

The nervous system and the endocrine system are integrated. The nervous system regulates the secretion of hormones from the endocrine glands. Some hormones (e.g. thyroid hormone) act on the nervous system to modify its function. Together they efficiently maintain homoeostasis.

- *Renin, thyroid hormone, insulin,* and *glucagon,* via postganglionic sympathetic nerves. These hormones are mainly regulated by non-neural mechanisms but neural control is important as it causes rapid changes in blood flow and secretory activity, allowing a faster response to stressful stimuli (insulin and glucagon secretion is also stimulated by parasympathetic nerves via the vagus nerve).
- *Adrenaline* from the adrenal medulla, via preganglionic sympathetic nerves (the adrenaline-secreting cells are modified postganglionic neurons that have become endocrine cells).

Endocrine control of neural function

Indirect effects include:
- Insulin can produce changes in mental function, sweating, nervousness, convulsions, coma, and death, by lowering blood glucose.
- Parathyroid hormone can cause tetany and mental dysfunction by changing calcium levels.

Direct effects include:
- Thyroid hormone increases sympathetic nerve activity and is important in brain development in early life.
- Insulin induces satiety in the hypothalamus.
- Steroid hormones pass through the blood–brain barrier and affect mental activity, sexual behaviour, and the control of body temperature.
- Adrenaline increases sympathetic nerve activity and affects mental activity.

Measuring hormones

Bioassay (not used in clinical practice) measures the amount of hormone required to produce a given response (i.e. measures the biological activity of a hormone). In-vivo bioassays quantify the response to a hormone that has been administered to an animal, e.g. measurement of blood glucose after injection of insulin. In-vitro bioassays measure the response when a hormone is added to an in-vitro preparation of the target tissue, e.g. the effect of ACTH on steroidogenesis in adrenal tissue. The disadvantages of bioassay are that it is insensitive and labour intensive, and results are often not reproducible.

Radioimmunoassay (RIA) is the most common assay. It measures the amount of hormone using monoclonal antibodies (derived from immunization of animals) that bind specifically to that hormone alone (Fig. 1.15). Some hormones and steroids are too small—in order to raise antibodies to them they need to be coupled with a carrier protein.

Enzyme-linked immunosorbent assay (ELISA) uses the same technique as RIA except hormones are labelled with enzymes instead of a radioactive marker—the enzyme activity is measured so that the amount of hormone can be calculated.

Radioreceptor assay is the same as for RIA except a preparation of hormone-specific receptors is used instead of a hormone-specific antibody.

High-performance liquid chromatography (HPLC) separates the hormone from a mixed solution (e.g. plasma) in a fractionating column; the amount of

hormone can then be measured. Its disadvantages are that it is expensive and slow.

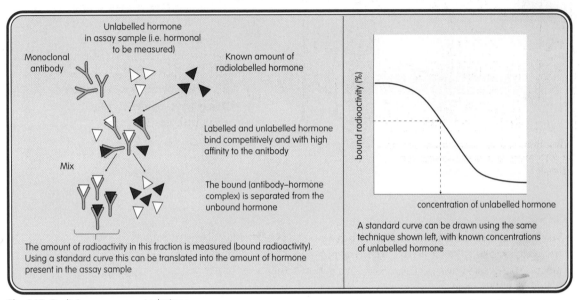

Fig. 1.15 Radioimmunoassay technique.

- Define a hormone and outline the effects of hormones on body function.
- List the various modes of hormone delivery to target cells.
- List the four main classes of hormones.
- Describe the types of hormone receptors and the second-messenger pathways.
- Explain methods of hormone antagonism.
- Describe the regulation and feedback control of hormone secretion.
- Summarize the similarities between the nervous and endocrine systems and how they are integrated.
- Outline the methods used to measure hormones.

2. The Hypothalamus and the Pituitary Gland

Structure of the hypothalamus and the pituitary gland

Macrostructure of the hypothalamus

The hypothalamus is located in the diencephalon (the posterior part of the forebrain), at the base of the brain (Fig. 2.1), where it forms the lower part of the lateral wall and the floor of the third ventricle (cavity carrying the cerebrospinal fluid).

Its relations are shown in Fig. 2.2 (its borders are arbitrarily defined by the structures surrounding it) and comprise:

- Anterior—the optic chiasma.
- Posterior—the mamillary bodies and the subthalamus.
- Superior—the third ventricle.
- Inferior—the pituitary stalk.

Its blood supply is from the middle cerebral artery (branch of the internal carotid artery). Blood drains into the intercavernous sinus and via portal veins (that pass through the anterior pituitary lobe) into the cavernous sinus.

There are numerous neural connections—with other regions of the brain and with the posterior lobe of the pituitary gland—that allow the hypothalamus to send and receive messages.

Macrostructure of the pituitary gland

The hypophysis cerebri—or pituitary body—was so named owing to the incorrect notion that it secreted the nasal mucus ('pituitary' means 'mucus'). It is an oval structure, about the size of a large pea, and consists of two lobes:

- The anterior (adenohypophysis).
- The posterior (neurohypophysis).

The anterior lobe is the larger and has three subdivisions:

- The pars distalis, which forms the major portion of the gland.
- The pars tuberalis.
- The pars intermedia, which adjoins the posterior lobe.

It is located in the sella turcica, under cover of the diaphragma sellae, and is connected with the tuber cinereum of the hypothalamus by means of the

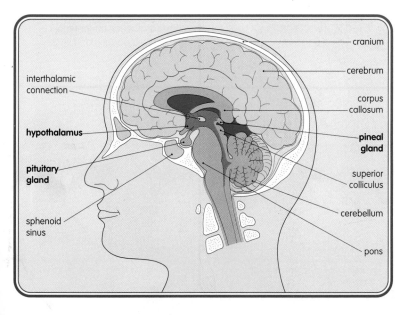

Fig. 2.1 Medial sagittal section of head showing the location of the hypothalamus and the pituitary gland (and the pineal gland).

cranium
cerebrum
corpus callosum
interthalamic connection
hypothalamus
pineal gland
pituitary gland
superior colliculus
cerebellum
sphenoid sinus
pons

pituitary stalk (the infundibulum), which passes through the aperture in the diaphragma sellae (see Figs 2.1 and 2.2).

Its relations are:

- Anterior—sphenoidal air sinuses.
- Posterior—dorsum sellae, the basilar artery, and the pons.
- Superior—diaphragma sellae, which separates the anterior lobe from the optic chiasma.
- Inferior—sphenoid bone and its sphenoid air sinuses.
- Lateral—cavernous sinuses and their contents (cranial nerves III–V).

The pituitary gland has a rich blood supply from the superior and inferior hypophyseal (pituitary) arteries (branches of the internal carotid artery). The anterior pituitary is also supplied by portal veins that arise from capillaries in the hypothalamus. *These partial veins provide a vascular link between the hypothalamus and the anterior pituitary.* There is retrograde (backwards) flow as well as antegrade (forwards) flow in these portal veins. The pituitary veins drain into the cavernous sinuses.

The proximity of the optic chiasma and of the cranial nerves in the cavernous sinus to the pituitary is important because pituitary tumours can compress the optic nerves and cause visual field defects (blindness in regions of lateral vision). Some rapidly expanding tumours extend sideways and can compress cranial nerves III, IV, and VI where they lie in the wall of the cavernous sinuses.

Microstructure of the hypothalamus

The hypothalamus is composed of nervous tissue and contains groups of specialized neurons called nuclei. The medial parts of the hypothalamus have a number of named nuclear groups, which include the preoptic,

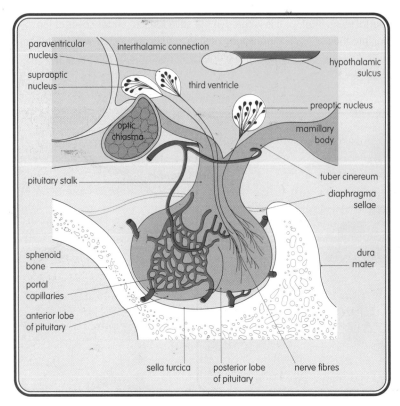

Fig. 2.2 Anatomical relationship of the pituitary gland and the hypothalamus to surrounding structures The paraventricular, peoptic, and suparoptic nuclei are within the hypothalamaus (hypothalamic hormones are carried to the posterior pituitary via nerve fibres and reach the anterior pituitary via portal blood vessels).

supraoptic, and paraventricular nuclei. These nuclei have axons which terminate in the posterior lobe of the pituitary and are involved in the regulation of hormonal secretions.

Microstructure of the pituitary gland

The two lobes of the pituitary are composed of different cell types.

The anterior pituitary is composed of a large number of epithelial cells arranged in clumps and cords, surrounded by many sinusoids (wide-diameter capillaries). Cell types comprise chromophils and chromophobes (see Fig. 2.3).

Chromophils are divided into acidophils and basophils according to how they stain.

Acidophilic cells include:
- Somatotrophs—synthesize growth hormone (GH).
- Lactotrophs—synthesize prolactin (PRL).

Basophilic cells include:
- Thyrotrophs—synthesize thyroid-stimulating hormone (TSH).
- Corticotrophs—synthesize adrenocorticotrophic hormone (ACTH) and melanocyte-stimulating hormone (MSH).
- Gonadotrophs—synthesize luteinizing hormone (LH) and follicle-stimulating hormone (FSH).

The posterior pituitary is composed of neural cells with a rich blood supply. Cell types, shown in Fig. 2.4, comprise pituicytes and axons of neurons (the cell bodies of the neurons are in the hypothalamic nuclei). *These nerves provide a direct neural link between the hypothalamus and the posterior pituitary.*

The hormones oxytocin and antidiuretic hormone (ADH; vasopressin) are synthesized in the cell bodies and travel down the axons into the posterior pituitary gland, where they are released. The sinusoids are in proximity to the end terminals of the axons to allow for efficient transfer of hormone.

Development of the hypothalamus and pituitary gland

The hypothalamus develops from the embryological forebrain and can be identified at week six of gestation.

The two lobes of the pituitary develop from different embryological tissues which fuse together:

Posterior pituitary

This is derived from the ectoderm of the primitive brain

In common with all protein-secreting cells, the anterior pituitary cells contain abundant rough endoplasmic reticulum and Golgi bodies, and are packed with secretory vesicles

Chromophil
- granular
- secretes hormone

Chromophobe
- smaller
- less granular
- could be depleted or resting stage of chromophil

fenestrated endothelium   sinusoid

Fig. 2.3 Histology of the anterior pituitary gland.

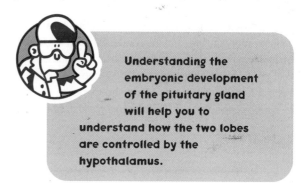

Understanding the embryonic development of the pituitary gland will help you to understand how the two lobes are controlled by the hypothalamus.

tissue, and is thus composed of neural tissue. It develops as a diverticulum (outgrowth) from the diencephalon, called the infundibulum, which extrudes downwards from the hypothalamus (see Fig. 2.5). The posterior lobe retains the vascular and neural supply with which it developed with (i.e. it is directly connected to the hypothalamus).

Anterior pituitary

This is derived from the ectoderm of the primitive mouth,

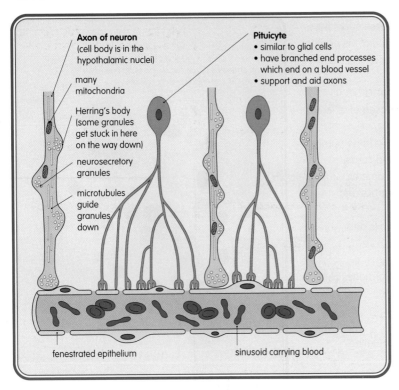

Fig. 2.4 Histology of the posterior pituitary gland.

Axon of neuron
(cell body is in the hypothalamic nuclei)

many mitochondria

Herring's body (some granules get stuck in here on the way down)

neurosecretory granules

microtubules guide granules down

Pituicyte
• similar to glial cells
• have branched end processes which end on a blood vessel
• support and aid axons

fenestrated epithelium

sinusoid carrying blood

and is thus composed of epithelial tissue. It develops as a diverticulum from the ectoderm of the primitive oral cavity, called Rathke's pouch, which grows upwards until it fuses with the infundibulum (see Fig. 2.5).

The stalk of Rathke's pouch regresses once it fuses with the infundibulum, and the connection with the roof of the pharynx is lost (occasionally, nests of squamous cells are retained in this area and these can give rise to cysts or tumours which may secrete hormones).

As the connection with the oral cavity is lost, so is the vascular supply from this region. Pituitary arteries from the internal carotid artery, and portal veins from the hypothalamus, grow down into the lobe during development (this rich vascular supply from the hypothalamus is important as it carries hypothalamic hormones directly to the pituitary gland; these hormones regulate pituitary hormone release).

There is no direct neural connection between the anterior pituitary gland and the hypothalamus (it communicates with the hypothalamus via portal veins).

 The hypothalamus is the main coordinator of the endocrine system—it is sometimes referred to as the 'conductor of the endocrine orchestra'.

○ Discuss the location, relations, and blood supply of the hypothalamus and the pituitary gland.
○ Describe the histology of the hypothalamus and the pituitary gland.
○ Outline the development of the hypothalamus and the pituitary gland.

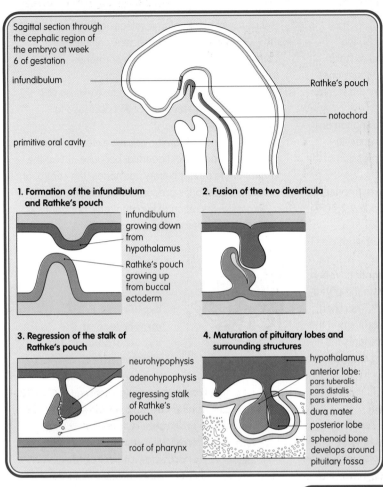

Sagittal section through the cephalic region of the embryo at week 6 of gestation

infundibulum

Rathke's pouch

notochord

primitive oral cavity

1. Formation of the infundibulum and Rathke's pouch

infundibulum growing down from hypothalamus

Rathke's pouch growing up from buccal ectoderm

2. Fusion of the two diverticula

3. Regression of the stalk of Rathke's pouch

neurohypophysis

adenohypophysis

regressing stalk of Rathke's pouch

roof of pharynx

4. Maturation of pituitary lobes and surrounding structures

hypothalamus

anterior lobe:
pars tuberalis
pars distalis
pars intermedia

dura mater

posterior lobe

sphenoid bone develops around pituitary fossa

Fig. 2.5 Embryological development of the anterior and posterior lobes of the pituitary gland.

HORMONES OF THE HYPOTHALAMUS

The hypothalamus secretes the following releasing and inhibiting hormones (see Fig. 2.6):

- GH-releasing hormone (GHRH).
- GH-inhibiting hormone (GHIH; somatostatin).
- Dopamine (prolactin-inhibiting hormone).
- Prolactin-releasing factors (PRF; one of which is TRH).
- Thyrotrophin-releasing hormone (TRH).
- Corticotrophin-releasing hormone (CRH).
- Gonadotrophin-releasing hormone (GnRH).

These hormones are peptides, synthesized by specialized hypothalamic neurons (different neurons secrete different hormones), and act on the anterior pituitary gland to regulate the release of pituitary hormones.

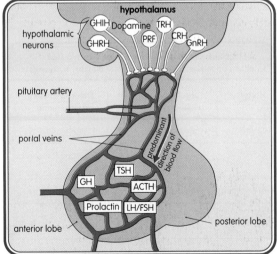

Fig. 2.6 Hormones of the hypothalamus and the portal veins that transport them directly to the anterior pituitary. (From *An Illustrated Review of the Endocrine System*, by Glenn F. Bastian. Copyright Glenn F. Bastian. Adapted with permission of Addison–Wesley Educational Publishers.)

Synthesis and secretion of hypothalamic hormones

As well as the hormones listed on page 21, the hypothalamus also synthesizes ADH and oxytocin (these are classified as posterior pituitary hormones—see Fig. 2.10—because this is where they are stored and secreted).

Each hormone is synthesized by transcription and translation of the gene that codes for its specific peptide, e.g. ACTH is synthesized by expression of the ACTH gene.

The episodic secretion of each of the hormones is controlled independently (see Figs. 4.8, 5.7, 9.2, 10.9, 10.19, 11.12).

The secretion of CRH has a circadian rhythm (see Fig. 5.8).

Once secreted, the hypothalamic hormones reach their target cells in the anterior pituitary via the portal veins (i.e. not via the systemic circulation). This short, direct connection between the hypothalamus and the pituitary allows a rapid response and prevents the tiny amount of hormone secreted from being diluted in the systemic circulation.

Effects of hypothalamic hormones

Each hormone stimulates or inhibits the secretion of specific anterior pituitary hormones (see Fig. 2.7). Some also have additional effects, e.g.: GHIH also inhibits the secretion of insulin, glucagon, gastrin, and secretin.

Deficiency/excess of hypothalamic hormones

Deficiency of hypothalamic releasing hormones (GHRH, TRH, CRH, GnRH) causes deficiency of the corresponding anterior pituitary hormones (hypopituitarism).

Deficiency of GHIH does not cause excess GH secretion because levels of GHRH decrease to compensate for it.

Deficiency of dopamine causes excess prolactin secretion (hyperprolactinaemia) because, unlike the control of the other pituitary hormones, the control of prolactin secretion is predominantly inhibitory.

Excessive secretion of hypothalamic hormones is very rare and does not tend to occur.

- Explain the importance of the hypothalamus in the control of the endocrine system.
- Describe the synthesis, secretion, and effects of the hypothalamic hormones.
- Define the importance of the portal veins that link the hypothalamus and the anterior pituitary gland.

Hormones secreted by the hypothalamus and their effects on the secretion of the anterior pituitary hormones		
Hormone	Target cells in anterior pituitary gland	Effect on anterior pituitary gland
GHRH	somatotrophs	↑ GH release
GHIH	somatotrophs and thyrotrophs	↓ GH and TSH release
dopamine	lactotrophs	↓ prolactin release
TRH	lactotrophs and thyrotrophs	↑ prolactin and TSH release
CRH	corticotrophs	↑ ACTH release
GnRH	gonadotrophs	↑ LH and FSH release

Fig. 2.7 Hormones secreted by the hypothalamus and their effects on the secretion of the anterior pituitary hormones.

HORMONES OF THE ANTERIOR PITUITARY GLAND

The anterior pituitary gland secretes the following trophic hormones (see Figs 2.8 and 2.9):
- GH —growth hormone.
- PRL —prolactin.
- TSH—thyroid-stimulating hormone.
- ACTH—adrenocoricotrophic hormone.
- MSH —melanocyte-stimulating hormone.
- LH —luteinizing hormone.
- FSH—follicle-stimulating hormone.

Anterior pituitary hormones are peptides or glycopeptides, synthesized by chromophils (different chromophil types secrete different hormones), and they

The anterior pituitary gland is the main controller of the endocrine system—in the analogy of the hypothalamus being the 'conductor of the endocrine orchestra', the anterior pituitary is the 'first violin'.

Hyperprolactinaemia is one of the most common endocrine disorders. It is caused either by dopamine deficiency from the hypothalamus or by prolactin-secreting tumours of the pituitary.

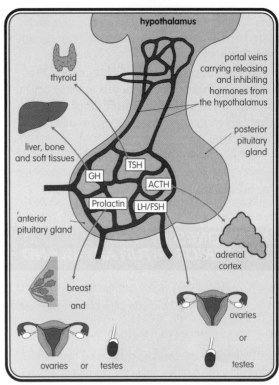

Fig. 2.8 Hormones of the anterior pituitary gland and their respective target organs. (From *An Illustrated Review of the Endocrine System,* by Glenn F. Bastian. Copyright Glenn F. Bastian. Adapted with permission of Addison–Wesley Educational Publishers.)

Anterior pituitary hormones, the cells that synthesize them, their effects, and the disorders caused by their deficiency and excess				
Hormone	Synthesized by	Effects	Deficiency	Excess
GH	somatotrophs	promotes growth in the muscles and bones and opposes the action of insulin (see Chapter 9)	dwarfism in children or adult GH deficiency syndrome	gigantism in children, acromegaly in adults
PRL	lactotrophs	initiates lactation and promotes the growth of the mammary glands and of the ovaries and testes (see Chapters 10 and 11)	hyperprolactinaemia (failure in postpartum lactation)	hyperprolactinaemia (impotence in males, amennorrhoea in females and decresed libido)
TSH	thyrotrophs	acts on the thyroid gland → release of thyroid hormones and changes to the thyroid gland (see Chapter 4)	hypothyroidism (decreased thyroid hormones)	extremely rare but causes hyperthyroidism (increased thyroid hormones)
ACTH	corticotrophs	acts on the adrenal cortex → release of glucocorticoids (e.g. cortisol) and adrenal androgens (see Chapter 5)	adrenocortical insufficiency (decreased cortisol and adrenal androgens)	Cushing's disease (increased cortisol and adrenal androgens)
MSH	corticotrophs	stmulates melanocytes in the skin	no effect	no effect
LH and FSH	gonadotrophs	acts on the reproductive organs → release of sex steroids and changes in the reproductive cycle (see Chapter 10)	gonadal insufficiency (decreased sex steroids)	extremely rare but causes infertility

Fig. 2.9 Anterior pituitary hormones, the cells that secrete them, their effects, and the disorders caused by their deficiency and excess.

either control the function of other endocrine glands (TSH, ACTH, LH, FSH) or have direct effects on distant organs (GH, PRL, MSH).

For more detail on each hormone, refer to the chapters on their respective target organs or action (i.e. see chapters covering growth, lactation, thyroid gland, adrenal cortex, and male and female reproduction).

For more detail on the deficiency and excess of anterior pituitary hormone secretion (hypopituitarism and hyperpituitarism), refer to Figs 15.1 and 15.2.

HORMONES OF THE POSTERIOR PITUITARY GLAND

The posterior pituitary gland secretes (see Fig. 2.10):
- ADH (anti-diuretic hormone, also called vasopressin).
- Oxytocin.

Both hormones are peptides comprising nine amino acids. They are synthesized in the cell bodies of specialized neurons in the hypothalamus, and travel down the axons to be stored/secreted by the posterior pituitary gland. This axonal communication is known as the hypothalamic–hypophyseal tract.

The actions of these hormones, and the effects caused by their deficiency or excess, are listed in Fig. 2.11.

For more detail on each hormone, refer to the chapters covering fluid balance and parturition.

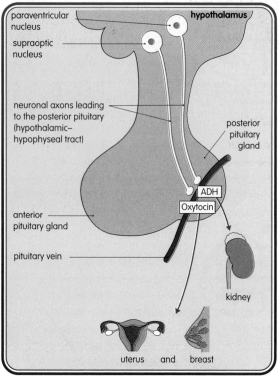

Fig. 2.10 Hormones of the posterior pituitary gland and their respective target organs. (From *An Illustrated Review of the Endocrine System,* by Glenn F. Bastian. Copyright Glenn F. Bastian. Adapted with permission of Addison–Wesley Educational Publishers.)

Posterior pituitary hormones, their effects, and the disorders caused by their deficiency and excess			
Hormone	Effects	Deficiency	Excess
ADH	increases water reabsorption in the kidney and modulates blood pressure	diabetes insipidus (polyuria, hypotension)	syndrome of inappropriate ADH secretion (SIADH)
oxytocin	stimulates uterine contractions during labour, stimulates postpartum milk ejection, elicits maternal behaviour	failure to progress in labour and difficulty with breast-feeding	no effect

Fig. 2.11 Posterior pituitary hormones, their effects, and the disorders caused by their deficiency and excess.

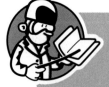

- Describe the importance of the anterior pituitary gland in the control of the endocrine system.
- List the hormones secreted by the anterior and posterior pituitary gland and, briefly, their effects.
- Name the disorders caused by the deficiency and excess of pituitary hormones.

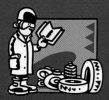

3. The Pineal Gland

STRUCTURE OF THE PINEAL GLAND

Macrostructure of the pineal gland

The pineal gland is an outgrowth of the roof of the diencephalon (the posterior part of the forebrain) in the posterior wall of the third ventricle. It can often be seen on X-rays as it starts to calcify in the second decade of life.

It is a pine-cone-shaped mass lying between the superior colliculi and below the posterior end of the corpus callosum (see Figs 2.1 and 3.1).

It has a very rich blood supply (from branches of the internal carotid artery) and a rich nerve supply (and therefore probably has a greater physiological role than is recognized). The pineal gland is not anatomically or functionally related to the pituitary gland.

Microstructure of the pineal gland

The gland is composed of two major types of neural cells:
- Pinealocytes (which synthesize and secrete melatonin).
- Glial cells.

ENDOCRINE FUNCTION OF THE PINEAL GLAND

The pineal gland synthesizes and secretes melatonin, which is derived from the amino acid tryptophan.

The secretion of melatonin is known as the 'chemical expression of darkness' because of its exclusive night-time synthesis and is modulated by the amount of light (stimulated by darkness and inhibited by light)— detection of light at the retina of the eye stimulates sympathetic nerves that innervate the pineal gland and inhibit melatonin secretion (Fig. 3.1).

The effects of melatonin are still obscure. In animals, it has a role in seasonal breeding and gonadal regression in the winter months. In humans, melatonin administration induces sleep and is said to lessen the symptoms of jet lag. It may also have a role in puberty (levels are low throughout this period) and in the regulation of biological rhythms.

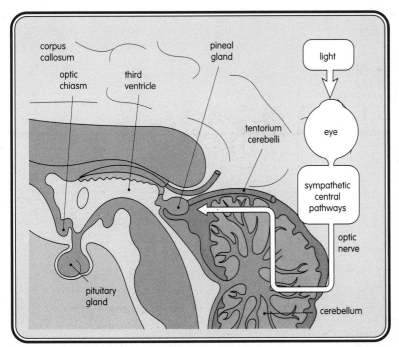

Fig. 3.1 Location of the pineal gland and the control of melatonin secretion. Melatonin secretion is inhibited by light detected by the retina of the eye.

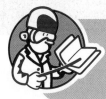

- Describe the location, relations, blood supply, and histology of the pineal gland.
- Outline the endocrine function of the pineal gland.

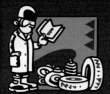

4. The Thyroid Gland

Structure of the thyroid and parathyroid glands

Macrostructure of the thyroid gland

The thyroid gland is a bilobed gland, weighing 10–25 g, that lies anterior to the trachea (see Fig. 4.1). The lateral lobes are each about 4 cm long and are connected by the communicating isthmus.

Relations are (see Fig. 4.2):

- Superficial —three strap muscles, pretracheal fascia, and sternocleidomastoid muscle.
- Medial—the larynx and trachea and, behind these, the pharynx and oesophagus.
- Posterior—the parathyroid glands, prevertebral fascia, and the contents of the carotid sheath.

The thyroid has a rich blood supply from the superior thyroid artery (a branch of the external carotid artery) and the inferior thyroid artery (a branch of the

subclavian artery). The superior and middle thyroid veins drain into the internal jugular vein and inferior thyroid vein drains into the brachiocephalic vein (Fig. 4.1). Blood flow is rapid (4–6 mL/min/g of tissue), which is indicative of an active secretory tissue.

Lymphatic drainage is to pretracheal, paratracheal, and inferior deep cervical nodes.

Macrostructure of the parathyroid glands

The parathyroid comprises four small glands—oval-shaped and about 5 mm across—situated behind the lateral lobes of the thyroid gland, within its capsule (Fig. 4.2). There is a superior and inferior gland in each lobe.

The parathyroids have a rich blood supply from the superior and inferior thyroid arteries (see Fig. 4.1).

Microstructure of the thyroid gland

The thyroid is composed of more than one million spherical follicles of varying sizes. Each follicle contains colloid and is lined by a layer of secretory epithelial cells (follicular cells), which secrete tri-iodothyronine (T_3), thyroxine (T_4), and thyroglobulin at the cell–colloid interface (Fig. 4.3). T_3 and T_4 are thyroid hormones that are stored in the colloid, bound to thyroglobulin.

Numerous microvilli project from the surface of the follicle cells into the lumen. These are involved in reuptake of the colloid to release T_3 and T_4 into the circulation. When the thyroid gland has been very actively secreting into the bloodstream, the lumina of the follicles are small (colloid released); when it has been underactive, the lumina are large.

A rich capillary network surrounds the follicles and is controlled by sympathetic and parasympathetic nerves.

Parafollicular cells (C cells) that synthesize and secrete calcitonin are found throughout the thyroid gland.

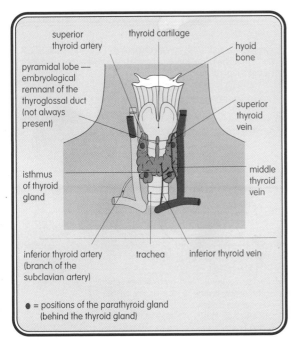

superior thyroid artery

thyroid cartilage

hyoid bone

pyramidal lobe — embryological remnant of the thyroglossal duct (not always present)

superior thyroid vein

isthmus of thyroid gland

middle thyroid vein

inferior thyroid artery (branch of the subclavian artery)

trachea

inferior thyroid vein

● = positions of the parathyroid gland (behind the thyroid gland)

Fig. 4.1 Anterior view of the neck, showing the location and blood supply of the thyroid gland. The 4 parathyroid glands, that secrete parathyroid hormone (see Chapter 8), are situated behind the lateral lobes of the thyroid gland.

The thyroid gland is the only endocrine gland that stores its hormone in an intracellular compartment.

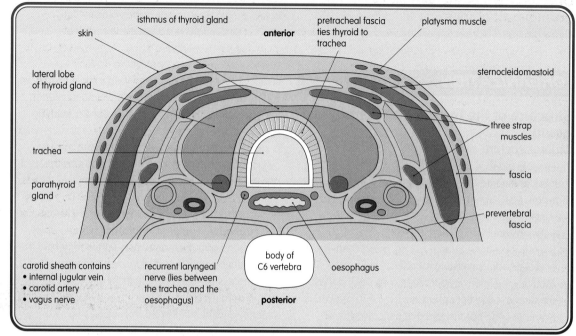

Fig. 4.2 Horizontal section of the anterior part of the neck at the level of the sixth cervical vertebra, showing the location of the thyroid and parathyroid glands and their surrounding structures. (The proximity of the recurrent laryngeal nerves is significant because they may be damaged during surgery on the gland or invaded by thyroid cancer—this may result in transient or permanent hoarseness and/or dysphagia because of paralysis of the laryngeal muscles.)

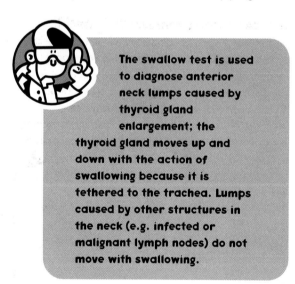

The swallow test is used to diagnose anterior neck lumps caused by thyroid gland enlargement; the thyroid gland moves up and down with the action of swallowing because it is tethered to the trachea. Lumps caused by other structures in the neck (e.g. infected or malignant lymph nodes) do not move with swallowing.

Microstructure of the parathyroid glands

The parathyroid glands are composed of two sorts of cells:

- Chief cells—secrete parathyroid hormone (PTH), which acts to increase plasma calcium levels (see Chapter 8).
- Oxyphil cells—function unknown, but their numbers increase throughout life.

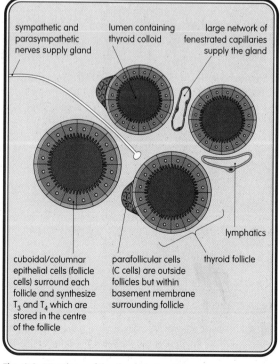

Fig. 4.3 Histology of the thyroid gland.

Development of the thyroid and parathyroid glands

These glands develop from embryological pharyngeal pouches. The pouches are formed at the cranial end of the foregut during weeks 4 and 5 of gestation owing to the formation of a series of pharyngeal arches (embryological 'gill-like' structures). They then separate from the lining of the pharynx and migrate downwards. By week 7 they are located in the regions where they are found in the adult, and where they continue their development.

Fig. 4.4 shows the development of these glands.

The thyroid develops from an endodermal outgrowth on the floor of the pharynx at the level of the first pharyngeal pouch. It grows downwards, becoming bilobed, and collects cells from the inferior part of the fourth pouch (may be responsible for C cells). As the thyroid grows down, the lower end proliferates and forms the glandular tissue; the rest (the thyroglossal duct) atrophies, but remnants may persist that are not connected to the thyroid gland (thyroglossal cysts). The site of origin of the thyroid becomes the foramen caecum of the tongue.

The thymus develops from the third pair of pharyngeal pouches, which migrate separately but fuse into one organ once in its definitive position.

Cells from the dorsal part of the third pouch migrate down with the developing thymus, but as they move past the thyroid they become embedded in it. They become the inferior parathyroid glands.

Cells from the superior part of the fourth pouch migrate down to the neck region, attached to the thyroid. They become the superior parathyroid glands.

The parathyroid glands exchange position as they migrate, i.e. the inferior parathyroids originate anterior to the superior glands in the pharynx, but end up inferior to them in their definitive position.

THYROID HORMONES

The thyroid gland secretes three hormones:
- Thyroxine (T_4).
- Tri-iodothyronine (T_3).
- Calcitonin (see Chapter 8).

Structure and synthesis of T_3 and T_4

T_3 and T_4 are iodinated derivatives of the amino acid tyrosine. T_3 contains three iodine molecules and T_4 contains four. Their structures are shown in Fig. 4.5.

The detailed steps in the synthesis and secretion of T_3 and T_4 are shown in Fig. 4.6 and comprise:
1. **Iodine trapping**—plasma iodide ions (I^-) are actively transported into the follicular cells from the plasma

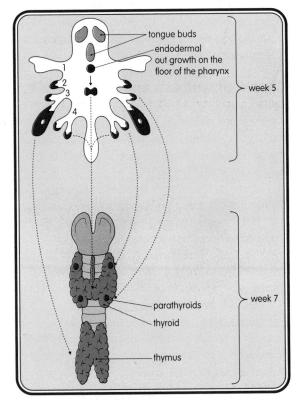

Fig. 4.4 Horizontal section through the pharynx (looking down on its floor) of a 5-week-old foetus, and the positions of the glands at 7 weeks. It shows the pharyngeal origins of the thymus, thyroid, and parathyroid glands. The pharyngeal pouches are numbered 1, 2, 3, 4. Arrows show the migration of the thyroid, parathyroid glands, and the thymus.

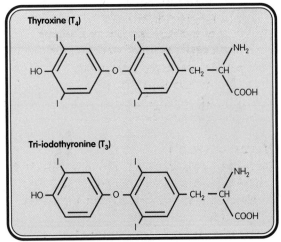

Fig. 4.5 Structures of T_3 and T_4.

against a concentration gradient (energy required for this process is supplied by Na^+/K^+ ATPase).

2. **Iodide oxidation**—I^- is rapidly oxidized into iodine (more reactive) by a peroxidase-catalysed reaction.

3. **Prethyroglobulin synthesis**—tyrosine is converted into prethyroglobulin (contains approximately 110 tyrosine residues).

4. **Iodination of prethyroglobulin** (occurs in the extracellular lumen of the thyroid follicle)—free iodine rapidly attaches to the prethyroglobulin molecules to form iodoprethyroglobulin (composed of iodinated units of T_1 and T_2).

5. **Coupling**—peroxidase enzymes convert the iodoprethyroglobulin into iodothyroglobulin (composed of iodinated units of T_3 and T_4), which is stored in the lumen. T_3 is made from $T_1 + T_2$; T_4 is made from $T_2 + T_2$.

6. **Secretion**—the iodothyroglobulin is taken up by the follicular cells by pinocytosis and broken down by lysosomal enzymes into T_3 and T_4, which diffuse down their concentration gradients into the blood.

Iodine

Iodine is a trace element in the body that is required by the thyroid gland to synthesize T_3 and T_4.

Normal iodine metabolism

Iodine is acquired from the diet. Dietary intake may be variable, as may the circulating quantities of iodide ions (I^-), but expected amounts in a normal person are

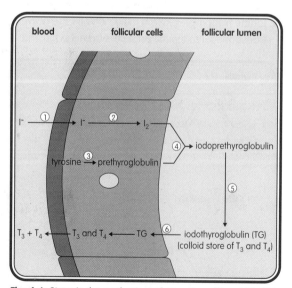

Fig. 4.6 Steps in the synthesis and secretion of T_3 and T_4. The numbers correspond with numbers in the text.

shown in Fig. 4.7. The recommended daily intake is 150 mg. Sources include meat, vegetables, iodized salt, and some bread preservatives (NB intensively farmed soils may yield vegetables that are deficient in iodine because of iodine supply in the soil becoming limited).

Plasma iodide levels are low; to compensate for this, the thyroid gland actively pumps iodide ions into its cells against a concentration and electrochemical gradient—this is known as the *iodine-trapping mechanism*. This mechanism is extremely efficient—the free-iodide concentration ratio of thyroid:plasma is normally about 25:1.

The uptake of iodide into the thyroid gland is enhanced by thyroid-stimulating hormone (TSH) and iodine deficiency, and inhibited by iodine excess and the drug digoxin.

Most iodine excretion is via the kidneys.

Iodine deficiency

Deficiency of iodine in the body results in:

- T_3 and T_4 deficiency (hypothyroidism), because the synthesis of T_3 and T_4 is iodine-dependent.
- Enlargement of the thyroid gland (goitre formation), under the influence of TSH (levels of TSH increase in response to T_3 and T_4 deficiency).

Control of synthesis and secretion of T_3 and T_4

As mentioned previously, T_3 and T_4 are synthesized by the follicular cells and stored as thyroglobulin colloid in the follicular lumen (there are several weeks/months supply of T_3 and T_4 stored).

T_3 and T_4 synthesis and secretion are controlled by the hypothalamus and the anterior pituitary gland (Fig. 4.8). TSH—released by the pituitary in response to thyrotrophin-releasing hormone (TRH) from the hypothalamus—binds to specific G-protein-linked receptors on the follicular cells (cAMP is the second messenger) and stimulates the thyroid gland to:

- Increase in size and vascularity.
- Increase iodide uptake.
- Increase protein synthesis and cellular metabolism.
- Increase intracellular volume and stores of colloid.
- Increase secretion of T_3 and T_4.

T_3 inhibits TSH secretion from the pituitary by negative feedback (NB it does not feed back on the hypothalamus). Plasma levels of T_3, T_4, and TSH are measured to determine thyroid function.

Deficient thyroid gland function leads to low circulating T_3 and T_4 concentrations (hypothyroidism), resulting in

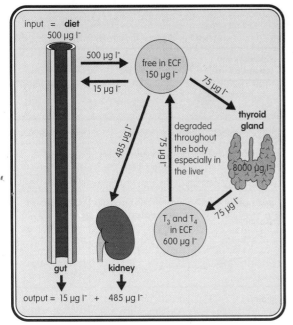

Fig. 4.7 Iodine metabolism. The amount of iodine in the thyroid is high because of the trapping mechanism and the large stores of thyroglobulin colloid that contain T_3 and T_4. (ECF = extracellular fluid.) (Adapted from *Basic & Clinical Endocrinology, 4th Ed.* by FS Greenspan. Courtesy of Appleton & Lange.)

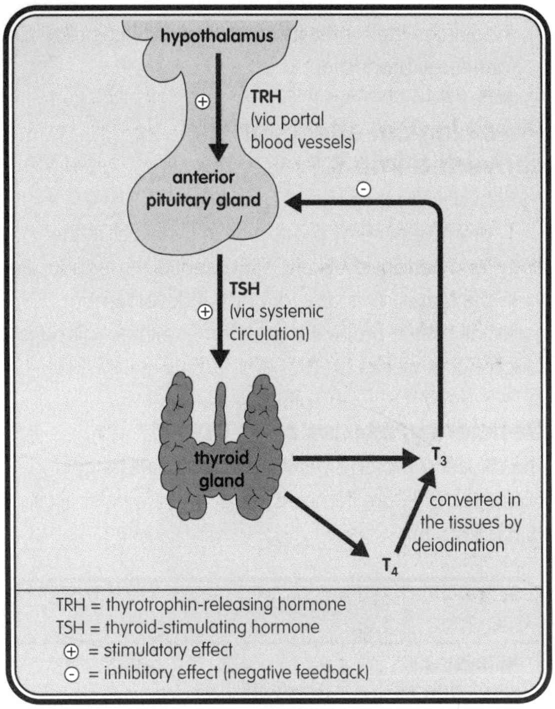

Fig. 4.8 Regulation of thyroid hormone secretion.

increased TSH secretion (pituitary gland increases TSH release to try to stimulate T_3 and T_4 secretion).

Excessive thyroid gland function leads to high circulating T_3 and T_4 concentrations (hyperthyroidism), resulting in decreased TSH secretion (high T_3 levels inhibit TSH release).

The rate of thyroid hormone secretion is normally 75–100 µg/day.

Once secreted, the thyroid hormones mainly circulate bound to plasma proteins, which are made in the liver:
- 70% is carried bound to thyroxine-binding globulin (TBG).
- 30% is carried bound to pre-albumin and albumin.

Only 0.04% of T_4 and 0.4% of T_3 are carried unbound—it is this free fraction (i.e. unbound) that is responsible for hormonal activity.

Deficiencies of the plasma proteins that carry T_3 and T_4 can cause symptoms of hyperthyroidism because there is too much unbound (and hence active) hormone circulating.

The concentration of circulating T_4 is much higher than that of T_3 (20:1). This is because the thyroid

secretes more T_4 than T_3, and T_4 is more stable (half-life of 7 days) than T_3 (half-life of 1 day).

T_4 (inactive hormone) is converted into T_3 (active) within its target cells by deiodination. This reaction is catalysed by deiodinase enzymes. Most tissues possess the type-1 deiodinase enzyme. The brain and pituitary also possess type-2 and type-3 deiodinase—these enzymes ensure that the CNS has a constant level of intracellular T_3.

T_3 is degraded by deiodination throughout the body or by conjugation in the liver.

Intracellular actions of T_3 and T_4

Free T_3 in the plasma enters cells by passive diffusion (or is derived from intracellular deiodination of T_4) and binds to intracellular T_3 receptors located in the membrane, mitochondria, and nucleus of the target cells.
- In the membrane, T_3 stimulates the Na^+/K^+ ATPase pump, resulting in increased uptake of amino acids and glucose (required as substrates for energy production).
- In the mitochondria, T_3 stimulates mitochondrial growth, replication, and activity, resulting in the increased production of energy molecules.
- In the nucleus, the hormone–receptor complex binds to the thyroid-response element of the DNA and

modulates the synthesis of enzyme proteins required for energy production.

Physiological effects of T_3 (T_4 is converted into T_3)

The physiological effects of T_3 are listed in Fig. 4.9.

T_3 promotes energy production in every cell in the body, and normal levels of it are essential throughout life.

In the foetus, T_3 is vital for normal development, especially of the brain and skeleton (the foetal gland is functional at weeks 10–11).

Deficiency/excess of T_3 and T_4

The clinical symptoms resulting from a deficiency and an excess of T_3 are itemized in Fig. 4.10 (see also Figs 15.5 and 15.6).

Physiological effects of T_3	
Processes and systems affected	**Effects of T_3**
rate of metabolism	stimulates mitochondria to generate more ATP, which is used to drive metabolic reactions — production of ATP requires oxygen, so by inducing the cell to make more ATP, T_3 causes increased oxygen consumption (i.e. increases the basal metabolic rate)
heat production	increases heat production (by increasing the basal metabolic rate)
carbohydrate and fat metabolism	stimulates: • lipolysis and glycolysis (catabolic processes) • gluconeogenesis in the liver, • glucose absorption from the gut, • insulin metabolism (— anabolic reactions stimulated by insulin are reduced) potentiates the glycogenolytic effects of adrenaline
development	essential for normal cell division, differentiation, and maturation in the developing foetus, especially in the brain and skeleton
growth	stimulates the production and action of growth hormone
cardiovascular system	increases heart rate and stroke volume
endocrine and nervous systems	increases the breakdown of cortisol and insulin; potentiates β-adrenergic effects; may be required for the production of prolactin

Fig. 4.9 Physiological effects of T_3.

Clinical symptoms caused by T_3 excess (hyperthyroidism) and T_3 deficiency (hypothyroidism)		
Processes and systems affected	**Effect of hyperthyroidism**	**Effect of hypothyroidism**
rate of metabolism	high basal metabolic rate	low basal metabolic rate
heat production	heat intolerance	cold intolerance
carbohydrate and fat metabolism	increased metabolism → weight loss	decreased metabolism → weight gain
development	may develop premature osteoporosis due to abnormal bone turnover	abnormal brain and skeletal development in the foetus → cretinism (mental retardation and dwarfism)
growth	pretibial myxoedema (thickening of the skin)	coarse dry skin and hair; hair loss
cardiovascular system	rapid pulse and palpitations	slow pulse
endocrine and nervous systems	increased sweating, irritability, restlessness, insomnia, menorrhagia	decreased sweating, slow thinking, lethargy, sleepiness, oligomenorrhoea

Fig. 4.10 Clinical symptoms caused by T_3 excess (hyperthyroidism) and T_3 deficiency (hypothyroidism).

○ **Discuss the anatomy, histology, and development of the thyroid and parathyroid glands.**
○ **Describe the structure and synthesis of the thyroid hormones (T_3 and T_4).**
○ **Explain the importance of iodine and outline its metabolism.**
○ **Outline the synthesis, secretion, regulation, metabolism, and effects of T_3 and T_4.**
○ **What are the effects of TSH on the thryoid gland?**
○ **List the effects of excess and deficiency of T_3 and T_4.**

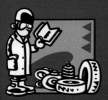

5. The Adrenal Glands

Structure of the adrenal glands

Macrostructure of the adrenal glands

There are two adrenal glands, each weighing about 5 g, which are situated in the retroperitoneum, on the upper poles of each kidney (Fig. 5.1). The right gland (pyramidal in shape) is located anterior to the right crus of the diaphragm, posterior to the vena cava and the right lobe of the liver. The left gland (crescent shaped) is located anterior to the left crus of the diaphragm, posterior to the splenic vessels and the pancreas, and inferior to the stomach.

Each gland has a yellow outer cortex and a inner medulla, the result of their different origins and different functions.

Blood is supplied from the adrenal arteries and drains towards the centre (medulla) of the gland and into the adrenal vein. Lymphatic drainage is to the lateral aortic nodes.

Nerves that supply the adrenal glands are predominantly *preganglionic* sympathetic fibres from the splanchnic nerves, and the nerve endings are in the adrenal medulla.

Microstructure of the adrenal gland

The adrenal gland is divided into the adrenal cortex and the adrenal medulla (Figs 5.2 and 5.3). The adrenal cortex is the paler, outer region of the adrenal gland and it is divided into three layers:

- The zona glomerulosa.
- The zona fasciculata.
- The zona reticularis.

The adrenal medulla is the darker, inner region of the adrenal gland and is composed of a loose meshwork of chromaffin cells (modified sympathetic ganglion cells). Chromaffin cells synthesize and secrete either adrenaline or noradrenaline (not both), dopamine, and some peptides. Secretory granules containing these hormones are stored in the cytoplasm. Chromaffin the cells are surrounded by sinusoids from cortical and medullary arteries (corticosteroids in the cortical arteries are essential for the formation of adrenaline from noradrenaline).

The adrenal medulla is richly innervated by preganglionic sympathetic fibres, which stimulate the chromaffin cells to secrete their hormones.

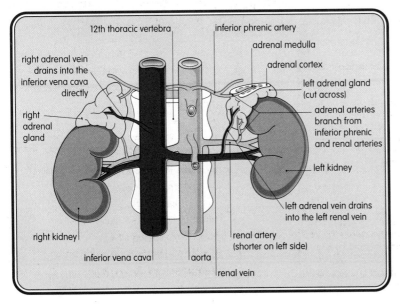

Fig. 5.1 Location and blood supply of the adrenal glands.

Microstructure of the adrenal gland and the major hormones secreted in each region			
Region	**Name**	**Cell structure**	**Hormones synthesized**
outer cortex	zona glomerulosa	cells arranged in clumps (Latin, glomerulus: blackberry)	mineralocorticoids (mainly aldosterone)
middle cortex	zona fasciculata	cells arranged in cords alongside blood sinusoids; cells contain abundant lipid, which is used in the synthesis of steroid hormone (Latin, fasciculus: bundle)	glucocorticoids (mainly cortisol)
inner cortex	zona reticularis	network of smaller cells (Latin, reticularis: network)	glucocorticoids and adrenal androgens (mainly DHEA and androstenedione)
centre of gland	adrenal medulla	loose network of chromaffin cells (modified sympathetic ganglion cells) surrounded by blood sinusoids	catecholamines (adrenaline and noradrenaline)

Fig. 5.2 Microstructure of the adrenal gland and the major hormones secreted in each region.

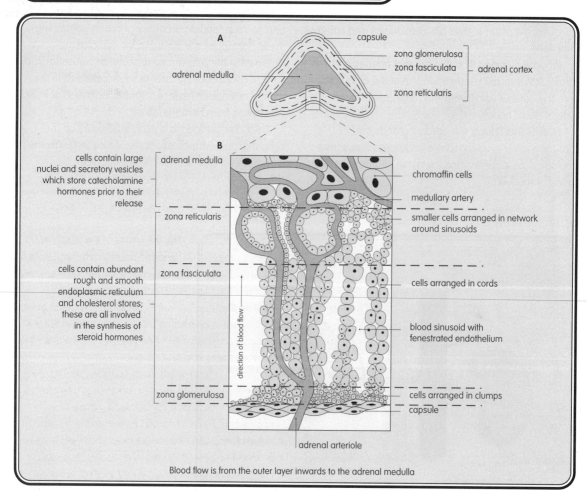

Fig. 5.3 (A) Cross-section through the adrenal glands. (B) Microstructure of the adrenal glands showing the different cell types found in each region and the direction of blood flow.

The adrenal medulla can be regarded as part of the sympathetic nervous system. It is in effect a sympathetic ganglion that lies in the adrenal gland. Preganglionic fibres from the sympathetic trunk synapse with the medullary cells and stimulate the release of adrenaline.

○ Outline the location, relations, and blood supply of the adrenal glands.
○ Describe the histology of the adrenal cortex and the adrenal medulla.
○ List the hormones secreted by the adrenal gland.
○ Explain the development of the adrenal glands.

Development of the adrenal glands

The formation of the adrenal glands is shown in Fig. 5.4.

The adrenal cortex

The adrenal cortex is derived from mesodermal tissue. At birth it is very large and is composed of two zones:
- the foetal zone, which gradually involutes after birth
- the definitive cortex, which produces steroid hormones (including cortisol) and is similar to the adult cortex.

The adrenal medulla

The adrenal medulla is a modified sympathetic ganglion derived from ectodermal tissue.

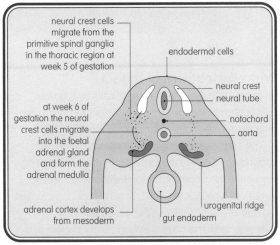

Fig. 5.4 Formation of the adrenal glands (detectable at week 8 of gestation).

HORMONES OF THE ADRENAL CORTEX

Glucocorticoids (cortisol)

Synthesis and secretion of cortisol

Cortisol is the major glucocorticoid. It is a steroid hormone, synthesized from cholesterol—by cells of the zona fasciculata region of the adrenal cortex—in response to stimuli that promote its secretion, e.g. adrenocorticotrophic hormone (ACTH) released by the pituitary in response to corticotrophin-releasing hormone (CRH) from the hypothalamus. Free levels of cortisol in the plasma feed back on the hypothalamus (and, to a lesser extent, on the pituitary) to inhibit CRH and ACTH release (Fig 5.5).

Once secreted, 95% of cortisol circulates bound to plasma proteins—80% bound to cortisol-binding protein (CBG) and 15% bound to albumin. The free (i.e. unbound) hormone is the biologically active component.

CBG synthesis in the liver is stimulated by oestrogens, therefore during pregnancy (when oestrogen levels are high) cortisol secretion increases in order to maintain the levels of free hormone in the blood.

Cortisol is degraded into α-cortol or β-cortol by the liver and conjugated to glucuronide or sulphate groups to make them more readily excreted by the kidney.

Approximately 1% of cortisol is excreted unmetabolized, and this can be measured over a 24-hour period to estimate levels of cortisol in the blood.

There is a circadian (diurnal) rhythm to plasma cortisol levels—levels are higher in the morning (peak at 6 a.m.) and lower at night (Fig. 5.6). This is due to a

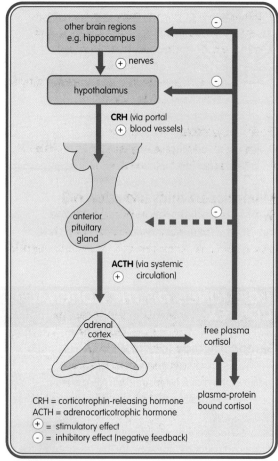

Fig. 5.5 Control of cortisol secretion.

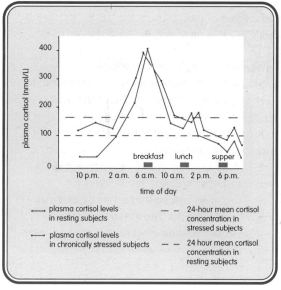

Fig. 5.6 Circadian variation in plasma cortisol in resting and chronically stressed subjects.

> **Prolonged steroid treatment with exogenous glucocorticoids drives down ACTH release, therefore endogenous cortisol production is extremely low—patients must be weaned off steroid treatment slowly to allow the rise of plasma cortisol to normal levels.**

change in the effectiveness of the negative feedback of cortisol on the hypothalamus.

- In the morning, cortisol feedback is less effective and ACTH secretion is high.
- In the evening, cortisol feedback is more effective and ACTH is secreted at its basal level, i.e. there is no hypothalamic drive.

During times of chronic stress, plasma cortisol is raised but still follows a circadian rhythm, as shown in Fig. 5.6. It is the area below the curve that is significant in determining increased plasma cortisol. There is no elevation in the peak of plasma cortisol in the morning, but levels are raised in the evening and at night. This causes disruption in sleep, as cortisol signals wakefulness.

Intracellular actions of cortisol

Free cortisol in the plasma enters cells by passive diffusion and binds to steroid receptors located in the cytoplasm or nucleus of target cells (see Fig. 1.10).

The cortisol–receptor complex binds to specific enhancer regions of the DNA, promoting or inhibiting the synthesis of specific proteins depending on the target cell type. For example: in some cells it increases the rate of transcription of the gene that codes for lipocortin, which is an anti-inflammatory protein that inhibits phospholipase A2 (topically applied glucocorticoid-containing creams act in this way to reduce skin inflammation); in the hypothalamus, cortisol binds to DNA and inhibits the transcription of CRH.

Physiological effects of cortisol

The physiological effects of cortisol are listed in Fig. 5.7. Cortisol is essential for life (bilateral adrenalectomy causes death within days). It allows other hormones to induce certain effects but in a controlled manner (i.e. it prevents over-response to a stimulus) and is important both in maintaining metabolic balance and in the body's response to stress.

The response to stress is called the general adaptation syndrome (GAS) and is divided into three phases:

- **Alarm reaction**—an initial stressful stimulus causes the secretion of adrenaline, noradrenaline, and cortisol (cortisol allows adrenaline and noradrenaline to exert their effect—the 'fight or flight' response).
- **Resistance**—cortisol acts more slowly than adrenaline and noradrenaline and is longer lasting, so the resistance to stress is maintained. It also counteracts the effects of other hormones, e.g. insulin, to maintain substrates required to combat stress.

- **Exhaustion**—prolonged stress causes continued cortisol secretion and results in muscle wastage, immune-cell atrophy, and hyperglycaemia.

Cortisol also prevents the body from over-responding to stress, e.g. suppresses inflammation.

Deficiency/excess of cortisol

The effects of cortisol deficiency and excess are listed in Fig. 5.8 (see also Figs 15.10 and 15.11)

Mineralocorticoids (aldosterone)
Synthesis and secretion of aldosterone

Aldosterone is the major mineralocorticoid. It is a steroid hormone synthesized from cholesterol—by cells

Cortisol modulates the body's response to stress and can be regarded as a 'stress hormone'.

Fig. 5.7 Physiological effects of cortisol.

Physiological effects of cortisol	
Process/system affected	**Effect of cortisol**
carbohydrate metabolism	maintains blood glucose during fasting by stimulation of glycogenolysis and gluconeogenesis
protein metabolism	increases breakdown of skeletal muscle protein into amino acids (which are used to make more glucose)
fat metabolism	stimulates lipolysis in the limbs and accumulation of fat in the trunk and face
immune system	inhibits antibody production and lymphoid-tissue growth
inflammatory responses	suppresses inflammation by reducing synthesis of prostacyclin
endocrine system	suppresses the secretion of the pituitary hormones ACTH, LH, FSH, TSH, and GH
nervous system	influences neuronal development in the foetal and neonatal brain; influences behaviour and cognitive function; augments the effect of catecholamines on the cardiovascular system
water metabolism	decreases sodium and water excretion by inhibiting glomerular filtration (i.e. has a weak mineralocorticoid-like action)
calcium metabolism	decreases calcium absorption from the gut; increases calcium resorption from bone and its loss from the kidney

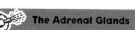

of the zona glomerulosa region of the adrenal cortex—in response to stimuli that promote its secretion (see Fig. 5.9). These include:

- Angiotensin II.
- Increased plasma K$^+$ levels.
- ACTH.

Aldosterone is secreted in very low concentrations and 60% circulates bound to plasma albumin (there is no specific binding protein). The 40% free (i.e. unbound) hormone is the biologically active component.

Aldosterone is rapidly inactivated by the liver (half-life = 15–20 minutes) and excreted by the kidney.

Intracellular actions of aldosterone

As shown in Fig. 5.9, free aldosterone (A) in the plasma enters cells by passive diffusion and binds to steroid receptors (REC) located in the cytoplasm or nucleus of target cells. The aldosterone–receptor complex binds to specific enhancer regions of the DNA, promoting the synthesis of specific proteins that mediate the effect of aldosterone.

Aldosterone increases the synthesis of:

1. Na$^+$ channels in the apical membrane, so increasing the rate of Na$^+$ entry into the cells from the collecting duct lumen.
2. Na$^+$/K$^+$ ATPase in the basal membrane, so

Fig.5.8 Effects of cortisol excess (Cushing's syndrome) and cortisol deficiency (e.g. Addison's disease).

Effects of cortisol excess (Cushing's syndrome) and cortisol deficiency (e.g. Addison's disease)		
Process/system affected	**Effect of cortisol excess**	**Effect of cortisol deficiency**
carbohydrate metabolism	tendency to hyperglycaemia (promotes insulin resistance)	tendency to hypoglycaemia (promotes sensitivity to insulin)
protein metabolism	thin skin and skeletal-muscle wasting (thin arms and legs), caused by increased proteolysis	reduced mobilization of protein
fat metabolism	'moon-face', 'buffalo-hump', protuberant abdomen, and striae (stretch marks), caused by increased fat deposition in the face and trunk	reduced lipolysis and hence reduced gluconeogenesis
immune system	increased susceptibility to infection	–
inflammatory responses	reduced wound healing and easy bruising	–
endocrine system	testicular atrophy or menstrual disturbances, caused by FSH and LH suppression	increased pigmentation of the skin and mucosa, caused by increased ACTH release
nervous system	depression, confusion, insomnia, occasional frank psychosis	lethargy
water metabolism	high blood pressure, swollen ankles, tendency to chronic cardiac failure; associated hypokalaemia due to water retention (but can also cause water depletion due to hyperglycaemia)	tendency to salt and water depletion; associated hyponatraemia and hyperkalaemia
calcium metabolism	tendency to hypocalcaemia and osteoporosis (tendency for collapse of lumbar spine, i.e. kyphosis)	tendency to hypercalcaemia

increasing the rate of Na+ reabsorption into the extracellular fluid (ECF).

3. ATP, so providing energy for the Na+/K+ ATPase molecules.
4. K+ channels in the apical membrane, so enhancing K+ secretion into the lumen.
5. Na+–H+ exchange proteins, so enhancing H+ secretion into the lumen and Na+ reuptake.

Physiological effects of aldosterone

Aldosterone regulates salt and water balance by controlling plasma electrolytes and water excretion in the kidney.

Other hormones that regulate salt and water balance include antidiuretic hormone (ADH), renin, angiotensin II, prostaglandins, atrial natriuretic peptides, and natriuretic hormone (see Chapter 7). Aldosterone also promotes sodium reabsorption from colonic and gastric glands, and from the ducts of sweat and salivary glands.

Deficiency/excess of aldosterone

The effects of aldosterone excess and deficiency are listed in Fig. 5.10.

Adrenal androgens
Synthesis and secretion of adrenal androgens

DHEA and androstenedione are the main adrenal androgens. They are synthesized from cholesterol in the zona reticularis region of the adrenal cortex. Synthesis and secretion of androgens only begins when the zona reticularis matures (adrenarche) at 7–9 years of age.

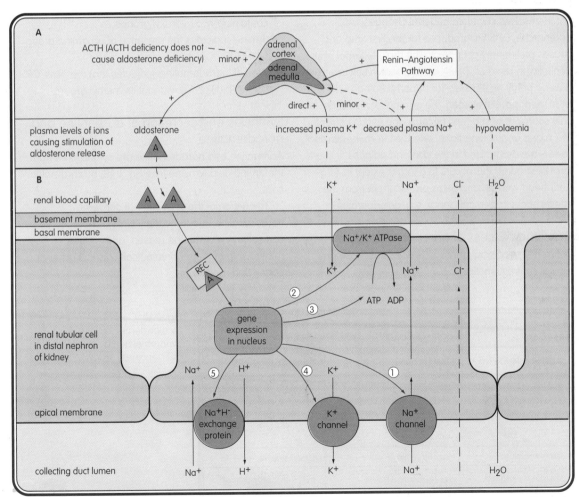

Fig. 5.9 (A) Control of aldosterone release. (B) Its intracellular effects that stimulate Na+, Cl-, and water reabsorption and K+ and H+ secretion into the renal collecting duct lumen. (The numbers correspond with the numbers in the text.)

Adrenarche preceeds sex-hormone release and occurs about one year before puberty and gonadal maturation (and menarche in females). It is not known what triggers adrenarche but ACTH may augment it once it has started.

Physiological effects of adrenal androgens

Adrenal androgens have minimal biological activity.

They are converted peripherally into testosterone and dihydrotestosterone (more potent androgens):

- In males, conversion of adrenal androgens accounts for only 5% of testosterone production, and its physiological effect is negligible.
- In females, conversion of adrenal androgens accounts for 40–65% of testosterone production.

Adrenal androgens may be involved in adrenarche by preparing the gonads for the onset of puberty (but do not themselves stimulate pubertal changes). At adrenarche, DHEA is produced for the first time and causes preliminary changes to the male external genitalia. In females, DHEA is important in sex drive and may be partly responsible for pubertal hair growth.

In menopausal women, the adrenal cortex is the only source of oestrogens because the ovaries atrophy. DHEA and androstenedione, released from the adrenal cortex, are aromatized in the skin and adipose tissue to form oestradiol. This occurs to a larger extent in Afro-Caribbean women and helps protect them from the effects of oestrogen deficiency, e.g. osteoporosis.

Deficiency/excess of adrenal androgens

Deficiency of adrenal androgens does not cause any clinical consequences.

Excessive secretion of adrenal androgens results in androgen excess.

- In males, androgen excess causes precocious puberty but has no clinical consequences in the adult.
- In females, androgen excess causes virilization/masculinization, characterized by temporal balding, a male-form body, muscle bulk, deepening of the voice, enlargement of the clitoris, and hirsutism.

HORMONES OF THE ADRENAL MEDULLA

Adrenaline and noradrenaline

Adrenaline and noradrenaline are catecholamine hormones and their structures are shown in Fig. 5.13:

- 'Catechol' indicates the presence of a benzene ring containing two hydroxyl groups.
- 'Amine' indicates the presence of an amino group ($-NH_2$).
- 'Nor' of 'noradrenaline' indicates that the 'N' is 'OR' ('ohne Radikal', i.e. without its methyl group).

Synthesis and secretion of adrenaline and noradrenaline

Adrenaline and noradrenaline are synthesized from the amino acid tyrosine (see Fig. 1.4B) by chromaffin cells.

The action of the enzyme that converts noradrenaline to adrenaline (PNMT) is potentiated by cortisol (this may be the reason for the close relationship of the embryologically distinct adrenal cortex and medulla).

Clinical symptoms caused by aldosterone excess (e.g. Conn's syndrome) and aldosterone deficiency (e.g. Addison's disease)		
Action of aldosterone	**Effect of excess**	**Effect of deficiency**
increases plasma Na^+	Na^+ retention rarely occurs because of other mechanisms regulating fluid volume — the 'escape' mechanism (see page 61)	loss of Na^+ is accompanied by loss of water (hence no change in plasma Na^+ concentrations)
decreases plasma K^+	hypokalaemia	hyperkalaemia
decreases plasma H^+	hypokalaemic alkalosis	mild metabolic acidosis
maintains ECF volume	hypertension	volume depletion and postural hypotension

Fig. 5.10 Clinical symptoms caused by aldosterone excess (e.g. Conn's syndrome) and aldosterone deficiency (e.g. Addison's disease).

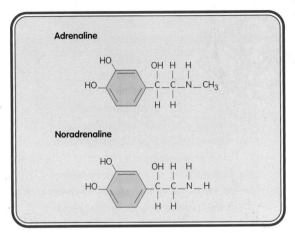

Fig. 5.11 Structure of adrenaline and noradrenaline.

The catecholamines are stored in vesicles in the cell cytoplasm, and released in bursts in response to nervous stimuli from the preganglionic sympathetic fibres during times of stress (e.g. during exercise, pain, fear, hypotension, hypoglycaemia, anoxia). Release is accompanied by generalized sympathetic discharge.

Once secreted into the blood, adrenaline and noradrenaline circulate bound to albumin.

They are rapidly metabolized (mainly in the liver, kidney, and nerve endings) by catecholamine-*O*-methyltransferase (COMT) and monoamine oxidase (MAO) into vanillylmandelic acid (VMA) and excreted in the urine.

Intracellular actions of adrenaline and noradrenaline (see Figs 1.5 and 1.6)

Adrenaline and noradrenaline bind to α and β receptors (linked to G proteins) present on the surface of many different cell types. The effect of adrenaline and noradrenaline in different tissues and organs varies depending on the type of α and β receptors exhibited by the tissue cells, e.g.:

- Adrenaline causes vasoconstriction in most tissues (gut, adipose, skin, kidney) because their arterioles exhibit α_1 receptors.
- Adrenaline causes vasodilatation in the lungs, heart, and muscles because their arterioles exhibit β_2 receptors.

Physiological effects of adrenaline and noradrenaline

Adrenaline is a stress hormone, called the hormone of 'flight or fight'. It prepares the body for increased physical and mental exertion (see Fig. 5.12). Circulating adrenaline reinforces the autonomic nervous system and exerts effects on tissues that are not directly innervated.

Noradrenaline exerts the same effects on the body as adrenaline, but mainly via the nervous system rather than the endocrine system (it is the major neurotransmitter of the sympathetic nervous system, which is activated by the same stressors that activate the adrenal medulla).

For more information on α and β receptors and on the role of the sympathetic nervous system in the 'flight or fight' response, see the *Crash Course! Nervous System and Special Senses*.

Deficiency/excess of adrenaline and noradrenaline (see also page 168)

The sympathetic nervous system compensates for deficiencies in the adrenal catecholamines and no clinical disability is detectable.

Excessive adrenaline secretion causes severe hypertension, pallor, pulsating headache, sweating, tremor, anxiety, nausea, vomiting, and weight loss.

- Describe the circadian rhythm of plasma cortisol levels.
- Define the role of cortisol as a stress hormone.
- List the hormones of the adrenal cortex and outline the control of secretion and the physiological effects of each.
- Discuss the effects of adrenal androgens and their role in adrenarche and during menopause.
- List the effects of excess and deficiency of the cortical hormones.

The Adrenal Glands

Catecholamines are secreted as true hormones by the adrenal medulla but also as neuro-transmitters by the autonomic (sympathetic and parasympathetic) nervous system. Adrenaline is mainly secreted by the adrenal medulla, whereas noradrenaline is mainly secreted by the autonomic nervous system (the adrenal medulla secretes very little noradrenaline).

- Describe the structure and synthesis of the catecholamines.
- Enumerate the secretion, intracellular actions, and physiological effects of adrenaline and noradrenaline.
- Discuss the importance of the α and β receptors in the response of different tissues to adrenaline and noradrenaline.
- List the effects of excessive adrenaline secretion.

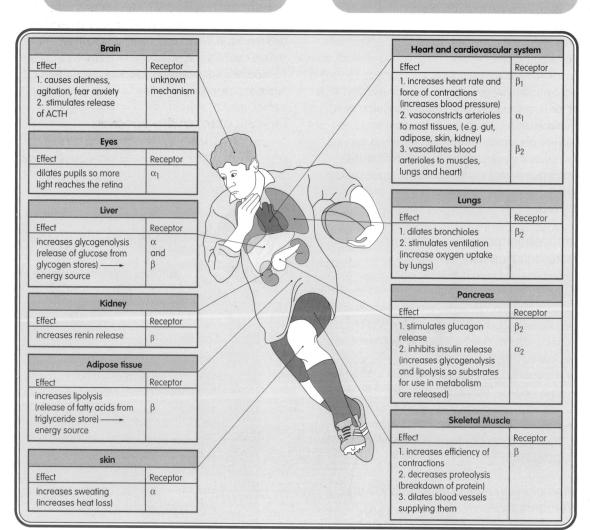

Brain

Effect	Receptor
1. causes alertness, agitation, fear anxiety 2. stimulates release of ACTH	unknown mechanism

Eyes

Effect	Receptor
dilates pupils so more light reaches the retina	α_1

Liver

Effect	Receptor
increases glycogenolysis (release of glucose from glycogen stores) $\longrightarrow$ energy source	α and β

Kidney

Effect	Receptor
increases renin release	β

Adipose tissue

Effect	Receptor
increases lipolysis (release of fatty acids from triglyceride store) $\longrightarrow$ energy source	β

skin

Effect	Receptor
increases sweating (increases heat loss)	α

Heart and cardiovascular system

Effect	Receptor
1. increases heart rate and force of contractions (increases blood pressure)	β_1
2. vasoconstricts arterioles to most tissues, (e.g. gut, adipose, skin, kidney)	α_1
3. vasodilates blood arterioles to muscles, lungs and heart)	β_2

Lungs

Effect	Receptor
1. dilates bronchioles 2. stimulates ventilation (increase oxygen uptake by lungs)	β_2

Pancreas

Effect	Receptor
1. stimulates glucagon release	β_2
2. inhibits insulin release (increases glycogenolysis and lipolysis so substrates for use in metabolism are released)	α_2

Skeletal Muscle

Effect	Receptor
1. increases efficiency of contractions 2. decreases proteolysis (breakdown of protein) 3. dilates blood vessels supplying them	β

Fig. 5.12 Physiological effects of adrenaline and noradrenaline, and the receptors present in each tissue/organ.

6. The Pancreas and the Gastrointestinal System

ORGANIZATION OF THE ENDOCRINE PANCREAS

Structure of the pancreas
Macrostructure of the pancreas
The pancreas is a long, flat, glandular organ, weighing about 80 g, that is situated in the retroperitoneum behind the stomach (Fig. 6.1). It extends across the posterior body wall from the curve of the duodenum to the hilus of the spleen.

It consists of:
- Head with an uncinate process.
- Neck.
- Body.
- Tail.

The head lies within the curve of the duodenum, in front of the vena cava; the tail reaches the hilus of the spleen.

Blood supply is from the branches of the splenic and superior and inferior pancreaticoduodenal arteries.

Nerves that supply the pancreas are from the splanchnic nerves and the vagi via the coeliac plexus.

Lymphatic drainage is to the coeliac group of pre-aortic nodes via the suprapancreatic nodes.

Microstructure of the pancreas
The pancreas contains both exocrine and endocrine cells.
- Exocrine cells (acinar cells) release digestive enzymes and bicarbonate into the duodenum via the pancreatic duct.
- Endocrine cells (comprise 1–2% of the wet weight of the pancreas) release hormones into the bloodstream.

Endocrine cells, grouped as clusters of cells called the islets of Langerhans, receive 5–10 times the blood flow of a comparable portion of exocrine pancreatic tissue.

There are 1–2 million islets in the pancreas. Each islet contains 2000–6000 cells of four distinct types (Figs 6.2 and 6.3).

Development of the pancreas
The pancreas develops from the foregut, from two discrete outgrowths from the duodenum which later fuse.

The stages of embryological development are illustrated in Fig. 6.4.

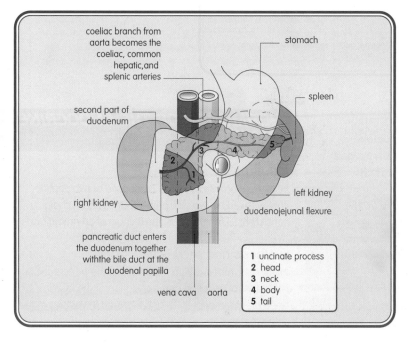

Fig. 6.1 Location of the pancreas in the upper part of the posterior abdominal wall, showing the labelled regions of the gland. (NB Each of the regions consists of the same cell types and structure.)

coeliac branch from aorta becomes the coeliac, common hepatic, and splenic arteries

stomach

second part of duodenum

spleen

right kidney

left kidney

duodenojejunal flexure

pancreatic duct enters the duodenum together with the bile duct at the duodenal papilla

vena cava   aorta

1 uncinate process
2 head
3 neck
4 body
5 tail

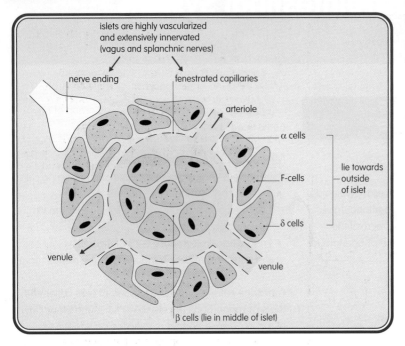

islets are highly vascularized
and extensively innervated
(vagus and splanchnic nerves)

nerve ending

fenestrated capillaries

arteriole

α cells

F-cells

lie towards
outside
of islet

δ cells

venule

venule

β cells (lie in middle of islet)

Fig. 6.2 Histology of the endocrine pancreas—the islets of Langerhans—showing the cell types and their locations.

Cell types, the hormones they secrete, and their relative numbers in the pancreatic islets

Cell type	Percentage of cells in islets	Hormone secreted	Role of hormone
alpha cells (α cells)	20 –25	glucagon	regulates anabolic pathways of metabolism
beta cells (β cells)	70 – 80	insulin	regulates catabolic pathways of metabolism
delta cells (δ cells)	<10	somatostatin	regulates gastric motility and the secretion of gut hormones
F cells (PP cells)	<10	pancreatic polypeptide	regulates digestive processes

Fig. 6.3 Cell types, the hormones they secrete, and their relative numbers in the pancreatic islets.

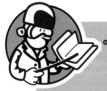

○ **Specify the location, relations, and blood and nerve supplies of the pancreas.**
○ **Describe the histology of the endocrine pancreas, including the relative proportions and distribution of the four different cell types.**
○ **Outline the development of the pancreas.**

HORMONES OF THE ENDOCRINE PANCREAS

Insulin

Insulin is a protein hormone composed of two peptide chains linked by two disulphide bridges (the A chain consists of 21 amino acids; the B chain of 30 amino acids).

Synthesis and secretion of insulin

Insulin is synthesized (in the β cells of the pancreatic islets) by transcription and translation of the insulin gene on chromosome 11, and is stored in vesicles in the cell cytoplasm.

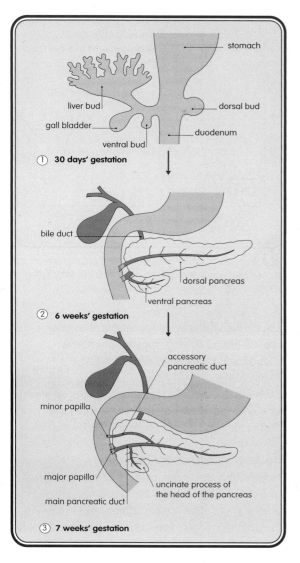

Fig. 6.4 Embryological development of the pancreas.
1. At 30 days' gestation, a ventral bud arises in common with the liver outgrowth from the duodenum, and a dorsal bud arises at the same level.
2. At 6 weeks' gestation, the ventral bud migrates posteriorly around the duodenum towards the dorsal bud and lies in close contact with it. Each bud has a discrete pancreatic duct at this stage.
3. At 7 weeks' gestation, the buds fuse, as do their pancreatic ducts to form the main duct that enters the duodenum in combination with the bile duct at the major papilla (the accessory duct is not always present and is derived from the dorsal duct).

C peptide (connecting peptide) is synthesized in the β cells together with insulin, and they are secreted in equimolar amounts.

Insulin is the only hormone in the body that decreases blood glucose levels (by increasing glucose uptake by cells), and therefore its secretion needs to be tightly controlled. Some factors initiate or potentiate insulin release, others inhibit it (Fig. 6.5).

Insulin secretion in response to a sudden rise in plasma glucose or to other stimulating factors occurs in a biphasic fashion (Fig. 6.6):

- First phase—stored insulin is rapidly released in a short burst lasting <1 minute.
- Second phase—stored and newly synthesized insulin is released until the stimulating factor subsides.

Fig. 6.5 Factors that control insulin secretion. NB Blood glucose is the most important factor in the regulation of insulin secretion.

Factors that control insulin secretion		
Primary stimulants (initiate insulin release)	**Secondary stimulants (potentiate insulin release)**	**Inhibitors (reduce insulin release)**
• increase in blood glucose concentration • basic amino acids • fatty acids and ketones (to a lesser extent) • diabetic drugs, e.g. sulphonylureas	• glucogen • growth hormone • parasympathetic innervation (acetylcholine) • gut hormones • other hormones (ACTH, TSH) • adrenaline (via β preceptors)	• hypolcalcaemia • somatostatin (GHIH) • sympathetic innervation (noradrenaline) • adrenaline (via α receptors)

Measurement of plasma C-peptide levels is sometimes useful in patients presenting with hypoglycaemia (low plasma glucose concentration). If blood tests show elevated plasma insulin and C-peptide levels, there may be an insulin-producing pancreatic β-cell tumour. If, however, blood tests show elevated insulin but suppressed C-peptide levels, then factitious hypoglycaemia should be suspected, i.e. the patient must have injected exogenous insulin—owing to either excessive treatment for diabetes or attempted suicide.

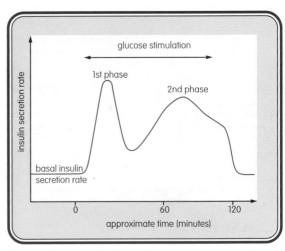

Fig. 6.6 Biphasic insulin secretion in response to prolonged glucose stimulation (e.g. after a meal) or other stimulating factors.

- In the liver, the enzyme hepatic phosphorylase, which breaks down glycogen to glucose, is inactivated by insulin by *phosphorylation*.

Insulin has different effects in specific tissues according to the enzymes present in different cell types and whether they are activated or deactivated by insulin.

Effects of insulin on metabolism

Insulin is an *anabolic hormone* in that it promotes the uptake of simple molecules into cells and their conversion into more complex storage molecules—i.e. glucose into glycogen, fatty acids into lipids, and amino acids into proteins (Fig. 6.8).

Deficiency/excess of insulin

Insulin deficiency (diabetes mellitus) causes hyperglycaemia.

Insulin excess causes hypoglycaemia. (See also page 50.)

Glucagon

Glucagon is a polypeptide hormone comprising 29 amino acids.

The cellular mechanism of insulin release is shown in Fig. 6.7.

Once secreted, insulin circulates unbound in the plasma and has a short half-life of about 5 minutes. It is degraded by virtually all the tissues of the body, but mainly by the liver and kidney.

Intracellular actions of insulin (see Fig. 1.9)

Virtually all cells have a cell membrane receptor that binds insulin. Insulin receptors can become internalized in the cell—this may provide a means of downregulating insulin action.

The insulin receptor has an intracellular tyrosine kinase region (but no second messenger for insulin has been identified). When insulin binds to the receptor, the tyrosine kinase causes an intracellular cascade of phosphorylation and dephosphorylation reactions that activate or deactivate specific enzyme proteins, e.g.:

- An important action of insulin is the conversion of glucose into glycogen—in most cells this reaction is controlled by the enzyme glycogen synthetase, which is inactive in the phosphorylated form and activated by *dephosphorylation*.

Diabetes mellitus is the most common endocrine disorder.

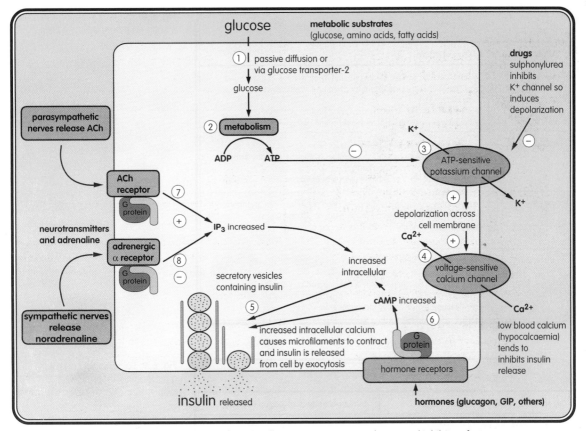

Fig. 6.7 Cellular mechanism of insulin release from β cells in response to stimulatory and inhibitory factors.
1. Glucose enters the pancreatic β cells by passive diffusion or via glucose transporter-2 protein (especially important during hyperglycaemia after meals).
2. Glucose metabolism causes an increase in intracellular ATP.
3. ATP inhibits the action of potassium channels in the cell membrane, causing the cell to depolarize.
4. The depolarization stimulates the calcium channels, so more calcium ions (Ca^{2+}) enter the cell.
5. Increased intracellular Ca^{2+} cause microtubules attached to the insulin-containing vesicles to contract and insulin is released from the cell into the bloodstream.
6. Glucagon, GIP, and other hormones bind to their respective receptors on the β-cell membrane and cause an increase in cAMP in the cell. cAMP causes an increase in Ca^{2+} and has a direct stimulatory effect on insulin release as well.
7. Parasympathetic nerves release acetylcholine (ACh), which causes an increase in inositol triphosphate (IP_3) in the cell. IP_3 causes an increase in Ca^{2+} and thereby stimulates insulin release.
8. Sympathetic nerves and adrenaline inhibit IP_3 release in the cell and thereby inhibit insulin release.

Synthesis and secretion of glucagon

Glucagon is synthesized—mainly in the α cells of the pancreatic islets, but also in gastrointestinal cells—by transcription and translation of the glucagon gene on chromosome 2, and is stored in vesicles in the cell cytoplasm.

Glicentin-related polypeptide fragment (GRPP; glicentin is an enteroglucagon hormone) is synthesized in the α cells together with glucagon, and they are secreted in equimolar amounts.

Glucagon is not the only hormone in the body that increases blood glucose levels (numerous other endocrine and nervous stimuli are also involved) and therefore its secretion is not as tightly controlled compared with that of insulin.

The factors that affect glucagon release are listed in Fig. 6.9. It should be noted that some factors (e.g. basic amino acids and gut hormones) stimulate both insulin and glucagon release together, which may allow protein synthesis and uptake of digested foodstuffs from the gut without upsetting the normal levels of glucose in the blood.

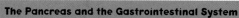

Major metabolic effects of insulin on different target cells	
Target cells	**Action of insulin**
body cells (including muscle)	• stimulates the uptake of glucose and its conversion into glycogen • activates enzymes important for glycolysis (breakdown of glucose produces ATP) • stimulates uptake of amino acids and protein synthesis • inhibits the enzymes that mediate protein and glycogen catabolism
adipose tissue	• facilitates the uptake of glucose by fat cells • stimulates lipogenesis (the conversion of glucose into fatty acids) • inhibits triglyceride catabolism • promotes fat storage (inhibits utilization of fats for ATP production)
liver cells	• stimulates glycogenesis (the conversion of glucose into glycogen) • inhibits glycogenolysis (the breakdown of glycogen) • inhibits gluconeogenesis (the conversion of non-carbohydrates into glucose)
other cells	• acts as a growth factor in the mammary gland during pregnancy and lactation • may influence satiety–insulin is not required by the brain for the uptake of glucose, but the cells of the hypothalamus (which contains the satiety centre) exhibit insulin receptors

Fig. 6.8 Major metabolic effects of insulin on different target cells.

Factors that control glucagon secretion	
Stimulants (promote glucagon release)	**Inhibitors (reduce glucagon release)**
• falling blood glucose concentration	• rising blood glucose concentration
• basic amino acids	• high levels of ketone bodies
• gut hormones	• high levels of fatty acids
• adrenaline and noradrenaline	• insulin
• sympathetic and parasympathetic innervation	• somatostatin

Fig. 6.9 Factors that control glucagon secretion.

Once secreted, glucagon circulates unbound in the plasma and has a short half-life of about 5 minutes. It is degraded by virtually all the tissues of the body, but mainly by the liver and kidney.

Intracellular actions of glucagon
Glucagon binds to a G-protein-coupled receptor on the target cell membrane, with cAMP as the second messenger.

Effects of glucagon on metabolism
Glucagon has opposite (antagonistic) effects to those exerted by insulin. It is a catabolic hormone in that it promotes the breakdown of complex storage molecules and the release of simple molecules into the blood (Fig. 6.10)

Major metabolic effects of glucagon on different target cells	
Target cells	**Action of glucagon**
body cells (including muscle)	• inhibits uptake of glucose and amino acids
adipose tissue	• stimulates lipolysis (breaks down triglyceride fat stores into fatty acids and glycerol)
liver cells	• stimulates glycogenolysis (conversion of glycogen into glucose) • stimulates gluconeogenesis (conversion of amino acids into glucose) • stimulates the synthesis of ketone bodies

Fig. 6.10 Major metabolic effects of glucagon on different target cells.

Deficiency/excess of glucagon

Glucagon deficiency does not tend to affect glucose homoeostasis because other factors—catecholamines, cortisol, growth hormone (GH), and the sympathetic nervous system—have the same action and compensate for it.

Glucagon excess (very rare) causes hyperglycaemia.

Somatostatin (GHIH) and pancreatic polypeptide

Although secreted by the endocrine pancreas, these hormones have actions on the gastrointestinal system and hence are dealt with later in this chapter.

Somatostatin is also secreted by the stomach and by neurons in the gut and hypothalamus.

- ° **Discuss the synthesis and control of secretion of insulin and glucagon.**
- ° **Explain the cellular mechanism of insulin secretion.**
- ° **Specify the intracellular actions of insulin and glucagon and their metabolic effects.**

ENDOCRINE CONTROL OF GLUCOSE HOMOEOSTASIS

Glucose homoeostasis is dealt with in greater detail in the *Crash Course! Metabolism and Nutrition*; this text concentrates on the endocrine aspects of control.

The importance of glucose homoeostasis

Glucose is the principal energy source in the body. All body cells require glucose to produce energy (ATP), which is needed to drive all the metabolic reactions within the cell.

Glucose is broken down to produce energy by a process called glycolysis.

Fatty acids and ketone bodies can also be used to produce energy in cells (except in the brain and red blood cells, although the brain can use ketone bodies during glucose deficiency).

Normal glucose homoeostasis

Glucose is supplied from the diet (food is digested in the gut and the resultant glucose molecules absorbed) and from the breakdown of amino acids (gluconeogenesis) and glycogen (glycogenolysis) in the liver.

Glucose is delivered to the cells via the bloodstream, hence the amount of glucose in the circulation must be strictly controlled to ensure that the cells have a constant supply.

Blood glucose concentrations do fluctuate (owing to absorption of glucose from the gut, uptake by and release from the liver, and uptake by peripheral tissues), but not by more than 2 mmol/L in the normal person.

- The normal range of fasting blood glucose concentration is 3.5–5.5 mmol/L.
- The 'safe' range for normal function is 3–10 mmol/L (concentrations outside this range cause severe morbidity—see section on disorders of the pancreas in Chapter 15).

Endocrine control of glucose homoeostasis

Hunger stimulates glucose intake when blood glucose concentrations are low. Following a meal, glucose is absorbed by the gut and circulated in the blood.

Excess glucose in the blood is stored in the form of glycogen (in the liver and muscle cells) or fat (in adipose cells). These stores can be broken down (by glycogenolysis or lipolysis) to provide glucose and fatty acids when they are needed.

Glucose homoeostasis is aimed at buffering the peaks and troughs in blood glucose concentrations that occur after and between meals, respectively.

The liver is the main regulatory organ of glucose homoeostasis.

Many hormones have an effect on blood glucose concentrations, but the five main hormones that regulate glucose homoeostasis are (Fig. 6.11):

- **Insulin**—when blood glucose concentrations are high, the pancreas secretes insulin, which removes glucose from the blood by stimulating its uptake into cells and its storage in the liver, muscles, and adipose tissue (glucose uptake by the brain is independent of insulin).

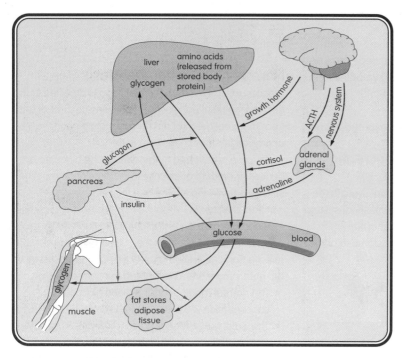

Fig. 6.11 Endocrine control of blood glucose concentrations.

- **Glucagon**—when blood glucose concentrations are low, the pancreas secretes glucagon, which stimulates the release of glucose from the liver.
- **Adrenaline**—this is secreted in response to stress and raises blood glucose concentrations and inhibits insulin secretion.
- **Cortisol** (secreted in response to ACTH) and **growth hormone**—stimulate the conversion of amino acids into glucose in the liver and induce insulin resistance (body cells become less responsive to insulin).

Insulin is the only hormone that removes glucose from the blood; the other hormones act to increase blood glucose concentrations (i.e. are antagonistic to insulin). Insulin and glucagon are the most important hormonal regulators of blood glucose—their relative levels in the blood at different glucose concentrations mirror each other (Fig. 6.12).

The effects of disordered glucose homoeostasis
Hyperglycaemia
Hyperglycaemia is an excess of glucose in the blood (diagnosed at a fasting blood glucose of >7.8 mmol/L) and can be caused by:
- Diabetes mellitus caused by impaired insulin secretion and/or insulin resistance by the tissues.

- Glucagonoma a very rare tumour of the α cells of pancreatic islets, resulting in excess glucagon secretion).

Effects of hyperglycaemia (Fig. 15.12) comprise:
- Glycosuria (glucose present in the urine)—resulting in polyuria.
- Salt and water depletion—causing thirst, dizziness, and cramps.
- Weight loss due to protein degradation to supply glucose.
- Vomiting.
- Tiredness and weakness.
- Tachycardia, hypotension, and hyperventilation.
- Infections (pruritis vulvae and boils).
- Impaired consciousness and visual acuity.

Insulin imbalance upsets the metabolism of carbohydrate, protein, and fat, but is most obvious in its distortion of glucose regulation. Diagnosis rests entirely on blood glucose levels.

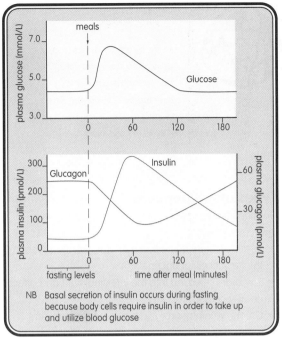

Fig. 6.12 Changes in blood levels of glucose, insulin, and glucagon after ingestion of a carbohydrate-rich meal.

NB Basal secretion of insulin occurs during fasting because body cells require insulin in order to take up and utilize blood glucose

In a non-diabetic patient who is becoming hypogycaemic during fasting, use the mnemonic EXPLAIN to list the possible causes:
EX—exogenous drugs (e.g. alcohol, insulin, sulphonylureas)
P—pituitary insufficiency
L—liver failure and liver enzyme defects
A—Addison's disease
I—islet-cell tumours (insulinoma) and immune hypoglycaemia (e.g. anti-insulin-receptor antibodies)
N—non-pancreatic tumours (some secrete insulin-like growth factor and all tumours are metabolically active and hence consume much glucose)

• Convulsions and coma (if severe).
Hyperglycaemia must be prevented even if symptoms are not evident as chronic hyperglycaemia damages the blood vessels, nerves, and eyes, and predisposes to infection (see Fig. 15.13).

Hypoglycaemia

Hypoglycaemia is a deficiency of glucose in the blood (diagnosed at a fasting blood glucose of <2.5 mmol/L) and can result:
• As a complication of treatment for diabetes mellitus (insulin overdose plus insufficient carohydrate intake in diabetic patients is the most common cause.
• During fasting in a patient with non-diabetic disorder (use the mnemonic EXPLAIN—see Hints & Tips box).
• As reactive (postprandial) hypoglycaemia after a meal (due to idiopathic excessive insulin secretion).

The effects of hypoglycaemia are:
• Adrenergic symptoms (due to increased catecholamine release)—hunger, sweating, pallor, palpitations, tachycardia, nervousness.
• Neuroglycopenic symptoms (due to deficiency of glucose to the brain)—headache, nausea, visual and speech disturbances, mental confusion, convulsions, coma.

○ Discuss the importance of glucose homoeostasis in the body.
○ What is the normal range of blood glucose concentrations?
○ Outline the importance of the liver in glucose homoeostasis.
○ List the hormones involved in the control of glucose homoeostasis.
○ State the relative changes of insulin and glucogon after the ingestion of a meal.
○ List the effects of disordered glucose homoeostasis.

THE ENDOCRINE ROLE OF THE GASTROINTESTINAL TRACT

The gastrointestinal tract is the largest endocrine organ in the body. It contains more endocrine cells than any other organ, but they are widely distributed throughout its length and secrete a number of different peptide hormones, which coordinate the digestion and absorption of food.

The first hormone ever described, in 1902 by Bayliss and Starling, was a gut hormone: secretin. Since then, many more gut hormones secreted by specialized enteroendocrine cells have been discovered.

Many of these gut hormones have also been isolated from the central nervous system and in enteric neurons, leading to the concept of the brain–gut axis.

Brain–gut axis

This concept describes the brain and the gut secreting similar peptide hormones to coordinate digestive processes together.

In the gut these peptides, released from enteroendocrine cells (hormones) and from the enteric nervous system (neurotransmitters), exert local control over absorption, secretion, motility, immune function, and blood flow.

In the central nervous system these 'gut peptides' are thought to be important in the regulation of bodily functions such as satiety (cholecystokinin; CCK), thermoregulation (bombesin), and growth (somatostatin).

APUD Concept

APUD cells are cells that have similar intracellular amine biochemical pathways (APUD = amine precursor uptake and decarboxylation). Such cells can actively absorb amine precursors and convert them into amines, which are used to make peptide hormones or neurotransmitters.

APUD cells are found not only in the gut (enteroendocrine cells and neurons in the gut wall) but also in the central nervous system (within the hypothalamus, pituitary, and pineal gland) and in other endocrine glands (thyroid, parathyroid).

APUD cells have similar embryological origins and characteristics. It was postulated that APUD cells originated from the primitve neural crest but it has now been shown that they are all derived from gut endodermal cells.

Pancreatic hormones can also be regarded as gastrointestinal hormones because the pancreas is an organ of the gastrointestinal system.

Types of gut peptides

Gut peptides are delivered to their sites of action in three main ways:
- Some circulate in the bloodstream in order to reach the target cell (endocrine).
- Some are released into the intestinal fluid and affect nearby cells (paracrine).
- Others, within neurons, act as neurotransmitters (neurocrine).

Some peptides have more than one mode of delivery, e.g. somatostatin exhibits all three modes.

Because of their various modes of delivery, it may be more correct to refer to them as regulatory peptides rather than as hormones. 'True' gut hormones include somatostatin, CCK, and gastric inhibitory peptide (GIP)—these reach their target cells via the bloodstream.

Fig. 6.13 shows the distribution of cells secreting gut hormones, together with the effects of gastrin, secretin, CCK, and GIP on gastric secretions and the secretion of bile, bicarbonate (HCO_3^-), and digestive enzymes.

The major gut hormones
Gastrin

This is a peptide hormone that exists in several forms e.g. gastrin (17 amino acids) and big gastrin (dimer of 34 amino acids).

It is secreted by G cells in the stomach antrum in response to:
- The presence of peptides and amino acids in the stomach.
- Vagal stimulation (parasympathetic).
- Distention of the stomach.

Gastrin acts on the gut to:
- Stimulate the parietal and chief cells of the

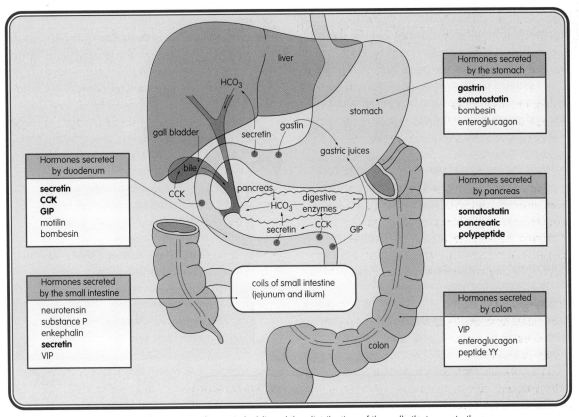

Fig. 6.13 Gut hormones (main hormones shown in bold) and the distribution of the cells that secrete them.

stomach to secrete enzymes required for protein digestion and hydrochloric acid.
- Increase gastric motility.
- Stimulate gastric mucosal growth.
- Stimulate insulin, glucagon, and secretin secretion after a protein meal.
- Relax the pyloric and ileocaecal sphincters.

An excess of gastrin release over a long period can cause gastric ulceration.

Cholecystokinin (CCK)

CCK is a peptide hormone comprising 33 amino acids.

It is secreted by I cells in the lining of the duodenum in response to the presence of digested fat and amino acids in the duodenum.

CCK acts to:
- Stimulate pancreatic enzyme secretion.
- Contract the gall bladder (bile released into common bile duct).
- Enhance the action of secretin by causing the release of bicarbonate from the pancreas.
- May influence satiety, i.e. reduce eating behaviour (action in the hypothalamus).

Secretin

Secretin is a peptide hormone comprising 27 amino acids.

It is secreted by S cells in the lining of the duodenum and small intestine in response to acid in the duodenum (low pH due to gastric HCl).

Secretin acts to:
- Stimulate pancreatic and liver secretion of bicarbonate.
- Inhibit gastric acid secretion.
- Potentiate the effect of CCK.

Glucose-dependent insulinotrophic peptide (GIP)

GIP is a peptide hormone comprising 42 amino acids. It used to be called gastric inhibitory peptide (new name devised to fit original acronym).

It is secreted by K cells in the lining of the duodenum in response to the presence of fats and carbohydrates in the duodenum.

GIP acts to:
- Inhibit gastric acid production and gastric motility.
- Stimulate insulin secretion (glucose dependent).

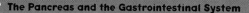
Somatostatin (also known as growth-hormone-inhibiting hormone; GHIH)

Somatostatin is a cyclic peptide hormone that exists in two forms: 14 and 28 amino acids.

It is secreted by δ cells of the pancreas and stomach and by neurons in the gut (and brain) in response to acid and amino acids in the stomach, increased levels of blood glucose, and CCK.

Somatostatin acts to:

- Inhibit the secretion of other hormones, e.g. insulin, glucagon, GIP, gastrin, CCK, vasoactive intestinal polypeptide (VIP), secretin, and motilin.
- Inhibit gastric motility.
- Inhibit the secretion of pancreatic enzymes and bile.

Pancreatic polypeptide

This is a peptide hormone comprising 36 amino acids.

It is secreted by PP cells of the pancreas in response to protein in the stomach, fasting, exercise, and low blood glucose.

Pancreatic polypeptide acts to:

- Slow the absorption of food.
- Regulate the release of pancreatic digestive enzymes.

Details of the other (non-major) gut peptides are listed in Fig. 6.14.

- Discuss the importance of the gastrointestinal tract as an endocrine organ.
- Explain the concept of the brain–gut axis.
- Outline the concept and origin of APUD cells.
- List the major gut peptides, their distribution, site of synthesis, stimulus for secretion, and their actions.

Fig. 6.14 The sites of secretion, stimuli for secretion, and actions of the gut peptides. NB The major gut peptides—gastrin, CCK, secretin, GIP, somatostatin, and pancreatic peptide—are included in the text.

The sites of secretion, stimuli for secretion, and actions of the gut peptides			
Gut peptide	Site of secretion	Stimulus for secretion	Action of peptide
enteroglucagon	A cells in the stomach and L cells in the colon	presence of glucose and fat in the stomach	reduces gastric-acid secretion and gut motility
bombesin	P cells in the stomach and duodenum	fasting	stimulates gastrin release
motilin	EC cells in the duodenum	absence of food in the duodenum	speeds gastric emptying and stimulates colonic motility
vasoactive intestinal polypeptide (VIP)	D1 cells and neurons in the small intestine and colon	gut distension	stimulates local gut secretion, motility, and blood flow
peptide YY (related to pancreatic polypeptide)	PYY cells of the colon	presence of intestinal fat	inhibits gastric motility and acid secretion (peptide YY is elevated in coeliac disease and cystic fibrosis)
substance P	enteric neurons in the small intestine	electrical stimulation, 5-HT, CCK	stimulates gut motility, secretion, and immune response; may have a role in inflammatory bowel disease
enkephalin	enteric neurons in the small intestine	unknown	inhibits gut motility and secretion
neurotensin	N cells of the small intestine	presence of intestinal fat	stimulates local gut motility, secretion, and immune response

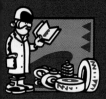

7. Endocrine Control of Fluid Balance

The importance of fluid balance

Fluid balance is essential to maintain overall hydration and to ensure an effective system of circulation (determined by the blood volume and pressure) in order to transport substances to and from the body cells in the correct concentrations to enable normal functioning.

Normal fluid balance

Water is the main component of the human body—total body water is approximately 42 litres and constitutes approximately 70% of body weight.

In any individual, the intracellular and extracellular water content stays remarkably constant from day to day (Fig. 7.1).

Water and sodium balance are closely linked because sodium ions are the main osmotically active solutes of the extracellular fluid (ECF). The normal plasma concentration of sodium ions is 135–145 mmol/L (Fig. 7.2).

Regulation of fluid balance

Water intake is controlled by thirst—osmoreceptors in the hypothalamus detect if the plasma osmolality (water concentration) is raised and stimulate the sensation of thirst. In contrast, there is no control over sodium intake.

The kidney is the main regulatory organ of fluid balance. Huge amounts of water and sodium are filtered into the renal tubules from the blood in the renal glomeruli, but most is reabsorbed back into the blood circulation—sodium ions are actively reabsorbed from the renal tubules, water follows sodium ions passively back into the blood owing to osmosis.

Hence, water reabsorption from the kidney is determined by the amount of sodium reabsorption.

The water and sodium not reabsorbed is excreted in the urine.

If the blood sodium ion content changes, the amount of water reabsorbed is altered—if the body is sodium depleted, water is excreted (from the kidneys); if the body is sodium overloaded, water is retained.

Water retention or excretion affects blood volume. If the blood volume does alter, the effective circulation (blood pressure) is maintained by changes in cardiac output and peripheral vasodilatation/vasoconstriction (controlled by the nervous and endocrine systems).

The hormones, nerves, and other chemical factors that control fluid balance do so by:
- Regulating the amount of water and/or salt excreted in the urine.
- Helping to maintain the blood circulation.
- Stimulating thirst.

Hormones that regulate fluid balance include:
- Antidiuretic hormone (ADH; vasopressin).
- Aldosterone.
- Renin.
- Angiotensin II.
- Atrial natriuretic factor (ANF).
- Natriuretic hormone.

Expected intake and output of water over a 24-hour period	
Water intake (mL)	**Water loss (mL)**
drinking: 1500	urine: 1500
food: 500	respiration: 400
metabolism: 400	skin evaporation: 400
	faeces: 100
total: 2400	total: 2400

Fig. 7.1 Expected intake and output of water over a 24-hour period.

Expected intake and output of sodium ions over a 24-hour period	
Na+ intake (mmol)	**Na+ loss (mmol)**
diet: 100–200 (very variable)	urine: 150
	faeces: 10
	sweat: 10
	skin: 10

Fig. 7.2 Expected intake and output of sodium ions over a 24-hour period.

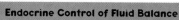

Nerves and chemical factors that regulate fluid balance include:

- Renal sympathetic nerves.
- Catecholamines.
- Kinins.
- Prostaglandins.
- Dopamine.

Being warm-blooded, land-living animals, our main problem is loss of salt and water by evaporation (via the skin and lungs), therefore most of the endocrine mechanisms are directed towards their conservation, e.g.: the renin–angiotensin–aldosterone system causes salt and water retention in the kidney; ADH conserves water only.

Counter-regulatory endocrine mechanisms prevent retention from proceeding unchecked, e.g. ANF and kinins increase salt and water excretion by the kidney.

Effects of disordered fluid balance

Dehydration occurs when the body is deficient of water; depending on the cause of the water loss, it may or may not be accompanied by sodium deficiency. The causes and effects of dehydration are listed in Fig. 7.3.

Fluid retention occurs when the body is overloaded with water; depending on the cause of the retention, it may or may not be accompanied by sodium overload. The causes and effects of fluid retention are listed in Fig. 7.4.

Causes and effects of dehydration		
	Deficiency of water and sodium	**Deficiency of water**
possible causes	↓ input, e.g. decreased ingestion in unconscious patient; ↑ output, e.g. diarrhoea, vomiting, burns, haemorrhage, *aldosterone deficiency* (Addison's disease)	↓ input, e.g. disorders of thirst; ↑ output, e.g. *ADH deficiency* (diabetes insipidus), *insulin deficiency* (diabetes mellitus - owing to the osmolar effect that excess glucose has in the kidney)
effect on plasma osmolality	no effect	raised — **hypernatraemia** (as the plasma sodium becomes more concentrated)
symptoms	thirst, weakness, apathy, postural dizziness, syncope, confusion, coma	
signs	hypotension, tachycardia, reduced skin turgor, cool peripheries, signs of shock, weight loss	

Fig. 7.3 Causes and effects of dehydration (the endocrine causes are shown in italic).

Causes and effects of fluid retention		
	Excess of water and sodium	**Excess of water**
possible causes	↑ input, e.g. overtransfusion of blood or saline; ↓ output, e.g. chronic cardiac or renal failure (*not due to aldosterone excess* because of the 'escape' phenomenon)	↑ input, e.g. psychogenic polydipsia (drinking excess); ↓ output, e.g. acute renal failure or *ADH excess* [syndrome of inappropriate ADH secretion (SIADH)]
effect on plasma osmolality	no effect on plasma osmolality; causes oedema (as the excess sodium and water are mainly distributed in the ECF only)	decreased plasma osmolality — **hyponatraemia** (as the plasma sodium becomes more diluted) **does not cause oedema** (as the excess water is distributed in the ECF and ICF)
symptoms	headache, apathy, nausea, vomiting, anorexia, muscle weakness, confusion, fits, may lead to coma and death	
signs	hypertension, cardiac failure	

Fig. 7.4 Causes and effects of fluid retention (the endocrine causes are shown in italic).

- Explain the importance of the kidney in fluid balance.
- Specify the importance of maintaining an effective blood circulation.
- Describe the normal daily intake and output of water and sodium ions.
- List the hormones and other factors involved in the control of fluid balance.
- What are the causes and effects of disordered fluid balance?

HORMONES INVOLVED IN FLUID BALANCE

ADH (vasopressin)

Anti-diuretic hormone (ADH) conserves water in the body via its action in the kidney. It increases water reabsorption in the collecting ducts and this results in the production of a concentrated urine.

Synthesis and secretion of ADH

ADH is a peptide hormone synthesized in the nerve cells of the hypothalamus by transcription and translation of the ADH gene. It is transported along axons and stored as neurosecretory granules in the nerve endings in the posterior pituitary.

It is released from its stores in response to raised plasma osmolality (decreased concentration of water in the blood) and other stimuli; release is inhibited by low plasma osmolality and alcohol (see Fig. 7.5).

The rapid release and metabolism (plasma half-life = 10–15 minutes) of ADH allows it to control water balance precisely.

ADH is degraded in the liver and kidney.

Intracellular actions of ADH

ADH binds to V receptors (linked to G proteins) present on the surface of its target cells.

In the blood vessels, ADH binds to V_1 receptors, resulting in smooth muscle contraction (via the release of IP_3 and the mobilization of intracellular calcium, which causes actin and myosin to bring about contraction).

In the kidney, ADH binds to V_2 receptors, resulting in the increased function of water-channel proteins. The steps involved are shown in Fig. 7.6.

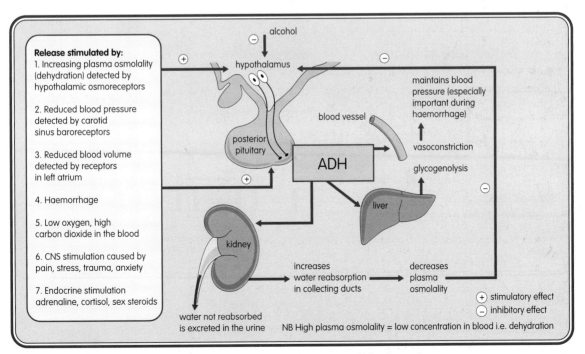

Release stimulated by:
1. Increasing plasma osmolality (dehydration) detected by hypothalamic osmoreceptors

2. Reduced blood pressure detected by carotid sinus baroreceptors

3. Reduced blood volume detected by receptors in left atrium

4. Haemorrhage

5. Low oxygen, high carbon dioxide in the blood

6. CNS stimulation caused by pain, stress, trauma, anxiety

7. Endocrine stimulation adrenaline, cortisol, sex steroids

alcohol

hypothalamus

posterior pituitary

ADH

blood vessel

maintains blood pressure (especially important during haemorrhage)

vasoconstriction

liver

glycogenolysis

kidney

increases water reabsorption in collecting ducts

decreases plasma osmolality

water not reabsorbed is excreted in the urine

NB High plasma osmolality = low concentration in blood i.e. dehydration

(+) stimulatory effect
(−) inhibitory effect

Fig. 7.5 The control of ADH secretion and its actions on the kidney, liver, and blood vessels.

Effects of ADH

ADH acts to:

Control water balance by increasing water reabsorption by the kidneys—increased ADH in the blood causes the production of concentrated urine; decreased ADH in the blood causes the production of dilute urine.

Regulate blood pressure (through its effects on blood volume)—very high ADH levels can promote smooth muscle contraction in the peripheral arterioles, which may be important during hypovolaemia, especially after haemorrhage; however, under normal conditions, ADH does not have an important effect on blood pressure.

Stimulate glycogenolysis in the liver.

Deficiency/excess of ADH (see Fig. 15.4)

ADH deficiency (diabetes insipidus) causes volume depletion and dehydration.

ADH excess (syndrome of inappropriate ADH secretion—SIADH) causes water retention.

The renin–angiotensin–aldosterone system

The renin–angiotensin–aldosterone system *controls sodium and water balance*, mainly by increasing the reabsorption of sodium ions in the kidney (water is reabsorbed passively along with sodium). The mechanism of interaction is shown in Fig. 7.7.

Synthesis and secretion of renin

Renin is a glycoprotein with enzymatic properties that is synthesized and stored in the juxtaglomerular granular cells in the walls of the renal afferent arterioles.

Renin is released into the blood in response to stimulation of the juxtaglomerular apparatus caused by:
- A fall in systemic blood pressure.
- A fall in renal blood pressure.
- A fall in the amount of sodium reaching the macula densa.

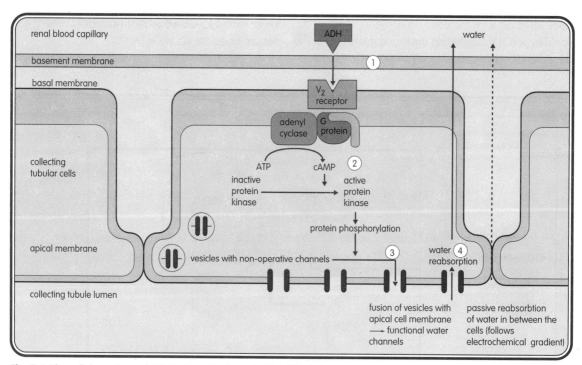

Fig. 7.6 The cellular actions of ADH in the collecting tubules of the kidney.
1. ADH binds to V_2 receptors in the basal membrane of the collecting-tubule cells.
2. Binding causes intracellular release of cAMP, which instigates a chain of reactions within the cell.
3. These reactions cause non-operative water-channel proteins in the cytoplasm to migrate to the apical membrane.
4. These channels become functional within the apical membrane and allow increased water reabsorption (in the absence of ADH the water channels are non-functional and the cells are relatively impermeable).

The control of renin release and the location and structure of the juxtaglomerular apparatus are shown in Figs 7.8 and 7.9, respectively.

Effects of renin

Renin acts on a plasma protein called angiotensinogen. This leads to an increase of angiotensin II in the blood (Fig. 7.10).

Effects of angiotensin II

The major effect of angiotensin II include:

- Stimulation of aldosterone secretion from the adrenal cortex (which increases sodium reabsorption in the kidney).
- Vasoconstriction of the systematic circulation. This increases the peripheral vascular resistance, resulting in increased blood pressure.
- Vasoconstriction of the intrarenal arterioles. This lowers the glomerular filtration rate by constricting afferent arterioles, resulting in increased sodium and water reabsorption.

It also stimulates other processing involved in salt and water balance:

- Inhibits renin release (negative feedback).
- Stimulates sensation of thirst via its effect on the hypothalamus.
- Stimulates ADH release (which increases water reabsorption in the kidney).

Deficiency/excess of renin and angiotensin II

An excess of plasma renin causes an excess of plasma angiotensin II, which produces hypertension and fluid

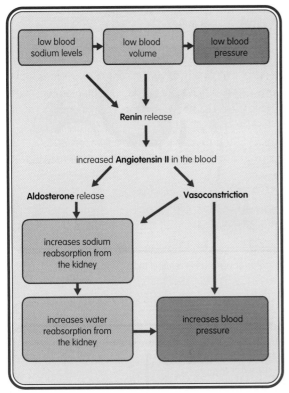

Fig. 7.7 Renin–angiotensin–aldosterone system.

Fig. 7.8 Control of renin release.

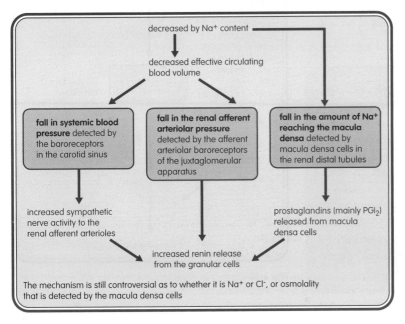

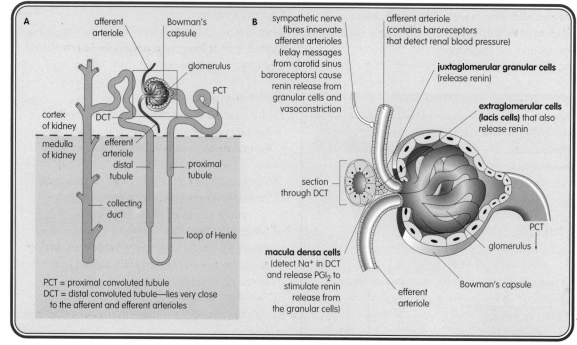

Fig. 7.9 (A) Kidney nephron showing the location of the juxtaglomerular apparatus in respect to its surrounding structures. (B) Juxtaglomerular apparatus (apparatus are shown in bold).

retention (by stimulating vasoconstriction and the release of ADH and aldosterone).

A deficiency of renin and angiotensin II does not have any recognized clinical consequences.

Aldosterone

Aldosterone is a mineralocorticoid steroid hormone synthesized by the zona glomerulosa cells of the

ACE inhibitors (e.g. the drug enalapril) are now widely used in the treatment of hypertension and congestive heart failure. By inhibiting the production of angiotensin II, they lower the blood volume and decrease the peripheral vascular resistance.
Hence they decrease blood pressure and make it easier for a failing heart to pump blood around the body.

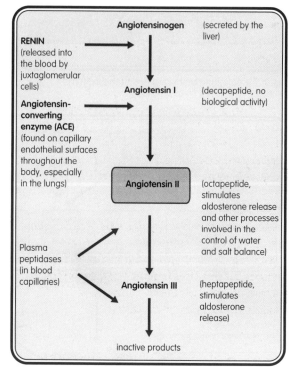

Fig. 7.10 Control of angiotensin formation in the blood and its degradation.

adrenal cortex (see Chapter 6 for more details).

Aldosterone acts on the kidney and is very important in the control of fluid balance. It was previously thought to be the regulator of sodium; however, when excess aldosterone is produced or administered, sodium retention rarely occurs, i.e. there is an 'escape' mechanism whereby sodium excretion returns to normal despite the raised aldosterone level. This phenomenon shows that body fluid regulation is complex and there are other regulators involved that antagonise the effects of aldosterone (i.e. natriuretic factors).

Natriuretic factors

Natriuretic factors increase sodium and water excretion in the urine and lower blood pressure, i.e. are antagonistic to the effects of the renal sympathetic nerves, the renin–angiotensin–aldosterone system, and ADH.

Atrial natriuretic factor (ANF)

ANF is a peptide hormone synthesized by the muscle cells of the atrium of the heart andsecreted in response to volume overload (detected as a stretch in cardiac muscle).

It acts to:
- Decrease sodium reabsorption by kidneys (increases sodium and water excretion).
- Inhibit the secretion of renin (causes angiotensin II and aldosterone levels to decrease).
- Inhibit the secretion of aldosterone from the adrenal cortex directly.
- Induce vasodilatation in the systemic circulation (minor) and in the renal afferent arterioles, which causes increased sodium and water loss.

Prostaglandins

Prostaglandins are lipid molecules synthesized in most body cells including kidney cells.

Renal prostaglandins do not function as circulating hormones, but they have important intrarenal effects:
- Inhibit the action of ADH and aldosterone.
- Induce vasodilatation in the kidney.

Kinins

Kinins are peptides synthesized in the kidney by the enzyme kallikrein.

They act to:

- Inhibit the action of ADH.
- Increase sodium loss.
- Induce prostaglandin synthesis in the kidney.
- Vasodilate the blood vessels of the kidney.

Dopamine

Dopamine is an amine synthesized in the proximal tubule cells. It:
- Reduces sodium reabsorption by inhibiting the Na^+/K^+ ATPase and by decreasing the activity of the $Na^+–H^+$-exchange protein in the renal tubular cells.
- Vasodilates the blood vessels of the kidney.

Natriuretic hormone

There is thought to be an as yet unidentified 'natriuretic hormone', probably of hypothalamic origin.

Summary

The endocrine control of fluid balance is summarized in Fig. 7.11.

- ○ **Describe the synthesis, secretion, and effects of ADH.**
- ○ **List the effects of deficiency and excess of ADH.**
- ○ **Itemize the components and effects of the renin–angiotensin–aldosterone system.**
- ○ **Name the five natriuretic factors that promote the excretion of sodium.**
- ○ **Discuss the integration of fluid balance control.**

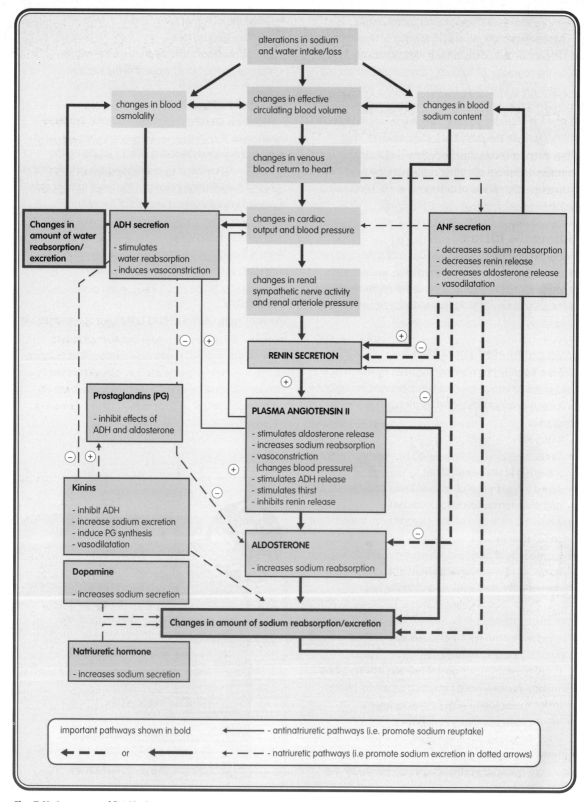

Fig. 7.11 Summary of fluid balance.

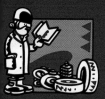

8. Endocrine Control of Calcium Homoeostasis

The importance of calcium homoeostasis

Calcium homoeostasis is essential in order for the body to function normally because calcium is necessary for many physiological processes, including:

- Bone mineral formation (i.e. bone growth and maintenance)—bone mineral is hydroxyapatite = $Ca_{10}(PO_4)_6(OH)_2$.
- Blood clotting—many clotting factors have calcium-binding sites and require calcium to make them active.
- Muscle contraction—troponin requires bound calcium before it can bind to actin.
- Activation and inhibition of enzymes—calcium acts as an intracellular second messenger; it is released from the endoplasmic reticulum in response to insotitol triphosphate (IP_3) (see Fig. 1.6)
- Release of hormones and neurotransmitters—stimuli promoting their release use calcium as their second messenger, e.g. insulin (see Fig. 6.7).
- Nerve function—calcium maintains the transmembrane potential and is essential for the normal depolarization of nerve cell membranes.
- Cell division and proliferation.

When measuring calcium in the blood it is important to correct for plasma albumin concentration.

A patient may have symptoms of hypercalcaemia (raised blood calcium levels) but have a plasma calcium within the normal range. This may be because they have deficient plasma albumin. Correcting for albumin will show the unbound (active) form to be raised, hence causing the symptoms.

Normal calcium homoeostasis

Calcium is a major constituent of all cells and there is a vast body pool of it (approximately 1.2 kg). Nearly all (99%) of the body calcium is in the bone.

The normal range of plasma calcium is 2.25–2.55 mmol/L. It must be kept within this range in order for the body to function normally.

- About 50% of plasma calcium circulates unbound (free ionic form) and is biologically active.
- About 40% is bound to plasma proteins, mainly albumin.
- About 10% is complexed, e.g. with citrate.

The normal distribution of calcium in the body is shown in Fig. 8.1. In an adult the daily input of calcium is equivalent to the daily output. Postive calcium balance, i.e. input is greater than output, occurs in children to allow for skeletal growth. Post menopausal women tend to be in negative calcium balance, i.e. output is greater than input.

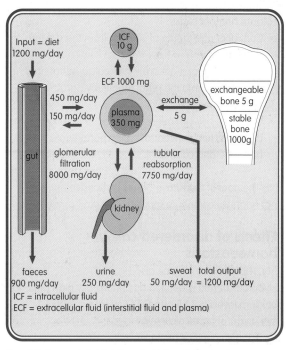

Fig. 8.1 Normal distribution of calcium in the body.

Calcium in the diet

The normal dietary requirement of calcium is about 1 g per day. It is abundant in food, especially dairy products (milk and cheese).

Calcium absorption from the gut is not very efficient (30% ± 15%) and is variable. It is increased in childhood and during pregnancy and lactation. It is decreased if calcium intake is high and with increasing age.

Other dietary factors can also affect absorption. The presence of basic amino acids and lactose in the gut enhances calcium absorption, e.g. lactose in milk complexes with the calcium and makes it more absorbable. Phytic acid, e.g. in unleavened or brown bread, chelates the calcium so it is not as easily absorbed, i.e. it decreases the bioavailability of calcium. (NB During the Second World War, rationed brown bread was fortified with calcium, a practice still carried out.)

Regulation of calcium homoeostasis

Calcium is normally ingested in excess and the surplus is excreted in the faeces and urine.

The role of calcium homoeostasis, therefore, is aimed at buffering the peaks and troughs that occur in the plasma calcium after and between meals, respectively.

There are three main mechanisms that control calcium homoeostasis:

- Control of absorption of calcium from the gut (mainly by vitamin D).
- Control of renal reabsorption of calcium that has been filtered into the renal tubule (by parathyroid hormone and calcitonin).
- Control of calcium release from bone to maintain the blood calcium concentration (by parathyroid hormone and calcitonin).

NB The pool of calcium in bones is massive but does not normally contribute much to calcium homoeostasis.

Effects of disordered calcium homoeostasis

Hypercalcaemia (see also Fig. 15.8)

Hypercalcaemia is defined as abnormally high plasma calcium levels (>2.55 mmol/L). Clinical signs and symptoms of hypercalcaemia include:

- Sluggish nervous response.
- *Bones*—painful and fragile, showing radiolucency

When investigating hypercalcaemia, remember: '*Bones, stones, groans, and psychic moans*'.

and erosions if hypercalcaemia is due to excessive bone resorption.
- *Stones*—ectopic calcification (e.g. of heart, pancreas, uterus, liver) and renal calculi.
- *Groans*—headache, abdominal pain, nausea, vomiting, anorexia, constipation, weight loss.
- *Moans*—weakness, tiredness.
- Fits, coma, mental confusion.
- Polyuria, dehydration, and renal failure.
- Short QT interval on ECG, cardiac arrhythmias.

NB Plasma calcium >3.75 mmol/L is lethal.

Hypocalcaemia (see also Fig. 15.9)

Hypocalcaemia is defined as abnormally low plasma calcium levels (<2.25 mmol/L). Clinical signs and symptoms of hypercalcaemia include:

- Hyperexcitable nervous response.
- Numbness and paraesthesia.
- Mood changes, e.g. depression.
- Tetany (due to uncontrolled contractions).
- Carpopedal spasm, especially with a blood-pressure cuff on the arm (Trousseau's sign).
- Neuromuscular excitability, e.g. tapping over the

- Why is calcium homoeostasis important?
- What is the normal distribution of calcium in the body?
- Identify the three main mechanisms that control plasma calcium levels.
- List the effects of disordered calcium homoeostasis.

parotid (facial) nerve causes the facial muscle to twitch (Chvostek's sign).
- Convulsions.
- Prolonged QT interval on ECG, cardiac arrhythmias.

NB Plasma calcium <1.5 mmol/L is lethal.

HORMONES INVOLVED IN CALCIUM HOMOEOSTASIS

Parathyroid hormone (PTH)
PTH is a peptide hormone (84 amino acids) that is essential to life.

Synthesis and secretion of PTH
PTH is synthesized by chief cells of the parathyroid glands (see Chapter 4) by transcription and translation of the PTH gene on chromosome 11.

It is stored in vesicles in the cell cytoplasm and released from its stores in response to low plasma calcium—simple negative feedback switches off its release as plasma calcium rises.

Intracellular actions of PTH
PTH binds to PTH receptors (linked to G proteins) and causes an increase in intracellular cAMP. PTH receptors are present on the surface of the renal tubule cells, osteoblasts (bone-synthesizing cells), and gut epithelial cells.

Effects of PTH
The effects of PTH are shown in Fig. 8.2.
In the kidney, PTH:
- Enhances calcium and hydrogen ion reabsorption in the distal tubules.
- Decreases phosphate and bicarbonate reabsorption in the proximal and distal tubules, i.e. increases their excretion.

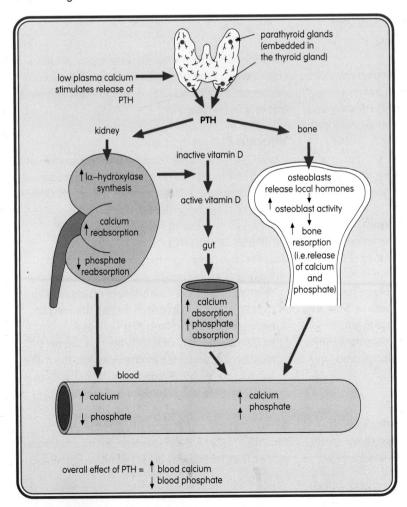

Fig. 8.2 Effects of PTH on the kidney, bone, and (indirectly) on the gut. NB PTH acts on the bone and gut to increase calcium and phosphate levels in the blood, however its overall effect is to increase plasma calcium and decrease plasma phosphate levels because of its effect in the kidney.

- Increases synthesis of 1α-hydroxylase, which is required for activation of vitamin D.

In bone, PTH acts on *osteoblasts* to stimulate decreased collagen synthesis. The release of prostaglandins (local paracrine hormones) that act on the *osteoclasts* (bone-resorbing cells) to stimulate:

- Increased osteolytic activity (i.e. erosion of bone matrix).
- Increased collagenase synthesis (required to erode bone).
- Increased hydrogen ion release—this acidifies the environment around the bone, and enhances bone erosion.

The overall effect of bone erosion by the osteoclasts is the demineralisation of the bone matrix and the release of calcium and phosphate into the blood.

In the gut, PTH indirectly (via activation of vitamin D) stimulates the uptake of dietary calcium and phosphate from the gut lumen.

Deficiency/excess of PTH

Deficiency of PTH (hypoparathyroidism) causes symptoms of hypocalcaemia. Excess of PTH (hyperparathyroidism) causes symptoms of hypercalcaemia. For symptoms and signs of hypocalcaemia and hypercalcaemia, see earlier in this chapter.

Calcitonin

Calcitonin is a peptide hormone (32 amino acids).

Synthesis and secretion of calcitonin

Calcitonin is synthesized by C cells of the thyroid gland (see Fig. 4.3) by transcription and translation of the calcitonin gene on chromosome 11.

It is stored in vesicles in the cell cytoplasm and rapidly released from its stores in response to a rise in plasma calcium and possibly in response to gut hormones (increased calcium in the gut capillaries causes calcitonin release before systemic plasma levels are raised).

Intracellular actions of calcitonin

Calcitonin binds to calcitonin receptors (linked to G proteins) and causes an increase in intracellular cAMP. Calcitonin receptors are present on the surface of the renal tubule cells and osteoclasts.

Effects of calcitonin

The effects of calcitonin are shown in Fig. 8.3.

In the kidney, calcitonin inhibits calcium and phosphate reabsorption.

In bone, calcitonin suppresses the activity of the osteoclasts, and in doing so inhibits the release of calcium and phosphate (but does not affect bone formation).

Deficiency/excess of calcitonin

Calcitonin does not appear to be essential to normal body function because no clinical consequences result from its deficiency or excess, e.g. thyroidectomy patients do not require calcitonin therapy; malignancy of the C cells can produce over 20 000 times the normal calcitonin with no effect on calcium balance.

Calcitonin *may* have an important role in:

- Protecting against threatened calcium loss during pregnancy and lactation, so the maternal skeleton is not eroded.
- Protecting against a sudden influx of calcium from the gut.

Calcitonin is used in the treatment of hypercalcaemia caused by hyperparathyroidism, osteoporosis, bone metastasis, Paget's disease, idiopathic hypercalcaemia, and vitamin D intoxication.

Vitamin D

Vitamin D is a steroid-like hormone (four-ring structure with one ring broken) derived from cholesterol. The structure of the active form—1,25-dihydroxycholecalciferol, also known as calcitriol—is shown in Fig. 8.4.

Synthesis and metabolism of vitamin D

Vitamin D can come from two different sources.

- It is mainly synthesized by photo-isomerization in the skin (vitamin D_3) under the influence of ultraviolet light.
- At least 10% is acquired from the diet (vitamin D_2). Endogenous production in the skin is often inadequate through lack of UV light, so vitamin D must be supplemented by dietary intake. The main natural sources are fish and eggs, therefore there is very little present in vegetarian or vegan diets.

Dietary vitamins are not generally considered to be hormones. 'Vitamin D' can be regarded as a misnomer, especially as the majority of the hormone is produced in the skin.

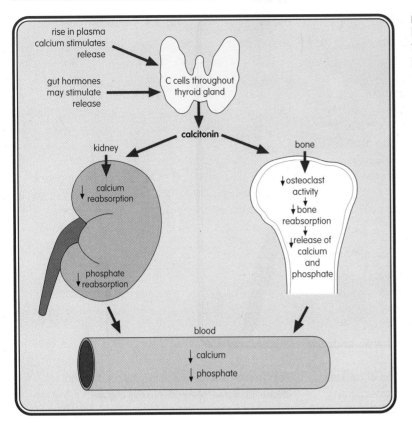

Fig. 8.3 Effects of calcitonin on the kidney and bone. Its overall effect is to decrease plasma calcium and phosphate levels.

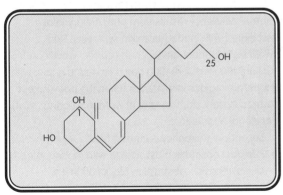

Fig. 8.4 Structure of 1,25-dihydroxycholecalciferol (1,25-diOHCC), the active form of vitamin D.

Vitamin D is activated in the kidney by the enzyme 1α-hydroxylase (Fig. 8.5). PTH increases the synthesis of 1α-hydroxylase and hence controls the amount of active vitamin D made (there is no direct feedback mechanism). Growth hormone (GH), cortisol, oestrogens, and prolactin also increase the synthesis of 1α-hydroxylase, therefore vitamin D must be important in growth, pregnancy, and lactation.

Intracellular actions of vitamin D

Active vitamin D binds to specific intracellular receptors found in the gut mucosal cells, osteoblasts, and epidermal cells. The receptor–hormone complex promotes the synthesis of proteins involved in calcium absorption.

Effects of vitamin D

The major effect of vitamin D is in the gut, where it increases the absorption of dietary calcium and phosphate. The mechanism by which it does so is unknown, but it has been shown to:

- Increase the synthesis of calcium-binding protein (calbindin). Calbindin buffers against mucosal-cell levels of calcium rising too high; however, as its production is maximal hours after maximal calcium absorption, it is unlikely that it has a primary effect on the increase of calcium absorption.
- Activate calcium channels (not proven).
- Promote mucosal-cell division and growth.

In bone, vitamin D increases the release of calcium and phosphate (i.e. demineralizes/resorbs bone) via the

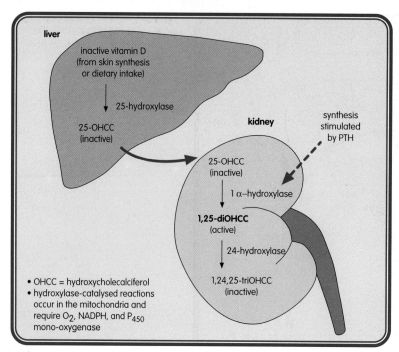

Fig. 8.5 Metabolism of vitamin D.

osteoblasts, by increasing the production of calcium-binding proteins (e.g. osteocalcin, and osteopontin). These proteins may help mobilize the calcium released.

In the kidney, vitamin D increases calcium and phosphate reabsorption.

The effects of vitamin D on the gut, bone, and kidney are shown in Fig. 8.6. Vitamin D also modulates:
- Levels of its precursors in the skin.
- Secretion of PTH, calcitonin, prolactin, and insulin.
- Cell differentiation in haematopoietic, lymphopoietic, bone, and epidermal cells.

Deficiency/excess of vitamin D
Deficiency causes impaired intestinal calcium absorption, hence plasma calcium levels decrease (hypocalcaemia). This causes PTH levels to rise, resulting in bone demineralization. Bone demineralization causes rickets in children (rickets occurs as the newly woven, growing bone fails to calcify) and osteomalacia in adults (Fig. 8.7).

Vitamin-D-resistant rickets is a rare, X-linked, and dominantly inherited disorder. It is not caused by dietary deficiency but by mutant vitamin D receptors, so the renal tubules are unresponsive to vitamin D.

Excess vitamin D causes vitamin D intoxication and plasma calcium levels rise dangerously (hypercalcaemia).

For symptoms and signs of hypocalcaemia and hypercalcaemia, see earlier in this chapter.

Causes of vitamin D deficiency
Primary deficiency results from poor dietary intake associated with inadequate skin synthesis. Skin synthesis is inadequate when the correct wavelength of sunlight required (290–300 nm) is limited (e.g. in temperate regions in winter) or when the body is kept covered in dark clothing (e.g. in women wearing traditional Middle Eastern dress).

Secondary deficiency is caused by:
- Bile-duct obstruction associated with inadequate skin synthesis—obstruction blocks off the enterohepatic circulation.
- Coeliac disease—inhibits the absorption of fat and fat-soluble vitamins in the gut.
- Liver disease (e.g. cirrhosis)—can cause enzyme deficiencies (e.g. 25-hydroxylase).
- Renal disease can cause enzyme deficiencies (e.g. 1α-hydroxylase is deficient in renal osteodystrophy).

Groups at risk of vitamin D deficiency
These include people who are not receiving enough sunlight or enough vitamin D in their diets, e.g.:
- Breast-fed babies, especially those born in northern latitudes in winter.

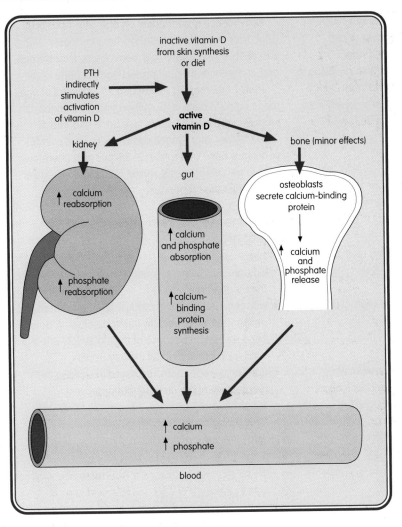

Fig. 8.6 Effects of vitamin D on the gut, bone, and kidney.

Fig. 8.7 Signs and symptoms caused by rickets and osteomalacia.

Signs and symptoms caused by rickets and osteomalacia	
Rickets	**Osteomalacia**
'knock-knees' or 'bow-legs' caused by bending of the long bones	bone pain
kyphosis, pigeon-chest, protruding forehead	bones appear 'thin' on X-ray, with localized lucencies (called Looser's zones)
features of hypocalcaemia	fractures (common in the neck of the femur)
	features of hypocalcaemia (e.g. proximal myopathy causes waddling gait)

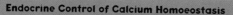

- Infants of mothers who are not receiving supplements—they may have defective dental enamel associated with low vitamin D status.
- Children and women of Asian origin who are living in temperate regions and who are vegetarian. Dark skin does not absorb enough sunlight in termperate climates and vegetarian diets tend to be low in calcium and high in phytates.
- The elderly and housebound.

Vitamin D supplements
Supplements are recommended for:
- Pregnant or lactating women.
- Children under 2 years old.
- Asian women and children, depending on their diets.
- Elderly persons.

Care should be taken to ensure against vitamin D intoxication, i.e. oversupplementation.

Osteoporosis
Osteoporosis is due to the reduced deposition of collagen matrix rather than the failure of calcification, hence the bone mass is abnormally reduced but mineralization is normal (compare with osteomalacia). The trabecular and/or cortical bone becomes fragile and susceptible to fracturing.

Its incidence is dependent on age, sex, and race: Caucasian postmenopausal women are most susceptible. Androgens (e.g. oestrogens, testosterone, and andrenal androgen) protect against bone loss.

Peak bone mass is reached at 25–30 years of age, then begins to decline. Both men and Afro-Caribbean women aged over 35 years lose bone at a rate of 0.3–0.5% per year; Caucasian women aged over 35 years lose bone at a rate of 2–5% per year (therefore tend to get osteoporosis earlier). Bone loss increases further after the menopause.

Hormone therapy and prevention of osteoporosis
This includes:
- Calcium supplements—not proved to be useful after the menopause.
- Hormone replacement therapy (HRT) in women—oestrogens are especially helpful in slowing down bone resorption because of their inhibitory effect on interleukin production by the osteoclasts.
- Calcitonin—appears to be useful in slowing the progression of the disease (but unproven).
- Weight-bearing exercise—decreases bone loss.
- Maximizing bone mass in mid-life—important to delay the onset of symptoms.

- Describe the synthesis, secretion, and effects of PTH, calcitonin, and vitamin D.
- List the effects of deficiency and excess of PTH and calcitonin.
- Discuss the causes and effects of vitamin D deficiency, including groups at risk and treatment.
- What hormones are used in the treatment of osteoporosis?

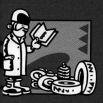

9. Endocrine Control of Growth

NORMAL GROWTH

Growth is genetically determined. However, its full potential depends on nutrition, health (illness and stress inhibit growth), and growth hormones.

The rate of growth varies at different ages. The maximal growth rate occurs in the foetus and is independent of hormones. The highest postnatal growth rate occurs just after birth (dependent on hormones), followed by a slower rate in mid-childhood. The growth rate increases again during puberty (onset: 8–13 years for girls; 9–14 years for boys). This is known as the pubertal growth spurt and is dependent on hormones, especially growth hormone (GH) and gonadal steroids. After puberty, the epiphyses of the long bones fuse, growth ceases and maximal height is achieved.

CELLULAR GROWTH AND PROLIFERATION

Cell division and differentiation depend on the actions of autocrine, paracrine, and endocrine hormones/factors. There are numerous growth specific hormones/factors, and other hormones (e.g. insulin, prolactin, thyroxine, vitamin D) that also affect growth. They all act on the G_1 phase of the cell cycle (Fig. 9.1) Growth hormones/factors promote growth either directly—via induction of cell proliferation, or indirectly, via their effects on cellular processes and metabolism required for normal growth.

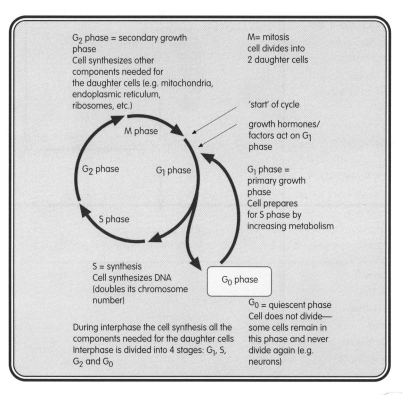

G_2 phase = secondary growth phase
Cell synthesizes other components needed for the daughter cells (e.g. mitochondria, endoplasmic reticulum, ribosomes, etc.)

M phase

G_2 phase G_1 phase

S phase

M= mitosis
cell divides into
2 daughter cells

'start' of cycle

growth hormones/
factors act on G_1 phase

G_1 phase =
primary growth phase
Cell prepares
for S phase by
increasing metabolism

G_0 phase

S = synthesis
Cell synthesizes DNA
(doubles its chromosome number)

G_0 = quiescent phase
Cell does not divide—
some cells remain in
this phase and never
divide again (e.g.
neurons)

During interphase the cell synthesis all the components needed for the daughter cells
Interphase is divided into 4 stages: G_1, S, G_2 and G_0

Fig. 9.1 Cell cycle. (The stages that a cell goes through in order to divide.)

HORMONES/FACTORS DIRECTLY INVOLVED IN THE CONTROL OF GROWTH

Growth hormone (GH; somatotrophin)

GH is a peptide hormone (191 amino acids) with an endocrine mode of delivery.

Synthesis and secretion of GH

GH is synthesized in the somatotroph cells of the anterior pituitary gland by transcription and translation of the GH gene on chromosome 17. It is stored in vesicles in the cell cytoplasm and secreted episodically in bursts. GH secretion is regulated by growth hormone-releasing hormone (GHRH) and growth hormone-inhibiting hormone (GHIH) from the hypothalamus, feedback inhibition by IGF-1 and other factors. See Fig. 9.2.

Effects of GH

GH acts on most body cells, but mainly the liver, chondrocytes, muscle, and adipose tissue. GH receptors have been located on target cell membranes, but its cellular mechanism of action is unknown.

- Indirect effects—it increases insulin-like growth factor (IGF) production in the liver, chondrocytes, fat cells, and muscle (IGF mediates the action of GH).
- Direct effects—it opposes the action of insulin (diabetogenic effect) in that it causes lipolysis in adipose cells and gluconeogenesis in muscle cells.

Deficiency/excess of GH

Deficiency of GH causes dwarfism (short stature) in children—but growth does continue at a basal rate in the absence of GH—and adult GH deficiency syndrome.

Growth hormone is the most abundant pituitary hormone, even in the adult. Therefore it must have important metabolic effects that are not related to growth—these are still not fully understood.

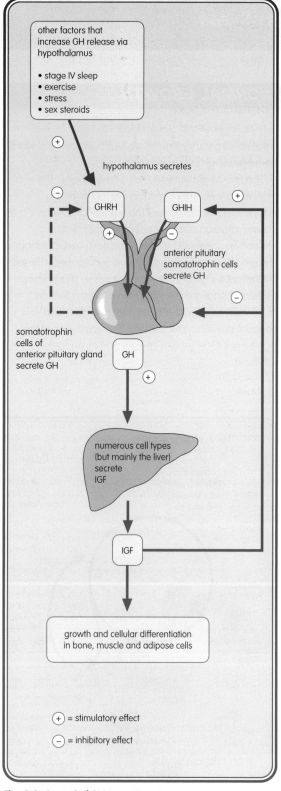

Fig. 9.2 Control of GH secretion.

Excess of GH causes gigantism in children and acromegaly in adults.

For symptoms and signs of adult GH deficiency syndrome and acromegaly, see Figs 15.1 and 15.3.

Insulin-like growth factors (IGFs; somatomedins)

IGF is a peptide hormone that exists as two forms: IGF-1 and IGF-2. Mode of delivery is endocrine and paracrine.

IGF is so called because its structure is similar to pro-insulin and it can bind to insulin receptors as well as its own receptors. It is also termed 'somatomedin', because it mediates the action of GH (old name somatotrophin).

Synthesis and secretion of IGFs

IGFs are synthesized by many cell types—but mainly by the liver and fibroblasts—by the expression of their respective genes (IGF-1 is found on chromosome 12, IGF-2 on chromosome 11). Secretion is stimulated by GH.

Plasma levels of IGFs are high in childhood with a peak at 12–17 years but fall to a constant basal level in adulthood.

Effects of IGF-1 and IGF-2

IGF-1 and IGF-2 act on the G_1 phase of the cell cycle to promote growth and cellular differentiation in:
- Bone—stimulate chondrocyte proliferation (promotes bone growth).
- Muscle—stimulate protein synthesis.
- Adipose cells—stimulate lipolysis in adipose cells.

IGF-1 induces cell division in already differentiated cells (clonal expansion), and its postnatal levels correlate with increasing body size; IGF-2 has an as yet unknown function, but its levels in childhood correlate with height velocity (cm/year).

Details of other major growth factors involved in cellular proliferation are listed in Fig. 9.3.

Other major growth factors involved in cellular proliferation			
Growth factor	Mode of delivery	Action on growth and development	Method and control of secretion
nerve growth factor (NGF)	paracrine	induces neuron growth and helps to guide growing sympathetic nerves to organs they will innervate (may also act on the brain and aid memory retention)	secreted by cells in path of growing axon; regulation of secretion not yet understood
epidermal growth factor (EGF)	paracrine and endocrine	promotes cell proliferation in the epidermis, maturation of lung epithelium, and skin keratinization	secreted by many cell types i.e. not only epidermal cells (EGF is also found in breast milk); regulation of secretion not yet understood
transforming growth factors (TGFα, TGFβ)	paracrine	stimulate growth of fibroblast cells; TGFα acts similarly to EGF; TGFβ especially affects chondrocytes, osteoblasts, and osteoclasts	secreted by most cell types but especially platelets and cells in placenta and bone; regulation of secretion not yet understood
fibroblast growth factor (FGF)	paracrine	mitogenic effect in several cell types; may induce angiogenesis (formation of new blood vessels), which is essential for growth and wound healing	secreted by most cell types; regulation of secretion not yet understood
platelet-derived growth factor (PDGF)	paracrine	potent cell-growth promoter; chemotactic factor (involved in inflammatory response)	secreted by activated blood platelets during blood vessel injury
erythropoietin	endocrine	stimulates the production of erythrocyte precursor cells	secreted by the kidney in response to falling tissue oxygen concentration
interleukins (8 known)	autocrine and paracrine	IL-1 stimulates B-cell proliferation and helper T cells to produce IL-2; IL-2 autoactivates helper T cells and activates cytotoxic T cells	IL-1 is secreted by activated macrophages; IL-2 is secreted by activated helper T cells

Fig. 9.3 Other major growth factors involved in cellular proliferation.

HORMONES INDIRECTLY INVOLVED IN THE CONTROL OF GROWTH

The effects of these hormones are summarized below.

Thyroid hormone
- Essential for normal cell division, differentiation and maturation in the developing foetus, especially in the brain and skeleton.
- Promotes the synthesis of myelin and axonal ramification in the developing brain, possibly by promoting a nerve growth factor.
- Stimulates the production of GH and enhances its effects.
- Stimulates metabolic processes that produce energy required for growth.
- Is involved in the closure of the epiphyses.
- Excess in children causes increased growth of soft tissues and bone, but final adult height is reduced owing to the premature closure of the epiphyses.

Cortisol
- Suppresses growth by inhibiting GH secretion— excess cortisol leads to decreased growth.

Insulin
- Controls metabolism of fats, carbohydrates, and amino acids.
- Enhances amino acid uptake into cells and protein anabolism, which acts to promote growth.

Antidiuretic hormone (ADH)
- Controls fluid balance (if fluid balance is abnormal, so is growth).

Parathyroid hormone and vitamin D
- Control calcium levels (normal calcium levels are required for normal growth).

LH, FSH, and sex steroids
- Are involved in the growth and maturation of the sex organs.
- The early onset of oestrogen or androgen secretion causes the early onset of the pubertal growth spurt, but the final adult height is reduced owing to the premature closure of the epiphyses.

Prolactin
- Promotes growth of the mammary glands and of the ovaries and testes [in conjunction with the gonadotrophins—luteinizing hormone (LH) and follicle-stimulating hormone (FSH)].

Placental lactogen
- Acts like prolactin in that it promotes the development of the maternal mammary glands.
- Stimulates cartilage growth and the incorporation of sulphur into it.
- Antagonizes insulin—promotes amino acid and glucose utilization in the foetus.
- Inhibits maternal growth hormone secretion.

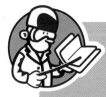

- What factors determine growth rate?
- Discuss the concept of the cell cycle and where growth factors act on it.
- Outline the synthesis, secretion, and effects of the hormones directly involved in the control of growth (i.e. GH and IGF).
- List the growth factors that stimulate proliferation of specific cell types.
- Name the hormones indirectly involved in the control of growth.

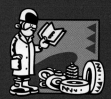

10. The Reproductive System

EMBRYOLOGICAL DEVELOPMENT OF GENDER

The first 6 weeks

The development of the reproductive structures follows an almost identical course in both males and females until week 6 of gestation. During this time, the following important processes take place (Fig. 10.1):

- From week 3, primordial germ cells migrate from the yolk sac, arriving in the mesenchyme of the posterior body wall by week 6. They induce formation of the genital ridges at the 10th thoracic segment. Cells of the mesonephros and coelomic epithelium aggregate into somatic sex cords, which later differentiate into Sertoli cells (male) and follicle cells (female).

- The mesonephric (wolffian) ducts develop in week 4. In males, the mesonephric ducts will develop into the epididymis and ejaculatory ducts (vasa deferentia); in females, they will regress.

- The paramesonephric (müllerian) ducts develop in week 6. In females, the paramesonephric ducts give rise to the fallopian tubes, the uterus, and the superior part of the vagina; in males, these ducts degenerate.

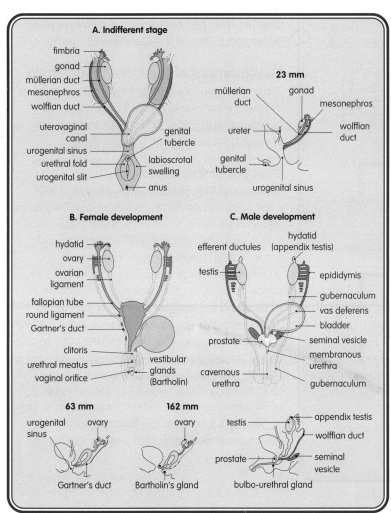

Fig. 10.1 Development of male and female reproductive tracts. (Adapted from *Basic & Clinical Endocrinology, 4th Ed.* by FS Greenspan. Courtesy of Appleton & Lange.)

Development of the male reproductive tract

By the end of week 6, expression of the sex-determining region (SRY) gene on the Y chromosome produces a protein, the testis-determining factor (TDF), which initiates a cascade of events causing the formation of the testes, male genital ducts, and associated primary sexual characteristics (Fig. 10.2).

Development of the female reproductive tract

In the female, absence of the SRY gene allows development of the female genital tract—the mesenchymal cells of the sex cord differentiate into stromal cells, coelomic cells become granulosa cells, and the genital ridge becomes an ovary.

Oogonia undergo mitosis, reaching maximum numbers (7 million) by the month 6 of gestation. There is a finite number of germ cells in the female as there is no stem-cell system. Thereafter the oogenia enter meiosis, but the process is arrested in prophase—probably by the follicle cells that surround the germ cells. Oogonia degenerate until there are 2 million at birth. By menarche, 400 000 remain.

The uterus and vagina begin formation as the paramesonephric ducts fuse inferiorly at week 9, near their attachment to the primitive urogenital sinus. From month 3 to month 5 of gestation, progressive 'zippering' of the ducts in a superior direction forms the uterus. Abnormalities of this process can result in a bifurcated uterus, and even a double vagina.

The broad ligaments are formed as a fold of peritoneum is dragged away from the posterior body wall. The lower part of the vagina is derived from the sinovaginal bulbs of the urogenital sinus (see Fig. 10.1).

Development of the external genitalia

The external genitalia develop from the same primitive structures in both sexes (Fig. 10.3). The indifferent genitalia arise in week 7 and appear similar in both sexes until the end of week 12 of gestation.

Descent of the testes

The testes and the ovaries both descend from their initial position in the 10th thoracic segment. The ovaries remain in the pelvis, whereas the testes migrate much further—into the scrotum (Fig. 10.4). Descent in both sexes depend on a ligamentous cord, the gubernaculum, which arises in week 7 from condensation of fascia in peritoneal folds that run on either side of the vertebral column.

The testes pass through the anterior abdominal wall via the inguinal canal in the last trimester of pregnancy. During this process a fold of peritoneum, the processus vaginalis, is pushed ahead of the descending testis. Later this becomes separated from the peritoneal cavity, and its remnant is termed the tunica vaginalis. Failure of this separation may lead to a patent processus, which is associated with inguinal hernia.

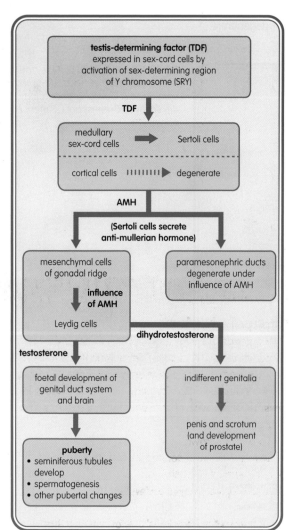

Fig. 10.2 Differentiation cascade of male genital development.

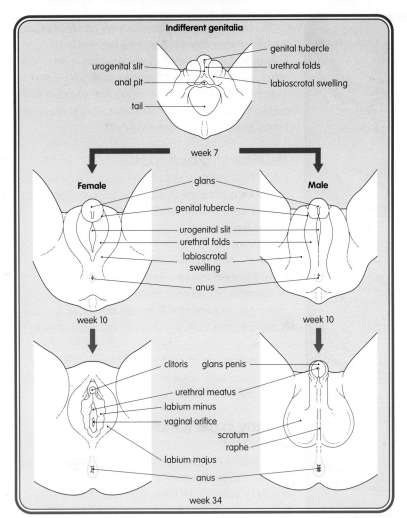

Fig. 10.3 Development of the external genitalia.

- List the primitive structures of the developing genital tracts and the structures that derive from them.
- Outline how and when differentiation of the male reproductive tract is initiated.
- Describe the origins of Sertoli, Leydig, and follicular cells.
- Outline the structures that give rise to the external genitalia.
- Describe the processes involved in testicular descent.

PUBERTY

Changes at puberty

After a period of steady growth in childhood, puberty is characterized by accelerated development and intense endocrine activity. The age of onset varies greatly, being between 8 and 13 years for girls, and 9 and 14 years for boys. There are a number of processes associated with puberty:

- Adolescent growth spurt.
- Development of secondary sexual characteristics.
- Achievement of fertility.
- Psychological and social development.

The initiation of puberty is not fully understood, but appears to be associated with maturation of the hypothalamus and increased secretion of releasing

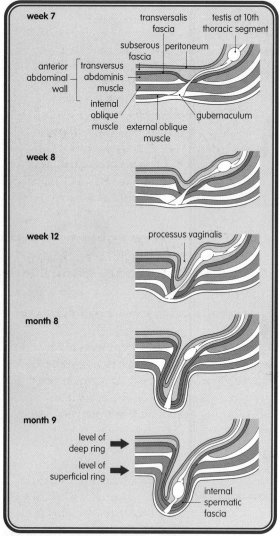

week 7
transversalis fascia
testis at 10th thoracic segment
subserous fascia peritoneum
anterior abdominal wall
transversus abdominis muscle
internal oblique muscle
external oblique muscle
gubernaculum

week 8

week 12
processus vaginalis

month 8

month 9
level of deep ring
level of superficial ring
internal spermatic fascia

Fig. 10.4 Descent of the testes during embryological development. (Adapted from *Human Embryology 2e,* by W Larsen. Courtesy of Churchill Livingstone.)

hormones. The resulting increase in pituitary activity (and pituitary enlargement) causes raised levels of growth hormone (GH), thyroid-stimulating hormone (TSH), and adrenocorticotrophic hormone (ACTH). The adrenal cortex produces sex steroids, which mediate the early changes of puberty; this is termed adrenarche, and takes place at about 7 years of age.

Later, pulsatile secretion of gonadotrophin-releasing hormone (GnRH) from the hypothalamus rises, initially at night, and stimulates gonadarche—the activation of the testes and ovaries. The main factor in this increase is the reduction in sensitivity of the hypothalamus to feedback inhibition by sex hormones.

The sex hormones produced by the gonads mediate the later stages of puberty and the onset of fertility (menarche being the start of menstruation in girls). The onset of puberty can be affected by body weight; for example, menarche may be delayed by malnutrition—it appears that a body mass of at least 47 kg is necessary for the initiation of the menstrual cycle.

The pubertal growth spurt
This is the earliest developmental event of puberty, but because the initial rise in growth velocity at adrenarche is slight, growth of the breasts or testes is usually noticed first. Onset is at 8–12 years in girls and 9–13 years in boys.

The pubertal growth spurt occurs in three stages:
* An initial increase due to adrenarche.
* The main growth spurt under control of GH, insulin-like growth factor (IGF-1), thyroid hormones, and sex steroids. This lasts 2–3 years in girls and 3–4 years in boys.
* Decreased growth and fusion of epiphyseal growth plates as adult levels of sex steroids are reached at the end of puberty.

Puberty in the female
Adrenarche
Adrenarche takes place between 7 and 8 years of age. Growth of pubic hair begins at 11–12 years, followed closely by axillary hair. These effects are mediated by the increasing production of adrenal sex hormones.

Thelarche
Development of the breast is the first sexual change to occur in girls, and is often noticed before the growth spurt. Nipple enlargement begins at 9–11 years, along with thickening of the ductal system. These changes are mediated by oestrogen.

Menarche
Initiation of menstruation occurs between the ages of 10 and 16 years, the mean being at age 13. The first ovulation occurs 10 months later on average. After mid-puberty, a positive feedback system develops whereby oestrogen can stimulate the release of gonadotrophins—luteinizing hormone (LH) and follicle-stimulating hormone (FSH). LH surges stimulate ovulation mid-cycle (see Fig. 10.14). The cycle may take some time to become regular, and 90% of all menstrual cycles are anovulatory in the first year after menarche.

Oestrogen-mediated changes

These include:

- Development of the breasts—maturation of the duct system; fat deposition and proliferation of connective tissue; nipple and areolar pigmentation.
- Development of the vagina—increased length; thickened mucosa; lactic acid production and decreased vaginal pH; secretion of clear discharge.
- Other genital changes—increase in the size of the clitoris and urethral meatus.

Progesterone-mediated changes

These include:

- Proliferation of secretory tissue in the breast.
- Contribution to vaginal and uterine growth.
- Initiation of cyclical changes in endometrium and ovary.

Puberty in the male

Adrenarche occurs between the ages of 8 and 9 years.

The testes

Growth of the testes is the first sign of puberty in boys and begins at 9–11 years of age. The right testis is larger than the left, which is usually lower. The increase is mainly due to proliferation of the seminiferous tubules, under the influence of FSH; however, stimulation of Leydig-cell function by LH also contributes.

Spermatogenesis begins between the ages of 11 and 15 years, and the first ejaculation may be expected around 13–14 years.

Other changes in the male

Pubic hair begins to develop at 10–13 years of age, under the influence of adrenal and testicular androgens. Axillary hair usually appears at 13 years. Facial hair growth starts somewhat later, at approximately 15 years of age. Sebaceous glands become active, causing acne in some boys.

The penis increases in length from (on average) 6.2 to 13.2 cm, and in thickness. The scrotum enlarges and thickens, and the scrotal skin becomes pigmented.

The larynx, cricothyroid cartilage, and laryngeal muscles enlarge. The voice breaks at about 13 years of age.

- List the main processes that occur in female puberty, with the ages at which they occur.
- Describe the role of oestrogen in female puberty.
- List the events that take place in male puberty, noting the ages at which they occur.

ORGANIZATION OF THE FEMALE REPRODUCTIVE ORGANS

The vulva

The macroscopic structure of the vulva is illustrated in Fig. 10.5.

The blood supply is rich, via branches of the pudendal arteries. Large venous plexuses drain the region and become engorged during sexual activity or pregnancy. Veins follow the corresponding arteries. Lymphatic drainage is to superficial and deep femoral nodes and iliac nodes.

The vagina

The vagina is a fibromuscular tube that extends from the vestibule of the vulva to the cervix. The muscular wall is folded into ridges (rugae) which allow great distension during childbirth. The relations of the vagina may be seen in Fig. 10.6.

The blood supply arrives via the vaginal and uterine arteries, which form plexuses around the vagina. The venous plexus is continuous with the vesical, pudendal, and haemorrhoidal plexuses. Lymphatic drainage of the lower third is to the inguinal nodes. The upper two-thirds drain to internal iliac, obturator, and sacral nodes.

The vagina is lined with non-keratinized, stratified squamous epithelium, which is continuous over the external part of the cervix. There are no mucus-secreting cells in the vaginal epithelium. However, interstitial fluid seeps between the cells. Vaginal lactobacilli digest glycogen from exfoliated squamous cells to produce the lactic acid which maintains the low vaginal pH of 5.0. Eradication of the vaginal flora by antibiotics interferes with this process, and predisposes to infection by the fungus *Candida albicans* (thrush). The glycogen

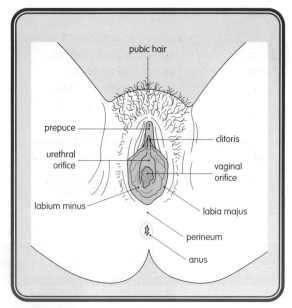

Fig. 10.5 Surface anatomy of the vulva.

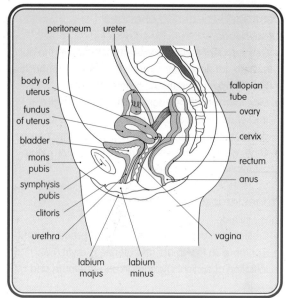

Fig. 10.6 Sagittal section of the female pelvis.

substrate is produced under the influence of oestrogen; hence thrush may also develop in women who are low in oestrogen, i.e. postmenopausal women or those taking the contraceptive pill, who have lower endogenous hormone levels.

The uterus and cervix

The uterus is a pear-shaped muscular organ that lies in the pelvis between the bladder and the rectum. Its lower part projects into the vaginal vault to form the cervix. The structure and relations of the uterus are shown in Figs 10.6 and 10.7.

Blood supply arrives via the uterine arteries (branches of the internal iliac), which anastomose with the ovarian arteries (directly from the aorta) and the vaginal plexus. Venous drainage is via the pampiniform plexuses. Lymphatic drainage runs to superficial femoral, sacral, iliac, and para-aortic nodes.

The uterus is composed of three tissue layers:
- The serosa.
- The myometrium.
- The endometrium.

The cervix is structurally and functionally distinct from the rest of the uterus. It is a cylindrical structure, approximately 3 cm in length. The superior end of the cervical canal is termed the internal os, and the inferior opening into the vagina, the external os (see Fig. 10.7).

The endocervical canal is lined with columnar mucous epithelium that is continuous with the endometrium. The ectocervix is lined with the stratified squamous epithelium of the vagina. The squamocolumnar junction, or transformation zone, is clinically important as it is the site of cell dysplasia that can give rise to cervical carcinoma. It is from this region that cells are scraped during a cervical smear so that they may be examined for signs of dysplasia. The consistency of cervical mucus is important in sperm transport. Oestrogen promotes watery mucus that facilitates transport, whereas progesterone promotes mucus hostile to sperm motility.

The fallopian (uterine) tubes

These muscular tubes project from the cornua of the uterus, curving over to embrace the ovaries. The tubes consist of four parts:
- The interstitial segment.
- The isthmus.
- The ampulla.
- The infundibulum.

The mucosa of the fallopian tubes secretes mucus and is ciliated. Mucus flows towards the uterus by peristalsis and ciliary activity. It serves to carry and nourish the fertilized ovum, and may play a role in the capacitation of sperm prior to fertilization.

The ovaries

These are paired ovoid structures that lie lateral to the uterus, attached to the broad ligament by a fold of peritoneum called the mesovarium. They are attached to the uterus by the ovarian ligaments (see Fig. 10.7).

Blood supply arrives via anastomosing branches of the ovarian and uterine arteries. Venous drainage is via the pampiniform plexus of veins. Lymphatic drainage runs to para-aortic nodes. The ovaries are richly innervated by the autonomic system, mainly sympathetic, from renal and hypogastric plexuses.

The microstructure of the ovary is illustrated in Fig. 10.8.

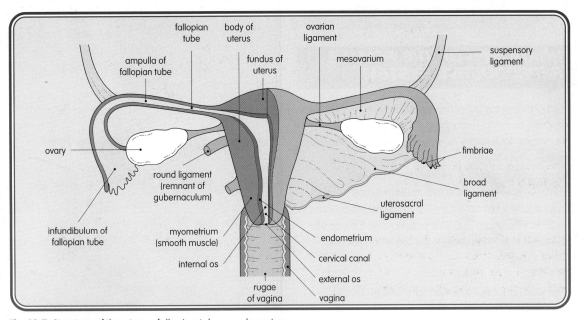

Fig. 10.7 Structure of the uterus, fallopian tubes, and ovaries.

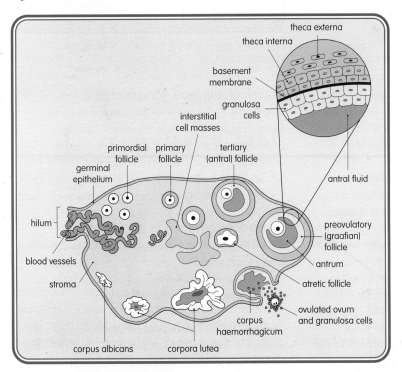

Fig. 10.8 Microstructure of the ovary.

° **Describe the anatomy of the vagina. How is vaginal pH maintained?**

° **Draw a diagram of the uterus, fallopian tubes, and ovaries.**

HORMONES OF THE FEMALE REPRODUCTIVE SYSTEM

The hormonal control of the reproductive system follows the motif common throughout endocrinology: the hypothalamic–pituitary axis controls ovarian hormone synthesis via releasing factors (GnRH) and trophic hormones (LH and FSH); ovarian steroids exert a feedback inhibition on the hypothalamus and pituitary. Other pituitary hormones (prolactin and oxytocin) are involved in lactation. Fig. 10.9 summarizes the overall hormonal regulation of reproduction in the female.

GnRH

GnRH is a linear decapeptide hormone produced by hypothalamic neurons. It stimulates the synthesis of LH and FSH by pituitary gonadotrophs.

Synthesis and secretion

GnRH-secreting neurons are located in the preoptic area of the anterior hypothalamus, and their axons terminate in the median eminence adjacent to the pituitary stalk. Thus, GnRH may be secreted from the terminal boutons into the portal vessels, which carry the hormone to its target cells in the anterior pituitary.

Control of secretion

Secretion of GnRH is pulsatile. During childhood, pulses are infrequent and erratic, and the hypothalamus is highly sensitive to feedback inhibition by circulating oestrogens. During puberty, sensitivity to inhibition falls, and the frequency of secretory pulses increases. After menarche, tonic pulses occur every 60–90 minutes, the frequency varying throughout the menstrual cycle. GnRH secretion is thus said to have two components:

• Tonic pulsatile secretion that maintains gonadotrophic function.
• Cyclical variation in pulse frequency throughout the menstrual cycle.

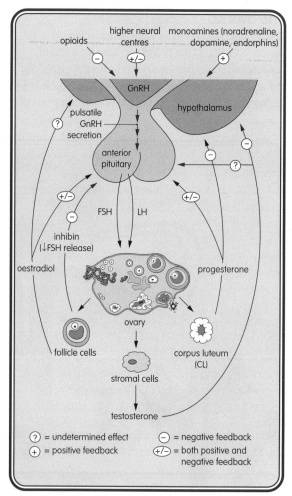

Fig. 10.9 Hormonal control of the female reproductive system.

Actions on pituitary gonadotrophs

GnRH binds to G-protein-coupled receptors on the surface of gonadotrophs in the anterior pituitary. Secretion of LH and FSH is stimulated via the cAMP second-messenger pathway. The sensitivity of gonadotrophs to GnRH is also subject to both positive and negative feedback effects of circulating sex steroids.

Gonadotrophins: LH and FSH

LH and FSH are both glycoprotein hormones comprising α and β subunits. The β subunit confers the specific hormone activity, while the α subunit is common to all pituitary glycoprotein hormones.

Control of synthesis and secretion

Secretion of both LH and FSH is controlled by GnRH: it maintains basal levels and regulates the cyclic variation that controls the menstrual cycle. Both hormones are synthesized and secreted by gonadotrophs of the anterior pituitary and act on the ovary (or testis in males). GnRH initiates secretion via activation of adenylate cyclase and the cAMP second-messenger system. The half-life in plasma of LH is 30 minutes; that of FSH is 3 hours.

Secretion of LH and FSH is subject to the following factors:

- Episodic secretion: pulsatile secretion every 60–90 minutes, following the pattern of GnRH.
- Positive feedback: just before ovulation, high levels of oestrogen exert a positive effect on LH and FSH production. This positive feedback stimulates the LH surge that causes ovulation.
- Negative feedback: FSH levels fall around day 5, as follicles begin to secrete oestradiol. Moderate levels of steroids inhibit LH and FSH production. This is the basis for the oral contraceptive pill. Danazol, a testosterone derivative, is used clinically to suppress gonadotrophin release in conditions such as dysmenorrhoea or endometriosis.
- Inhibin, a peptide hormone produced by ovarian granulosa cells, inhibits the secretion of FSH. However, subunits of inhibin (termed activin) have been shown to stimulate FSH production, so this mechanism appears to be complex!

Levels of LH and FSH are low before puberty, and high after the menopause. Nocturnal elevations indicate the onset of puberty.

Effects of the gonadotrophins

FSH receptors have been found only on granulosa cells of the ovary. LH receptors, on the other hand, are expressed on thecal, granulosa, interstitial, and luteal cells of the ovary. The actions on the various cell types are explained later in the discussion of steroid hormone synthesis.

Ovarian steroid hormones

The ovary synthesizes and secretes a number of steroid hormones:

- Oestrogens—oestrone, oestradiol (the most active), and oestriol (increased in pregnancy).
- Progesterone—produced during the luteal phase of the menstrual cycle.
- Androgens—androstenedione, testosterone, and dihydrotestosterone. These are precursors for oestrogen synthesis and are also secreted to act on the tissues.

Synthesis and secretion

As in the adrenal gland, steroid hormones are not stored in significant amounts in the ovary, and secretion is closely related to synthesis. Cholesterol is the precursor of steroid synthesis, and is present in the ovary in both free and esterified forms. Circulating lipoproteins maintain the supply. Cholesterol is first converted to pregnenolone: this is the rate-limiting step of steroid synthesis (see Chapter 1) and in the ovary this is regulated by LH.

Steroid synthesis takes place predominantly in the cells of the developing follicle. The thecal cells produce the androgenic precursors androstenedione and testosterone under the influence of LH. During the follicular phase of the menstrual cycle, these diffuse across the basement membrane to the granulosa cells, where they are converted to oestrogens by aromatase activity. This is stimulated by FSH.

This arrangement is referred to as the 'two-cell' model of oestrogen production in the follicle (Fig. 10.10). However, recent studies have shown that aromatase activity may also be important in the thecal cells.

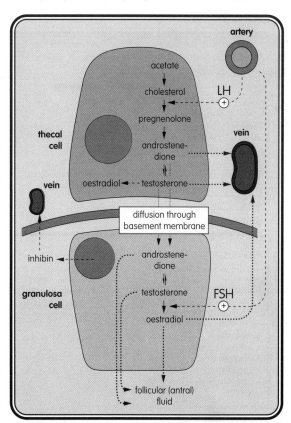

Fig. 10.10 The 'two-cell' model—production of steroid hormones in follicle cells.

After ovulation, LH stimulates the remaining follicular cells to synthesize progesterone. These cells form the corpus luteum, which stimulates the glands of the endometrium in preparation for implantation of the fertilized ovum. Expression of LH receptors on granulosa cells is stimulated by FSH and oestradiol during the follicular phase.

Stromal cells of the ovaries are also active, producing androstenedione, testosterone, and dihydrotestosterone under the influence of LH. Only testosterone and dihydrotestosterone have significant androgen activity on the tissues, but androstenedione may be converted to testosterone in the periphery.

Transport of the sex steroids

The sex steroids are transported in the blood bound to plasma proteins:

- Oestradiol binds to sex-hormone-binding globulin (SHBG) and—less avidly—to albumin.
- Progesterone binds to corticosteroid-binding globulin (CBG) and—less avidly—to albumin.

Synthesis of SHBG is stimulated by oestrogens and inhibited by androgens—levels are twice as high in women as in men.

Intracellular action of the ovarian steroids

In common with all steroid hormones, the ovarian steroids diffuse through the membrane of the target cell and bind to intracellular receptors and the hormone-receptor complexes then attach to sites on chromosomal DNA. A variety of cellular effects may then be induced by manipulation of DNA transcription.

The physiological effects of the steroid hormones are outlined in Fig. 10.11.

Other ovarian hormones
Inhibin and activin

These are dimeric glycoprotein hormones that have a common α subunit but different β subunits. Inhibin is produced by the granulosa cells and acts upon pituitary gonadotrophs to suppress FSH production. Activin stimulates FSH production.

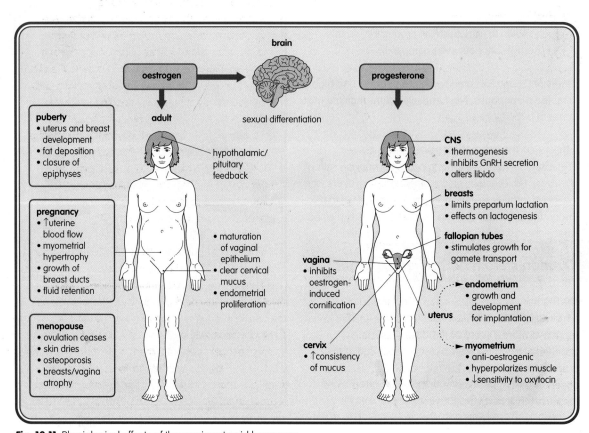

Fig. 10.11 Physiological effects of the ovarian steroid hormones.

Relaxin

This is a polypeptide hormone featuring disulphide bonds linking its two chains, a structure similar to that of insulin. It has been shown in some species to cause cervical softening and relaxation of pelvic ligaments in preparation for birth. However, its role in humans is not yet fully understood.

The 'two-cell' model of steroid synthesis in the ovarian follicle is important to know. Fig 10.10 is worth learning because it not only summarizes the sites of steroid synthesis in the follicle but will also help you to remember where LH and FSH act in the ovary.

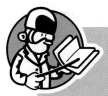

○ What are the factors involved in regulation of gonadotrophin secretion and where do they act?
○ Explain the 'two-cell' model of ovarian steroid synthesis.
○ List the principal actions of oestrogens, progesterone, and androgens in the female.

HORMONAL CHANGES AND THE MENSTRUAL CYCLE

The menstrual cycle is the series of events during which a mature ovum is released from the ovary into the reproductive tract every 28–32 days. Associated changes occur throughout the reproductive tract to prepare for fertilization. The hormonal variations observed during the cycle (see Fig. 10.14) orchestrate these changes and possible pregnancy.

Ovarian follicles

In the female, the germinal cells (ova) exist in a state of suspended meiosis in the outer cortex of the ovary. By the time puberty is reached, there are about 400 000 remaining, although probably less than 400 of these will develop fully and be ovulated.

Stages of the ovarian cycle

The menstrual cycle is characterized by follicular development and expansion (the follicular phase), release of the ovum (ovulation), and secretion of progesterone by the remaining follicle cells or corpus luteum (luteal phase). Menstruation itself occurs when the luteal body degenerates and progesterone production ceases.

Development of the ovarian follicle

The stages of follicular development are as follows (Fig. 10.12):

• Primordial follicle—the dormant stage. This consists of an ovum arrested in the first prophase of meiosis surrounded by a single layer of immature granulosa cells and by a basement membrane.
• Primary follicle—the ovum increases in size. The granulosa cells become cuboidal and undergo mitosis, expanding to three layers. A membrane called the zona pellucida develops around the ovum.
• Secondary follicle—proliferation of granulosa cells produces multiple layers surrounding the ovum. Adjacent stromal cells align with the basement membrane to become the thecal cells. Fluid begins to collect between the granulosa cells.
• Tertiary (antral) follicle—a fluid-filled cavity, or antrum, forms within the granulosa cell layer. Growth to this point is independent of gonadotrophins, but antrum formation requires stimulation by FSH.
• Preovulatory (graafian) follicle—the follicle reaches a diameter of 2.5 cm before ovulation.

Development occurs in a cohort of follicles, which are initiated in the last days of a preceding luteal phase. The dominant follicle, which will go on to ovulate, is the one that is most responsive to FSH. Development to the antral phase takes about 3 months, so there are always a number of follicles at different stages of development within the ovary. During this stage, there is increasing expression of FSH and LH receptors on follicular cells.

The follicular phase (days 1–13)

At the start of each menstrual cycle, several developing follicles (which have reached the antral stage) are stimulated into rapid growth by LH and FSH (days 1–4). Selection of one of these takes place between days 5 and 7 of the cycle through an unknown mechanism, and this becomes predominant. The others degenerate and are termed atretic. It takes 2 weeks (days 1–13) to develop from the antral follicle to the graafian follicle, ready for ovulation. During this stage, the follicle secretes increasing amounts of oestrogen, and LH receptors are induced on the granulosa cells by FSH and oestradiol.

Ovulation (day 14)

By day 12 of the cycle, oestradiol levels exceed 700 pmol/L and continue to rise. This precipitates a surge of LH (via positive feedback), which peaks 10–12 hours before ovulation occurs on day 14. Ovulation occurs randomly in only one ovary through mechanisms that are not understood.

Ovulation involves the rupture of the follicle wall, which releases the ovum and surrounding granulosa cells (the cumulus oophorus) into the peritoneum, adjacent to the opening of the fallopian tube. The ovum is then swept into the fallopian tube by ciliary activity on the fimbriae. The mechanisms of ovulation are poorly understood, but many vascular and metabolic factors are active in this process.

The luteal phase (days 15–28)

After ovulation, the remaining follicular cells form the corpus luteum, which synthesizes progesterone under the influence of LH.

Progesterone stimulates the endometrial glands to produce a glycogen-rich secretion that supports the fertilized ovum. If implantation occurs, human chorionic gonadotrophin (hCG) produced by syncytiotrophoblast maintains the corpus luteum, and progesterone levels continue to rise, maintaining the endometrium and preventing follicular growth. High levels of progesterone have a negative feedback effect on the pituitary, inhibiting the release of LH and FSH.

The corpus luteum has a preprogrammed (and fairly constant) life of about 10 days. Unless implantation occurs, it degenerates after this time, and progesterone and oestradiol levels fall dramatically over 1–2 days. This releases the inhibition of LH and FSH production, and levels rise, promoting follicle development (FSH). The fall in progesterone and oestradiol triggers breakdown of the endometrium and menstruation.

The endometrium
Microstructure of the endometrium

The endometrium consists of two distinct layers (Fig. 10.13):

- The basal layer (stratum basale), which is not shed at menstruation and undergoes little cyclic change.
- The functional layer (stratum functionale), which arises from the basal layer each month and is shed at menstruation. The stratum functionale is further divided into a thin superficial layer called the

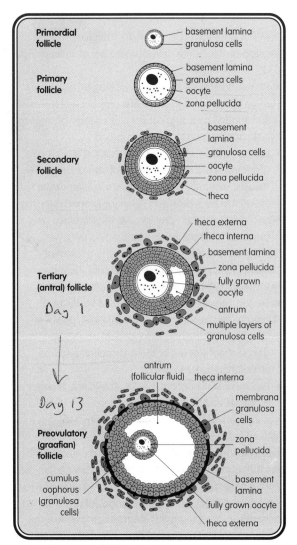

Fig. 10.12 Stages of follicular development.

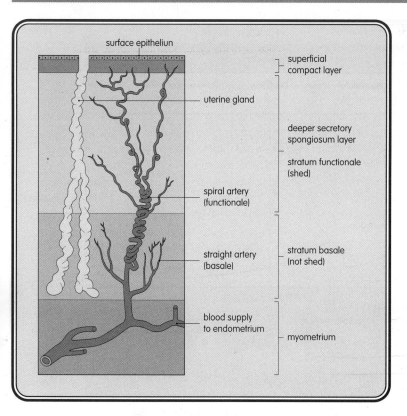

surface epitheliun

uterine gland

spiral artery
(functionale)

straight artery
(basale)

blood supply
to endometrium

superficial
compact layer

deeper secretory
spongiosum layer

stratum functionale
(shed)

stratum basale
(not shed)

myometrium

Fig. 10.13 Structure of the endometrium.

compact layer, and the deeper spongiosum layer where the secretory glands of the endometrium lie.

The vasculature of the endometrium is highly specialized. Spiral arteries arise from branches of the uterine artery in the myometrium. In the stratum basale, these arteries remain straight, and are not influenced by changes in plasma levels of oestrogen and progesterone. The distal, spiral portion in the stratum functionale responds to the end of the luteal phase by constricting, causing hypoxia, ischaemia and subsequent necrosis—menstruation.

Endometrial changes throughout the menstrual cycle

The endometrial cycle has three stages (Fig. 10.14):
- Proliferative.
- Secretory (the latter part of which is sometimes referred to as the ischaemic phase).
- Menstrual.

The proliferative phase (days 4–13)

After the end of menstruation, the stratum functionale regenerates from the basal layer, under the influence of oestrogens from the ovarian follicle. Glandular epithelium proliferates and covers raw areas of stroma until the stratum functionale is thick and undulated. Glands become more tortuous, and the stroma is dense and rich in mitotic figures.

The secretory phase (days 14–28)

After ovulation, progesterone from the corpus luteum stimulates the secretory phase, and glands become highly tortuous. Glycogen-rich vacuoles appear in the glandular epithelium. Glandular activity is greatest at day 21, when progesterone levels also peak. Implantation would occur around day 21. From days 22–24, decidual changes begin to appear, especially in the region of the spiral arteries, and leucocyte infiltration of the stratum functionale is apparent by day 26.

The menstrual phase (days 1-4)

In the absence of hCG secreted by an embryo, decreasing progesterone levels from the corpus luteum cause vasoconstriction of the spiral arteries, beginning on day 25 or 26. This causes ischaemia, infarction, and necrosis of the stratum functionale. Sloughing of the layer occurs, with the passing of menstrual blood.

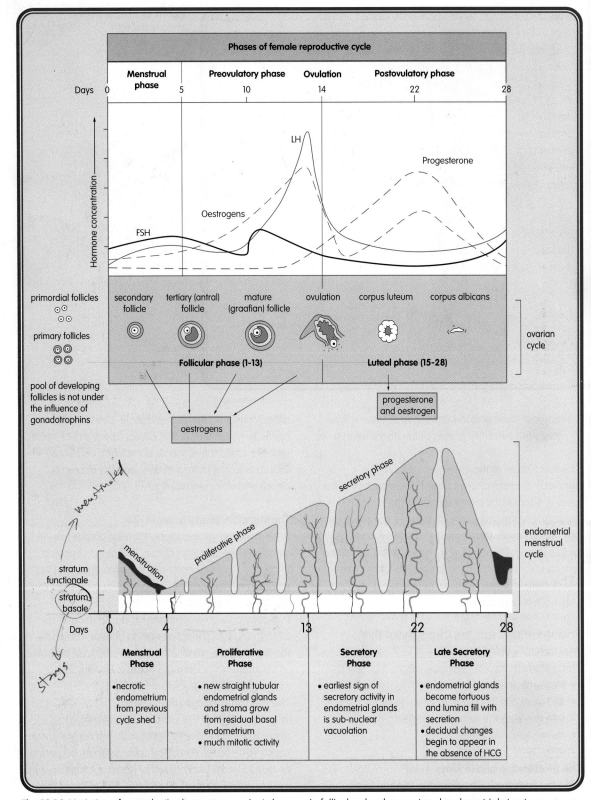

Fig. 10.14 Variation of reproductive hormones against changes in follicular development and endometrial structure.

Other changes in the menstrual cycle
Cervical mucus
Cervical mucus varies in consistency throughout the menstrual cycle. During the late follicular phase of the cycle, around the time of ovulation, oestrogen stimulates copious secretion of watery mucus, which is ideal for penetration by sperm. However, during the luteal phase, progesterone reduces secretion and increases its viscosity. Throughout the majority of the menstrual cycle, therefore, the mucus is scant and viscous, and the change at the time of ovulation can be used clinically to assess fertility.

Vaginal epithelium
The distribution of cell types in the vaginal epithelium changes throughout the cycle.

- List the stages of the ovarian cycle and describe the hormone production by the follicle in each.
- List the stages of the endometrial cycle and the hormonal influences on each.

THE MALE REPRODUCTIVE ORGANS

The male external genitalia
The penis
The anatomy of the penis is illustrated in Fig. 10.15.

Blood supply arrives via the cavernous arteries and the superficial and deep dorsal arteries (branches of the pudendal artery). Venous drainage is via the dorsal veins. Innervation by the terminal branches of the pudendal nerve carries sensation and autonomic fibres. Lymphatic drainage runs to superficial inguinal nodes.

Erectile function
Relaxation of vascular smooth muscle in the erectile tissue allows vasodilatation and engorgement of the sinusoidal spaces with blood at arterial pressure. The fascial sheaths and tunica albuginea of the penis resist

Fig. 10.15 Structure of the penis.

Labels: glans penis, Colles' fascia, superficial dorsal vein, Buck's fascia, deep dorsal vein and artery, corpus cavernosum, cavernosal artery, tunica albuginea, urethra, corpus spongiosum

expansion, and internal pressure rises until it occludes venous drainage. This vascular occlusion maintains the rigidity necessary for sexual intercourse to take place, without placing excessive demands on cardiac output.

Control of erection depends upon adequate neurological control, arterial flow, and functioning venous drainage. Neurological control is exerted in the following ways:

The mechanism by which erection takes place is often misunderstood. It is important (for instance, in a viva) to mention that the venous drainage is occluded by the increase in pressure within Buck's fascia. A common mistake is to assume that engorgement of the cavernous spaces due to arterial dilation is the only factor involved.

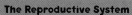

- Non-adrenergic, non-cholinergic (NANC) innervation and nitrergic (nitric oxide) innervation promote erection.
- Parasympathetic activation relaxes helicine arteries in erectile tissue.
- Sympathetic stimulation is required for ejaculation.

Other factors modify the neurological controls—prostaglandins, vasoactive intestinal polypeptide (VIP), histamine, and 5-hydroxytryptamine (5-HT) all have effects on the smooth muscle of the corpora cavernosa.

 Remember 'Point and Shoot!' to recall the roles of parasympathetic and sympathetic innervation in the penis.

The scrotum

The scrotum is a pendulous, sac-like structure that contains the testes and distal part of the vas (ductus) deferens, and the spermatic cords. It allows the testes to remain 2–3°C cooler than the core temperature, which is necessary for spermatogenesis. There are a number of important tissue layers to consider. From the outside, they are:

- Skin and superficial fascia—contains the dartos muscle, which contracts in response to cold.
- External spermatic fascia—outer coat of the spermatic cord. It is continuous with the external oblique aponeurosis of the anterior abdominal wall, from which it is embryologically derived.
- Cremasteric muscle and fascia—continuous with the internal oblique muscle. The cremasteric reflex causes retraction of the testes.
- Internal spermatic fascia—continuous with the transversalis fascia and the internal lining of the spermatic cord.
- The spermatic cord—contains the vasa deferentia and the neurovascular bundle supplying each testis.

The testes, accessory ducts, and glands

The structures of the male reproductive tract are illustrated in Fig. 10.16.

The testes

These are paired, ovoid structures with a mean volume of 19 mL in the adult. The testicular capsule consists of three layers:

- The tunica vaginalis (deriving from peritoneum).
- The tunica albuginea (fibrous connective tissue).
- The internal tunica vasculosa.

Blood supply arrives via the testicular arteries, which like the ovarian arteries are direct branches of the abdominal aorta. Venous drainage is via the pampiniform plexus of veins, then to the vena cava on the right, and the renal vein on the left. Lymphatic drainage runs along the arteries to para-aortic nodes.

The male ductal system

The ductal system produces and stores spermatozoa and seminal fluid; it allows the spermatozoa to mature and propels them from the body on ejaculation.

The ducts consist, in functional order, of the following structures:

- The seminiferous tubules—these empty into …
- The rete testis, a convoluted network of ducts.
- Ten to twelve efferent ductules—spermatozoa are transported by pressure, ciliary activity, and duct contraction into …
- The epididymis—spermatozoa take 12 days to pass through this highly convoluted tube. During this time they undergo final stages of maturation and become potentially fertile and motile.
- The vas (or ductus) deferens, a muscular tube 35–50 cm long.
- Seminal vesicles—adjacent to the prostate gland, these structures produce seminal fluid rich in fructose, providing nutrition for the spermatozoa. They produce about 60% of the total ejaculate.
- The prostatic urethra—the prostate gland also adds fluid to the semen (about 20%).
- The penile urethra—seminal fluid is added by bulbo-urethral and urethral glands.

The prostate

This is a small gland that surrounds the urethra as it leaves the bladder. It consists of tubuloalveolar tissue with a fibromuscular stroma, and secretes fluid into the duct. The prostate is important clinically because it enlarges in later life (benign prostatic hypertrophy) and may cause urinary obstruction. It is also a common site of carcinogenesis in men.

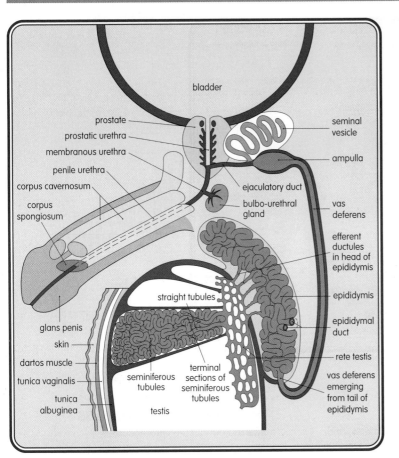

Fig. 10.16 Schematic representation of the male reproductive tract.

○ **Draw a diagram showing the cross-sectional structure of the penis. What are the physical factors involved in erection?**

○ **List the layers of the scrotum and their derivation from abdominal wall structures.**

○ **List the structures of the ejaculatory duct in order, with notes as to their function.**

TESTICULAR HORMONES AND SPERMATOGENESIS

Spermatogenesis and the microstructure of the testis

The testis consists of two compartments separated by a basement membrane (Fig. 10.17):

- The seminiferous tubules—these (about 250 million per testis) are the site of spermatogenesis.
- The interstitium—this contains androgen-secreting Leydig cells, blood vessels, lymphatics, and nerves.

Leydig cells and the interstitium

Leydig cells are dispersed throughout the testes in the interstitium between the seminiferous tubules. They synthesize the testicular steroid hormones under the influence of LH. Leydig cells also release small amounts of protein hormones such as oxytocin, endorphins, angiotensin, and prostaglandins, which may be involved in local regulation of testicular function.

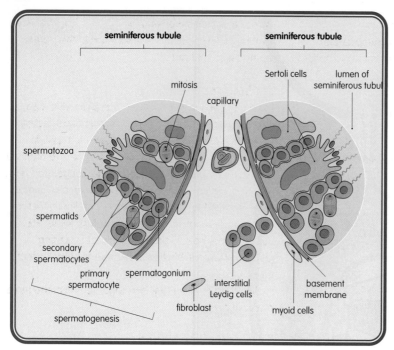

Fig. 10.17 Microstructure of the testis, showing seminiferous tubules and the interstitial cells.

The seminiferous tubules and spermatogenesis

These are approximately 170 μm in diameter, and comprise a basement membrane lined with Sertoli cells and germinal cells. Sertoli cells perform a variety of functions:

- They are linked to each other by tight junctions and form the blood–testis barrier. This prevents the passage of proteins and maintains the tubules as a site of immunological privilege, protecting spermatogenic cells from immune response.
- They extend cytoplasmic processes to surround and support developing germ cells.
- They phagocytose residual bodies (leftover cytoplasm from the formation of spermatozoa).
- They secrete androgen-binding globulin (ABG)—this has a high affinity for testosterone and maintains high tubular levels of this hormone for the benefit of the germ cells. ABG production is stimulated by FSH via the cAMP pathway.
- They synthesize other protein hormones, including inhibin, which suppresses FSH secretion by the pituitary.

The germ cells progress through a number of stages during spermatogenesis. There are two main functions which must be served:

- Production of haploid spermatozoa (23 chromosomes) by meiosis from diploid spermatogonia (46 chromosomes).
- Maintenance of the germ-cell pool by mitotic divisions of the precursor cells.

The sequence of spermatogenesis and the cell types involved are detailed as follows:

- Spermatogonia—these are the diploid stem cells that undergo mitotic division to maintain the germ-cell population. They lie on the basement membrane of the seminiferous tubules.
- Primary spermatocytes—these are diploid cells that undergo the first division of meiosis, to form …
- Secondary spermatocytes—these are haploid cells undergoing the second division of meiosis to form …
- Spermatids—these are haploid cells that undergo physical modification and cytoplasmic reduction (spermiogenesis) to produce residual bodies and …
- Spermatozoa (Fig. 10.18)—these are gametes that are released into the lumen of the seminiferous tubule. They do not become motile until after storage in the epididymis.

This whole process takes approximately 64 days and is dependent on testosterone secreted by Leydig cells in the interstitium.

Hormonal control of the testis

There are three testicular steroid hormones that are important in the function of the male reproductive system:

- Testosterone.
- Dihydrotestosterone.
- Oestradiol.

Synthesis and secretion

The sex steroids are synthesized predominantly in the Leydig cells of the testicular interstitium. The precursor

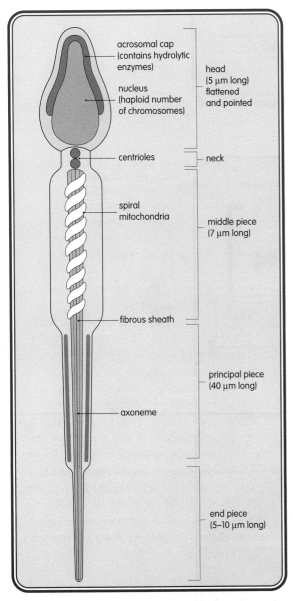

Fig. 10.18 Microstructure of a mature spermatozoon. Lengths not shown to scale.

molecule is cholesterol, and the biochemical pathway involved is described in the description of the steroid hormones (see Chapter 1).

Control of secretion

The hypothalamic–pituitary axis is explained in full in the earlier section regarding the female reproductive system. GnRH stimulates pituitary gonadotrophs to secrete LH and FSH. LH activates Leydig cells to produce testosterone via the cAMP second-messenger pathway. Feedback inhibition of GnRH by testosterone regulates this pathway. Prolactin (PRL) has an inhibitory effect on testosterone production if present at high levels. FSH acts on Sertoli cells to produce androgen-binding globulin (ABG). Inhibin has a negative feedback effect on FSH.

Fig. 10.19 illustrates the hormonal control of the male reproductive system.

Transport of the steroids

In the plasma, testosterone is mostly bound to SHBG and ABG (60%), and to albumin (38%). The free 2% is able to diffuse into cells and exert its effect.

Effects of testicular steroids

The testosterone receptor is intracellular and is found in the cytoplasm of the target cells. Once a molecule of testosterone or dihydrotestosterone has bound, the complex migrates to the nucleus and binds to specific sites on the DNA. The effects of the androgens are mediated via modification of DNA transcription.

The physiological effects of the androgens are outlined in Fig. 10.20.

- **What are the two compartments of the testis and the function of each?**
- **List the types of cell found in the seminiferous tubule and state their role in spermatogenesis.**
- **Describe the hormonal control of testicular function.**

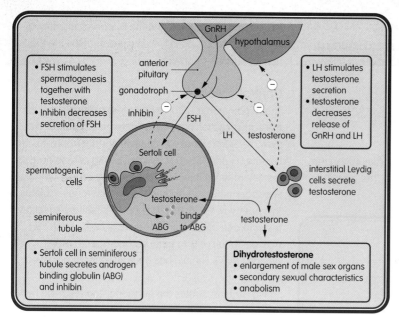

Fig. 10.19 Hormonal control of testicular function.

• FSH stimulates spermatogenesis together with testosterone
• Inhibin decreases secretion of FSH

GnRH

hypothalamus

anterior pituitary

gonadotroph

inhibin

FSH

LH

testosterone

• LH stimulates testosterone secretion
• testosterone decreases release of GnRH and LH

Sertoli cell

spermatogenic cells

seminiferous tubule

testosterone

binds to ABG

ABG

interstitial Leydig cells secrete testosterone

testosterone

• Sertoli cell in seminiferous tubule secretes androgen binding globulin (ABG) and inhibin

Dihydrotestosterone
• enlargement of male sex organs
• secondary sexual characteristics
• anabolism

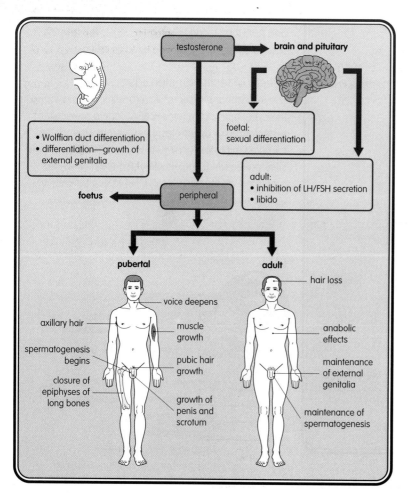

Fig. 10.20 Physiological effects of testicular androgens.

testosterone

brain and pituitary

• Wolffian duct differentiation
• differentiation—growth of external genitalia

foetal:
sexual differentiation

adult:
• inhibition of LH/FSH secretion
• libido

foetus

peripheral

pubertal

adult

voice deepens

hair loss

axillary hair

muscle growth

anabolic effects

spermatogenesis begins

pubic hair growth

maintenance of external genitalia

closure of epiphyses of long bones

growth of penis and scrotum

maintenance of spermatogenesis

COITUS

Coitus is the act of sexual intercourse. It results in the deposition of the male gametes (spermatozoa) in the female reproductive tract, at the level of the cervix. Genital and systemic changes (e.g. increased blood pressure) occur during sexual excitement.

The sexual response can be described by the 'EPOR' model (Fig. 11.1):

- Excitement phase—the process of increasing sexual arousal involves both psychological and tactile stimuli and causes penile erection, vasocongestion of the labia, secretion of cervical mucus, and transudation of fluid through the vaginal epithelium, which aids lubrication.
- Plateau phase—sexual arousal becomes intensified.
- Orgasmic phase—the climax of sexual excitement is accompanied by ejaculation in the male.
- Resolution phase—genital and systemic changes revert to normal and sexual arousal decreases. This phase is normally followed by a short absolute refractory period in the male during which rearousal is not possible.

○ **Failure of the excitatory response in the male may cause infertility.**
○ **Failure of the excitatory response in the female does not cause infertility but may cause superficial dyspareunia.**

FERTILIZATION

At ejaculation, semen containing approximately 60 million mature spermatozoa is deposited at the cervix. The semen coagulates in the vagina and this protects the spermatozoa against the hostile acidic environment of the vagina. Approximately 10% of the spermatozoa enter the uterus via the cervical os. In the oestrogen-primed uterus, capacitation occurs. This involves the removal of glycoproteins from the sperm head and the influx of calcium ions, causing the spermatozoa to become more motile (whiplash movements of the tail

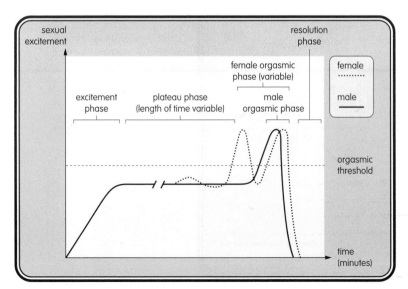

Fig. 11.1 EPOR model, showing the changes in the level of sexual excitement that occur during sexual intercourse.

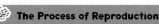

propel spermatozoa) and to be able to undergo the acrosomal reaction (see below).

The spermatozoa reach the fallopian tubes 2–7 hours after coitus. When they reach the ampulla of the fallopian tube they may encounter an oocyte (if ovulation occurs when the spermatozoa are present in the tubes). Chemical signals from the oocyte induce a further change in the spermatozoa, called the acrosomal reaction. This reaction allows the spermatozoa to:

- Bind to the zona pellucida of the oocyte, by making holes in the acrosomal membrane.
- Penetrate the oocyte, by increasing the strength of the whiplash movement of the tail.

The transport of a released oocyte and the process by which it is fertilized is shown in Fig. 11.2.

IMPLANTATION

Once the diploid fertilized egg (zygote) begins to divide,

it is called an embryo. It continues dividing as it is transported down the fallopian tube towards the uterine cavity. Fig. 11.3 shows the stages that the embryo goes through and the steps in the implantation of the blastocyst.

Pre-eclampsia is a pregnancy-specific disorder that causes intrauterine growth retardation and maternal hypertension, and predisposes to eclampsia. It is believed to be caused by an immunological disturbance that prevents the invasion of the trophoblast into maternal blood vessels.

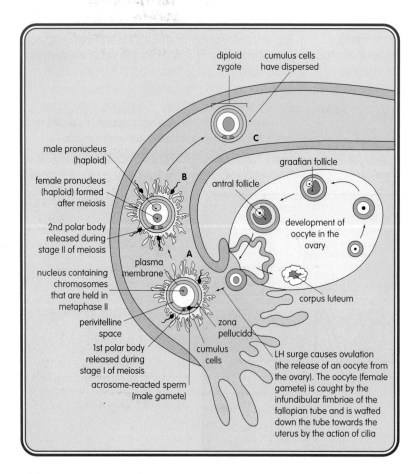

Fig. 11.2 Process of fertilization (fusion of the male and female gametes) in the fallopian tube.
(A) Spermatozoa release hyaluronidase which helps them to penetrate the zona pellucida (only one spermatozoon enters the perivitelline space).
(B) Fusion of the sperm to the oocyte plasma membrane causes calcium ions to flux across the oocyte. The calcium flux induces the release of cortical granules and the resumption of meiosis in the oocyte. Cortical granules lead to the release of a perivitelline space factor that prevents other sperm from entering. The fused sperm enters the oocyte without its tail.
(C) The pronuclei fuse to form a diploid egg, called a zygote, which starts to divide within a few hours.

diploid zygote | cumulus cells have dispersed

C

male pronucleus (haploid)

female pronucleus (haploid) formed after meiosis

2nd polar body released during stage II of meiosis

plasma membrane

nucleus containing chromosomes that are held in metaphase II

perivitelline space

1st polar body released during stage I of meiosis

acrosome-reacted sperm (male gamete)

B

antral follicle

A

zona pellucida

cumulus cells

graafian follicle

development of oocyte in the ovary

corpus luteum

LH surge causes ovulation (the release of an oocyte from the ovary). The oocyte (female gamete) is caught by the infundibular fimbriae of the fallopian tube and is wafted down the tube towards the uterus by the action of cilia

Implantation is affected by levels of oestrogen and progesterone. Oestrogen levels are highest at ovulation—this induces endometrial proliferation and promotes the transport of the embryo to the uterus. Postovulation, levels of progesterone (secreted by the corpus luteum) increase, which induces secretory (decidual) changes in the endometrium—this enables the blastocyst to be successfully implanted. The emergency pill contains high levels of oestrogen and inhibits implantation (rapid transport of the embryo means that it reaches the uterus before the secretory phase of the endometrium).

CONTRACEPTION

The aim of contraception is to prevent unplanned pregnancies. Every contraceptive method is evaluated according to its:

- Effectiveness—no method is 100% effective owing to inherent deficiencies in the method and to user failure. If motivation is low, methods that are instigated away from the act of coitus may be more successful.
- Acceptability—the individual's preference of contraceptive method depends on lifestyle, relationship, age, and religion.

- Safety—the risks and benefits of each method should be considered for each patient, e.g. a female aged over 35 years who smokes should not be recommended the combined oral contraceptive pill.
- Reversibility—most methods are rapidly reversible, others may take some time to reverse (e.g. depot injection), while sterilization is irreversible.

The emergency pill and the intrauterine contraceptive device (IUCD) act to prevent implantation of the fertilized ovum, i.e. they act after conception has occurred, but are considered as methods of contraception. Both can be used as postcoital contraception. Therapeutic abortion is the termination of a pregnancy (once it has been established) and should not be regarded as a method of contraception.

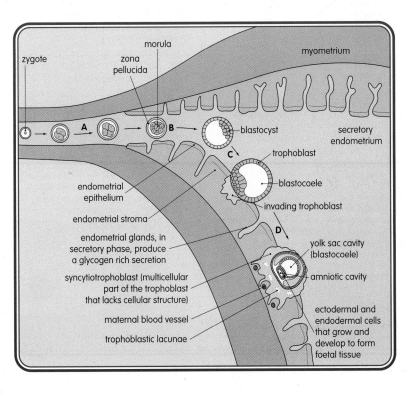

Fig. 11.3 Growth and development of the embryo after fertilization and the process of implantation.
(A) Embryo is transported along the fallopian tube by ciliary action.
(B) Morula (intermediate embryological stage between the zygote and the blastocyst) reaches the uterine cavity approximately 3 days after fertilization.
(C) Trophoblast (cells that form the wall of the blastocyst) attaches to the secretory endometrium and begins to invade (approximately 8 days after fertilization).
(D) Trophoblast grows rapidly into the endometrium. The syncytiotrophoblast erodes the endometrium and engulfs endometrial blood vessels—these blood vessels communicate with the trophoblastic lacunae. The lacunae become the future maternal blood spaces of the placenta.

Methods of contraception

Hormonal contraception

The principal action of hormonal methods of contraception is to suppress ovulation. They also assist contraception by:

- Suppressing the migration of sperm through the cervix, by inhibiting the changes in cervical mucus that normally occur around the time of ovulation.
- Increasing the activity of the smooth muscle in the fallopian tubes and uterus, so that the ovum is

transported to the endometrium before the secretory phase and therefore it cannot implant.

- Inhibiting the implantation of a fertilized ovum, by preventing the proliferation of the endometrium that normally occurs around the time of ovulation.

All hormonal contraceptives contain synthetic progestogens, e.g. norethisterone (Fig. 11.4). The combined oral contraceptive pill (COCP) and the emergency pill also contain synthetic oestrogens, e.g. ethinyloestradiol. The increased risk of

Types of hormonal contraceptive					
	Combined oral contraceptive pill (COCP)	Progestogen-only pill (POP)	Emergency pill	Depot (contraceptive injection)	Implants
Composition	synthetic oestrogens and progestogens	synthetic progestogens	high dose of synthetic oestrogens and progestogens	synthetic progestogens (medroxy-progesterone)	synthetic progestogens
Administration	oral, daily for 21 days with a 7-day gap before the next course of pills (during the 7 day gap a withdrawal bleed occurs)	oral, daily without a break between packs, and must be taken at the same time every day	oral, must be taken within 72 h of coitus if no other contraception was used	intramuscular injection, lasts 8–12 weeks	small soft tubes inserted under the skin, lasts up to 5 years
Mode of action	principal action = suppression of ovulation	does not reliably suppress ovulation	inhibits implantation	does not reliably suppress ovulation	prevents ovulation
Effectiveness if taken/applied according to instructions	>99%	99% (less effective in young women and if >70 kg)	>95%	>99%	>99%
Advantages	often decreases menstrual bleeding, pain, premenstrual tension, and acne, and may protect against ovarian cancer	useful for women who cannot use the COCP (because POP contains no oestrogen)	postcoital contraceptive	do not have to remember to take pills, may protect against endometrial cancer	same as for depot
Disadvantages	increased risk of thromboembolic disease (e.g. deep vein thrombosis, pulmonary embolism, cerebral thrombosis), dyslipidaemia, hypertension	side effects include: irregular uterine bleeding ('breakthrough bleeding' or amenorrhoea), breast discomfort, premenstrual tension, skin reactions, increased risk of ectopic pregnancy	same as for COCP, although risk is increased owing to high dose of oestrogen, often cause nausea and vomiting	side effects are same as for POP, plus: weight gain, loss of bone density	same as for depot, plus: often difficult to remove owing to fibrosis
Comments	not reliable if taken >12 h late, or after vomiting/diarrhoea	not reliable if taken >3 h late, or after vomiting/diarrhoea	should not be used as a regular form of contraception	not immediately reversible	

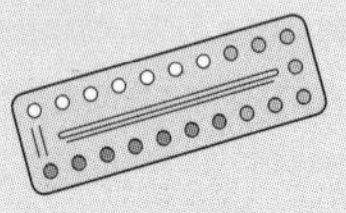

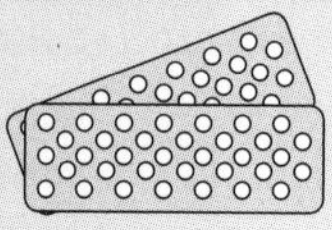

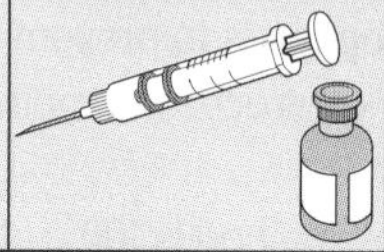

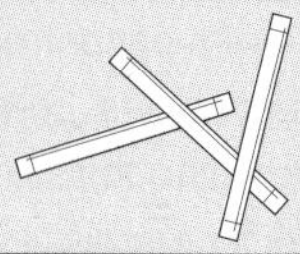

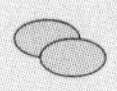

Fig.11.4 Types of hormonal contraceptive.

thromboembolism, dyslipidaemia, and hypertension associated with the COCP and emergency pill are related to their oestrogen component. Lower-dose oestrogen pills carry a smaller risk, equivalent to one-tenth of that associated with pregnancy. However, because of these risks, the COCP is not suitable for smokers who are over 35 years old or for women who are breastfeeding, diabetic, obese, hypertensive, or prone to thromboembolic disease.

Non-hormonal contraception

Barrier methods include the male condom and the diaphragm (Fig. 11.5). Female condoms, although available, have not proved to be a popular method, and the diaphragm remains the most commonly used and safest female barrier method. Spermicidal creams must be used with barrier methods. Spermicides alone are not recommended.

Copper-containing intrauterine contraceptive devices (IUCDs) act by causing a mild inflammatory reaction in the uterus. Progestogen-containing IUCDs release hormone locally so that systemic effects of progestogens are reduced.

The natural (symptothermal) method requires monitoring of:
- Changes in body temperature (rises 0.2–0.4°C at ovulation).
- Changes in cervical mucus.
- Calendar recordings: cycle length is recorded for at least six months to estimate the timing of ovulation—e.g. in a 28-day cycle the high-risk time is days 10–17 of the cycle—but the information obtained must be used in combination with mucus and temperature changes.

NB Coitus interruptus is not an effective method

	Male condom	Diaphragm or cap with spermicide	Intrauterine contraceptive device (IUCD)	Natural (symptothermal) method
Description	rubber sheath, lubricated with spermicidal cream	flexible rubber device used with spermicide	small plastic or copper device (some contain progestogen)	avoid ovulation—unprotected sexual intercourse confined to the 'safe' infertile times of the menstrual cycle
Administration	put over the erect penis during intercourse	device is inserted into the vagina before intercourse and covers the cervix; it must stay in for at least 6 h after sex	inserted into the uterus and can stay there for 5 years	the fertile and infertile times of the menstrual cycle are identified by measuring monthly changes in body temperature and cervical mucus
Mode of action	prevents sperm from entering vagina	prevents sperm from entering uterus	inhibits sperm migration and prevents implantation	prevents sperm from encountering ovum
Effectiveness if taken/ applied according to instructions	98%	92–94% depending on the type of device used	98–99% depending on the type of device used	98% (although much lower if the menstrual cycle is irregular)
Advantages	may protect both partners from sexually transmitted diseases, and may protect female against cervical cancer	female is in control of contraception (important if male is not motivated); reusable	immediately effective, requires little follow-up; hormone-containing IUCD cause lighter periods	no side effects
Disadvantages	requires high motivation and may interrupt spontaneity and sensitivity	less protection against sexually transmitted disease	may cause heavy, prolonged, painful periods and predispose to pelvic inflammatory disease	need to use alternative method during fertile days; requires close attention to symptoms of cycle

Types of non-hormonal contraceptive

Fig. 11.5 Types of non-hormonal contraceptive.

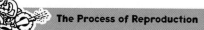
because pre-ejaculatory secretions also contain spermatozoa.

Sterilization

Sterilization is an irreversible, highly effective (>99%) method of contraception. It should not be chosen if there is any doubt that future fertility is not required; hence, counselling is important. The male or female partner can be sterilized.

Male sterilization (bilateral vasectomy) may be performed under local anaesthesia. The vas deferens are cut and tied off to prevent the transport of sperm into the ejaculatory fluid. The ejaculate is not spermfree for 3–4 months and alternative contraception is required until examination of the semen shows it to be spermnegative.

Female sterilization is usually performed by laparoscopy but requires general anaesthesia. The fallopian tubes are occluded with clips to prevent the oocytes from encountering sperm or reaching the uterus.

- ○ Describe the phases of sexual excitement according to the 'EPOR' model.
- ○ Outline the changes that must occur to the spermatozoa before they can successfully fertilize an oocyte.
- ○ Draw diagrams to show the process of fertilization and implantation.
- ○ List the different methods of contraception.

THERAPEUTIC ABORTION

Both surgical and medical methods are used. Up to 8 weeks, abortion can be induced using a combination of oral Mifepristone (an antiprogesterone drug) and a prostaglandin vaginal pessary. Surgical termination is relatively safe and simple up to week 12 of gestation and is legal up to week 24.

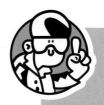

The maternal and foetal circulations do not mix. Foetal blood in the capillary networks of the chorionic villi flows in proximity to the maternal blood in the intervillous space. The proximity allows efficient exchange of gases, nutrients, and metabolites to occur.

THE PLACENTA

Structure of the placenta

Fig. 11.6 shows the structure of the placenta and describes the maternal and foetal blood circulations. There is a high rate of maternal blood flow through the placenta—500 mL/min.

Functions of the placenta

The placenta does not merely nurture the foetus but also has the following functions:

- Synthesis of hormones involved in the maintenance of pregnancy and the preparation of the breasts for lactation (see Reproductive hormones in pregnancy). Hormones are produced by the trophoblast of the placenta.
- Respiratory-gas exchange (oxygen and carbon dioxide passively diffuse across the placenta).
- Nutrient transfer and waste-product excretion (cross the placenta by facilitated diffusion).
- Heat transfer.
- Protection of the foetus from rejection by the maternal immune system (unproven). Maternal immune cells and immunoglobulin M (IgM) cannot cross the placenta, although IgG can cross via pinocytosis.

REPRODUCTIVE HORMONES IN PREGNANCY

During pregnancy, the corpus luteum in the ovary is maintained (it normally regresses 10 days after ovulation if conception does not occur). It develops from the collapsed

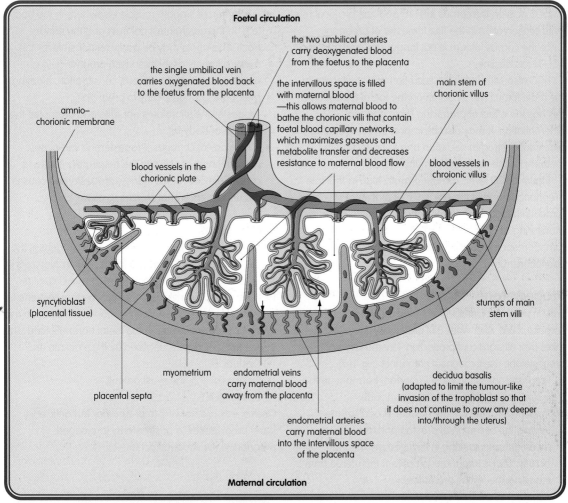

Foetal circulation

the two umbilical arteries
carry deoxygenated blood
from the foetus to the placenta

the single umbilical vein
carries oxygenated blood back
to the foetus from the placenta

the intervillous space is filled
with maternal blood
—this allows maternal blood to
bathe the chorionic villi that contain
foetal blood capillary networks,
which maximizes gaseous and
metabolite transfer and decreases
resistance to maternal blood flow

main stem of
chorionic villus

amnio–
chorionic membrane

blood vessels in the
chorionic plate

blood vessels in
chroionic villus

syncytioblast
(placental tissue)

stumps of main
stem villi

myometrium

endometrial veins
carry maternal blood
away from the placenta

decidua basalis
(adapted to limit the tumour-like
invasion of the trophoblast so that
it does not continue to grow any deeper
into/through the uterus)

placental septa

endometrial arteries
carry maternal blood
into the intervillous space
of the placenta

Maternal circulation

Fig. 11.6 Schematic representation of the structure of the placenta. (Adapted from *The Developing Human, Clinically Oriented Embryology, 5e,* by KL Moore and TVN Persaud. Courtesy of WB Saunders.)

postovulatory follicle and is composed of theca lutein and granulosa lutein cells. It has an important endocrine function during pregnancy. Hormones secreted by the corpus luteum are crucial for the maintenance of pregnancy in the first 7–8 weeks, after which time the placental hormones take over this function. The main hormones secreted by the corpus luteum are:

- Progesterone.
- Inhibin.
- Relaxin.

The placenta has an important endocrine function. It secretes numerous steroid and peptide hormones that act locally (i.e. within the placenta) or systemically (e.g. on other endocrine organs). The main placental hormones are:

- Human chorionic gonadotrophin (hCG).

- Progesterone.
- Oestrogens (mainly oestradiol and oestriol).
- Human placental lactogen (hPL).
- Relaxin.

Placental hormones are essential to maintain pregnancy and to bring about the maternal adaptations that are necessary during pregnancy (see Maternal adaptations to pregnancy).

hCG

hCG is a peptide hormone that is structurally and functionally similar to luteinizing hormone (LH). The developing trophoblast begins to secrete hCG following implantation, and plasma hCG levels rise progressively, peaking at week 10 of pregnancy (Fig. 11.7).

hCG acts on the corpus luteum and has a critical role in its conservation in the first trimester of pregnancy. Once the corpus luteum is not longer required, plasma hCG levels decline.

hCG also stimulates the secretion of testosterone in the male foetus (via its action on the foetal testes) and this has the effect of producing male gonadal differentiation. It may also be important in regulating placental oestrogen secretion and in protecting the foetus from the maternal immune system.

Plasma hCG levels are abnormally high in multiple pregnancies and in the presence of placental tissue tumours (hydatidiform moles and choriocarcinomas). Monitoring of hCG levels can be used to assess the tumour response to chemotherapy in the treatment of choriocarcinoma.

Progesterone

Early in pregnancy, progesterone is mainly produced by the corpus luteum. After week 8 of pregnancy, the placenta takes over all significant production. Plasma levels of progesterone rise throughout pregnancy (Fig. 11.7).

Progesterone is the most important hormone in the maintenance of pregnancy. Effects include:

- Relaxation of the uterine muscle. Progesterone inhibits the secretion of prostaglandins in the myometrium, resulting in reduced myometrial activity. This is important to prevent the uterus from expelling the foetus prematurely.

- Relaxation of smooth muscle elsewhere in the body (e.g. in the gastrointestinal tract and the urinary tract). This effect may be partly responsible for the minor ailments associated with pregnancy (e.g. nausea, vomiting, heartburn, constipation, bloating).
- Metabolic changes. Early in pregnancy, progesterone stimulates appetite and promotes the storage of body fat.
- Physiological changes. Progesterone stimulates respiration by sensitizing the respiratory centre to carbon dioxide. In the kidney, progesterone causes the ureters and renal calyces to dilate.

Oestrogens

During pregnancy, the main source of oestrogens is the placenta. Cholesterol, required for oestrogen synthesis in the placenta, is provided from the maternal circulation. However, the placenta lacks the enzyme that converts pregnenolone into DHEA (see Fig. 1.6) and this step in the synthetic pathway occurs in the foetal adrenal gland. The three main oestrogens secreted by the placenta are:
- Oestriol (E3).
- Oestradiol (E2), the most potent.
- Oestrone (E1).

Oestrogens are not vital to pregnancy but deficiency (rare) predisposes to postmaturity (prolonged pregnancy). Oestrogens act to:

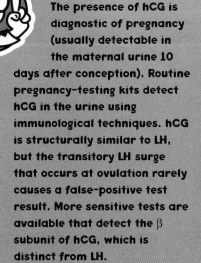

The presence of hCG is diagnostic of pregnancy (usually detectable in the maternal urine 10 days after conception). Routine pregnancy-testing kits detect hCG in the urine using immunological techniques. hCG is structurally similar to LH, but the transitory LH surge that occurs at ovulation rarely causes a false-positive test result. More sensitive tests are available that detect the β subunit of hCG, which is distinct from LH.

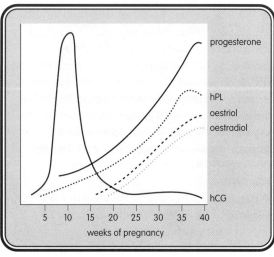

Fig. 11.7 Plasma levels of the reproductive hormones during normal pregnancy. (Hormones return to non-pregnant levels by day 3 of post-delivery.) (Adapted from Fundamentals of Obstetrics and Gynaecology, 6e by Dr Llewellyn-Jones, Mosby, 1994.)

- Increase the blood flow to the uterus and stimulate the growth of the myometrium.
- Soften the cervix and relax the pelvic ligaments (by loosening the collagen fibres in connective tissue).
- Stimulate breast growth and development directly and indirectly (oestrogens stimulate prolactin secretion).
- Enhance water retention.
- Stimulate the production of oxytocin receptors in the myometrium in late pregnancy (oxytocin is involved in parturition).

hPL

hPL is a peptide hormone secreted by the placenta. Plasma hPL levels rise from week 5 of pregnancy until term (Fig. 11.7).

hPL has a diabetogenic effect that is similar to that of growth hormone (GH). This is important to ensure that the placenta (and the foetus) has an adequate supply of glucose, fatty acids, and amino acids. It causes the following metabolic changes:

- Enhancement of lipolysis in maternal adipose tissue. This is important in pregnancy as it reduces utilization of maternal glucose (free fatty acids released by lipolysis provide an alternative substrate for energy production), so glucose is spared and more is available for foetal energy requirements.
- Enhancement of amino acid transfer across the placenta.
- Inhibition of maternal GH secretion.

hPL also has prolactin-like effects in that it stimulates the growth and development of the breasts.

Inhibin

Inhibin is a peptide hormone secreted by the ovary in the pregnant and non-pregnant state. It may have a role in pregnancy to suppress FSH secretion by the pituitary gland and to stimulate progesterone production.

Relaxin

Relaxin is a peptide hormone secreted by the corpus luteum and—late in pregnancy—by the placenta. It relaxes the myometrium (important to allow the uterus to enlarge) and relaxes the pelvic ligaments (important to allow the foetus to pass through at birth). It acts by stimulating enzymes in connective tissue (e.g. ligaments) which dissolve collagen. It may also have an effect on cervical dilatation during parturition.

Prolactin

Prolactin secretion rises throughout pregnancy and at term plasma levels are 20 times the non-pregnant level. The placental oestrogens stimulate the anterior pituitary gland to synthesise and secrete prolactin. During pregnancy, prolactin stimulates the growth and development of the breasts and helps regulate fat metabolism. The most important effect of prolactin is to promote postpartum lactation. Lactation is suppressed during pregnancy by the high oestrogen levels.

- Describe the maternal and foetal blood circulations within the placenta.
- List the functions of the placenta.
- Discuss the placental and ovarian hormones that are secreted during pregnancy.
- How is pregnancy diagnosed?

MATERNAL ADAPTATIONS TO PREGNANCY

Physiological and structural changes occur in pregnancy to nurture the foetus and to prepare for parturition and lactation. Most body systems undergo adaptations during pregnancy (Fig. 11.8):

- Cardiovascular system—modifications ensure that the transport of gases and nutrients to the foetus is sufficient.
- Respiratory system—adaptations maintain an adequate supply of oxygen to the foetus and the rapid removal of carbon dioxide.
- Metabolism—adaptations ensure that the foetus has sufficient amounts of glucose, amino acids, and fatty acids required for growth and development.
- Endocrine system—changes in hormone levels maintain maternal homoeostasis and adjust the effects caused by the placental and ovarian hormones.

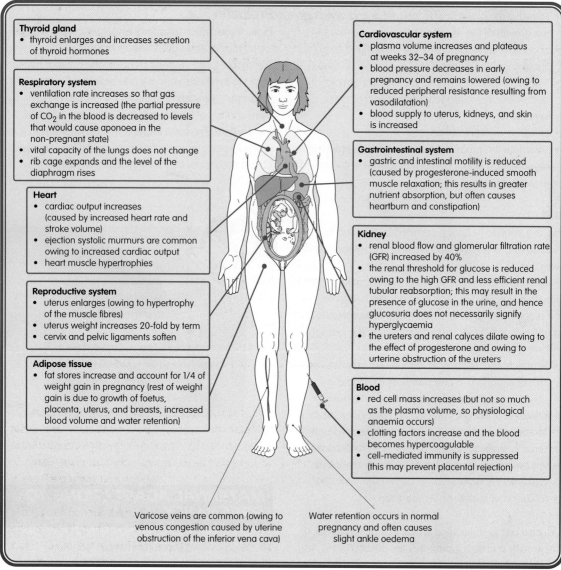

Thyroid gland
- thyroid enlarges and increases secretion of thyroid hormones

Respiratory system
- ventilation rate increases so that gas exchange is increased (the partial pressure of CO_2 in the blood is decreased to levels that would cause aponoea in the non-pregnant state)
- vital capacity of the lungs does not change
- rib cage expands and the level of the diaphragm rises

Heart
- cardiac output increases (caused by increased heart rate and stroke volume)
- ejection systolic murmurs are common owing to increased cardiac output
- heart muscle hypertrophies

Reproductive system
- uterus enlarges (owing to hypertrophy of the muscle fibres)
- uterus weight increases 20-fold by term
- cervix and pelvic ligaments soften

Adipose tissue
- fat stores increase and account for 1/4 of weight gain in pregnancy (rest of weight gain is due to growth of foetus, placenta, uterus, and breasts, increased blood volume and water retention)

Cardiovascular system
- plasma volume increases and plateaus at weeks 32–34 of pregnancy
- blood pressure decreases in early pregnancy and remains lowered (owing to reduced peripheral resistance resulting from vasodilatation)
- blood supply to uterus, kidneys, and skin is increased

Gastrointestinal system
- gastric and intestinal motility is reduced (caused by progesterone-induced smooth muscle relaxation; this results in greater nutrient absorption, but often causes heartburn and constipation)

Kidney
- renal blood flow and glomerular filtration rate (GFR) increased by 40%
- the renal threshold for glucose is reduced owing to the high GFR and less efficient renal tubular reabsorption; this may result in the presence of glucose in the urine, and hence glucosuria does not necessarily signify hyperglycaemia
- the ureters and renal calyces dilate owing to the effect of progesterone and owing to uterine obstruction of the ureters

Blood
- red cell mass increases (but not so much as the plasma volume, so physiological anaemia occurs)
- clotting factors increase and the blood becomes hypercoagulable
- cell-mediated immunity is suppressed (this may prevent placental rejection)

Varicose veins are common (owing to venous congestion caused by uterine obstruction of the inferior vena cava)

Water retention occurs in normal pregnancy and often causes slight ankle oedema

Fig. 11.8 Major maternal changes that occur during pregnancy.

- Gastrointestinal system—changes increase nutrient absorption.
- Renal system—adaptations increase the excretion of the waste products produced by maternal and foetal metabolism.
- Immune system—suppression may help prevent maternal rejection of the placenta.
- Reproductive system—enlarges and becomes prepared for parturition.

Multiple pregnancies cause more marked physiological changes as the demands on the mother are greater.

Changes in the endocrine system during pregnancy

Endocrine function is altered in pregnancy because of the trophic hormones secreted by the placenta. The placental hormones:
- Alter the secretion of the pituitary hormones (Fig. 11.9).
- Stimulate the synthesis of plasma binding proteins that bind to circulating hormones.

Oestrogens stimulate the synthesis of plasma binding proteins including thyroxine-binding globulin (TBG) and

Changes that occur in pituitary hormone secretion during pregnancy, and the effects caused by these changes		
Secretion of anterior pituitary hormone	Hormone secretion in pregnancy (compared with non-pregnancy)	Effect of altered plasma hormone level in pregnancy
prolactin ↑↑↑	enhanced by placental oestrogens	promotes growth and development of the breasts and regulates fat metabolism
FSH ↓ and LH ↓	FSH secretion is suppressed by inhibin and placental oestrogens LH secretion is suppressed by the combined effect of progesterone and oestrogen	prevents further follicular development and ovulation during pregnancy
GH ↓	suppressed by hPL	unknown (hPL has similar effect to GH)
ACTH ↑	enhanced indirectly by the reduction in free cortisol levels in the blood	stimulates increased cortisol secretion from the adrenal cortex
TSH	no change	although TSH levels do not change in pregnancy, thyroid gland function is altered (thyroid hormone secretion increases)

Fig. 11.9 Changes that occur in pituitary hormone secretion during pregnancy, and the effects caused by these changes. (ACTH, adrenocorticotrophic hormone.)

corticosteroid-binding globulin (CBG). The increase in these plasma proteins means that a greater proportion of the circulating thyroid and corticosteroid hormones are bound. In consequence, secretion of thyroid hormone and cortisol is grossly elevated to maintain the free hormone levels. Free tri-iodothyronine (T_3) and thyroxine (T_4) levels are normal, but free cortisol levels are mildly elevated compared with the nonpregnant state. The increased free cortisol may account for the development of abdominal striae (stretch marks), glycosuria, and hypertension that can occur in pregnancy.

Aldosterone synthesis and secretion rise slowly throughout pregnancy to reduce the sodium loss caused by progesterone.

Changes in metabolism during pregnancy

Early in pregnancy, progesterone stimulates appetite and promotes the storage of body fat. As pregnancy continues, hPL levels rise and promote the breakdown of these stores (lipolysis). Lipolysis provides fatty acids that are utilized by the mother for energy. Fatty acids are important as an energy source because during pregnancy the maternal tissues become progressively insulin resistant. Increasing levels of hPL and, to a lesser

extent, cortisol, may cause this diabetogenic effect. Insulin resistance means that the maternal tissues take up less glucose and so there is more glucose available for placental transfer to the foetus. Insulin resistance is usually mild but can cause impaired glucose tolerance or gestational diabetes in some women.

Amino acid metabolism is altered in pregnancy in order to supply the foetus. The availability of amino acids is increased owing to the inhibition of their breakdown in the liver. This effect is due to progesterone.

- Outline the physiological and metabolic changes that occur in the mother in response to pregnancy.
- Give examples of how the placental hormones affect the maternal endocrine system.

PARTURITION

Parturition (labour) is the process by which the foetus, the placenta, and the membranes are expelled from the uterus by coordinated myometrial contractions. Labour at full term normally occurs between weeks 37 and 42 of gestation. Premature labour occurs before week 37, and postmaturity occurs after week 42.

Events of parturition

The onset of labour is recognized by the presence of regular, painful uterine contractions and progressive cervical ripening (cervix softens, shortens, and dilates to allow the foetus through). Labour is divided into three stages.

First stage of labour

This is the time from the onset of labour until full cervical dilatation. Uterine contractions increase in strength and become progressively more frequent. As the uterine muscle contracts it also retracts (the muscle does not relax to its original length, but stays at a shortened length). This helps to expel the foetus and allows the uterus to contract down after birth to prevent postpartum haemorrhage. The foetal head gradually descends into the pelvis. This stage lasts 8–10 hours in first labour (nulliparous women/ 'primips') and 2–6 hours in subsequent labours (multiparous women/'multips').

Second stage of labour

This is the time from full cervical dilatation until the birth of the foetus. It usually lasts 40–60 minutes in primips and 10–15 minutes in multips.

Third stage of labour

This is the time from the birth of the foetus until the delivery of the placenta and membranes. The uterus continues to contract and retract, to dehisce and expel the placenta, and then the contractions slowly subside. This final stage is usually accelerated by the injection of an oxytocic agent or ergometrine.

Factors involved in the initiation of parturition

Prostaglandins and oxytocin are believed to be important in the stimulation of uterine contractions, but the factors that actually trigger the onset of labour are not fully understood. A number of contributory factors are involved, including:

- Foetal adrenal activity. The increase in foetal adrenal gland activity is probably due to the maturation of the foetal hypothalamus and the decreasing efficiency of the placenta (insufficient gas and metabolite exchange stimulates the stress response in the foetus). Foetal cortisol is secreted and stimulates oestrogen and prostaglandin release from the placenta and myometrium, respectively. However, abnormal cortisol secretion or exogenous hydrocortisones do not alter the onset of labour.
- Foetal hypothalamus maturation. As well as stimulating the foetal adrenal gland, the mature hypothalamus has been found to secrete oxytocin at term. Foetal oxytocin may act on the myometrium via the placenta.
- Uterine distension. Distension of the uterus, caused by foetal growth, stimulates the synthesis of oxytocin receptors in the myometrium. During labour, the stretching of the cervix and vaginal stimulation stimulate oxytocin synthesis in the hypothalamus (see Fig. 11.10). However, denervation of the uterus does not stop the normal onset of labour.

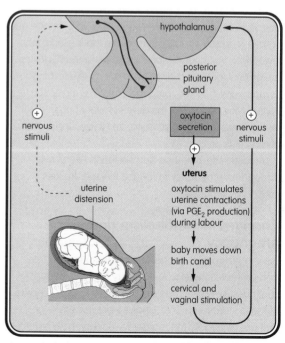

Fig. 11.10 Control of oxytocin secretion during labour and its actions on the uterus.

- Local alterations in the oestrogen:progesterone ratio. The increase in the oestrogen:progesterone ratio is important in the stimulation of prostaglandins from the myometrium. Oestrogens also stimulate the production of oxytocin receptors in the myometrium prior to labour.
- Circadian rhythm. There are probably a number of factors involved in the initiation of parturition. Labour may only commence when a number of factors/hormones are at optimal levels. Labours that are not actively managed in hospital have been found to show circadian rhythmicity. The secretion of many hormones follows circadian rhythms and so it is believed that labour may be triggered by hormones.

Hormonal control of parturition
Oxytocin and prostaglandins
Oxytocin stimulates uterine contractions during labour. It is a peptide hormone synthesized in the hypothalamus and secreted by the posterior pituitary gland.

Non-pregnant concentrations of oxytocin are normally very low, but levels are elevated during parturition and lactation. Oxytocin secretion is increased during labour owing to a positive feedback mechanism (the Ferguson reflex) shown in Fig. 11.10—oxytocin secretion is stimulated by uterine distension and vaginal stimulation; oxytocin causes the uterus to contract, which in turn stimulates more oxytocin release (as it causes the foetus to descend and stimulate the vagina).

The numbers of oxytocin receptors in the myometrium are increased in late pregnancy. The binding of oxytocin to these receptors stimulates prostaglandin production (especially PGE_2) in the myometrium.

Prostaglandins (unsaturated long-chain fatty acids) are cytokines that have innumerable actions in the body. In labour they are synthesized mainly in the myometrium, but also in the cervix and placenta. PGE_2 stimulates the release of calcium ions in the myometrial cells, which binds to actin and myosin and brings about muscle contraction. PGE_2 also stimulates cervical ripening.

Prostaglandins are important in the initiation of labour. Labour can be induced at term using vaginal pessaries containing PGE_2 that ripen the cervix and subsequently stimulate myometrial contractions. Oxytocin is not important in the initiation of labour. The onset of regular uterine contractions precedes the rise in plasma oxytocin, and high oxytocin levels are reached only at the end of labour. Oxytocin is believed to augment the strength of the uterine contractions. Oxytocic agents are used in the active management of labour to stimulate contractions in order to speed up delivery once it has commenced (oxytocic agents do not induce labour).

Relaxin
Relaxin promotes the relaxation of the pelvic ligaments prior to parturition and may soften the cervix. It is important to prepare the pelvis for parturition. The pelvic ligaments must stretch to allow the foetus to pass down through the pelvis.

- Outline the stages of labour.
- List the factors that contribute to the initiation of parturition.
- How are oxytocin, prostaglandins, and relaxin involved in parturition?

LACTATION

Structure of the female breast
Macrostructure of the breast
The mammary glands are specialized accessory glands of the skin, situated on the front of the thorax. In the male and prepubertal female, the breasts are rudimentary organs. In the adult female, they develop into soft hemispherical structures.

The base of each breast extends from the side of the sternum to the midaxillary line, and from the second to the sixth rib (Fig. 11.11). The majority of the breast tissue lies in the superficial fascia (the axillary tail pierces the deep fascia). The nipple is situated on the apex of the breast and is surrounded by the pigmented areola.

Blood supply is mainly from the internal thoracic and intercostal arteries. The axillary tail is supplied by the lateral thoracic artery (a branch of the axillary artery).

Lymphatic drainage is to an anastomosing network that links both breasts in the midline. From here the lymph drains laterally to the pectoral nodes in the axilla, superiorly to the infraclavicular and cervical nodes, inferiorly to the diaphragmatic nodes, and medially to the parasternal nodes. These details are important to know because malignant breast tumours are common and lymphatic spread of malignant cells means that the lymph nodes frequently become involved.

Microstructure of the breast

The mammary glands consist of glandular tissue and a variable amount of fat. The gland is divided into 15–20 lobes by the superficial fascia in which it lies. Each lobe contains lobules consisting of clusters of acini whose ducts join up to form a lactiferous duct that terminates at the nipple. The nipple and areola contain some smooth muscle and modified sebaceous glands (Montgomery glands that lubricate the nipple during suckling). The acini synthesize and secrete milk during lactation. They are surrounded by contractile myoepithelial cells that contribute to the ejection of milk.

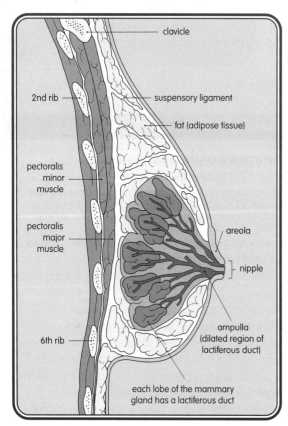

Fig. 11.11 Location and structure of the mature female breast.

Development of the mammary glands

In the embryo, mammary glands develop from modified skin glands. At birth, the breasts are the same in the male and female, containing very few acini. Further development does not occur until puberty in the female. Oestrogens stimulate the lactiferous glands to branch, and lobules containing abundant acini develop. The breasts increase in size owing to fat deposition and connective-tissue growth.

Cyclic breast changes occur in the non-pregnant woman owing to the fluctuations of oestrogens and progesterone. Premenstrually, the breasts become swollen and tender.

During pregnancy the breasts enlarge owing to fat deposition around the acini, ductal proliferation, and acinous development.

Endocrine control of lactation

During pregnancy the main hormones that stimulate breast growth and development are oestrogens, progesterone, prolactin, and hPL. Cortisol, insulin, and GH are also necessary for optimal breast development in pregnancy.

The secretion of milk during pregnancy is inhibited by the high levels of circulating oestrogens, but late in pregnancy colostrum is secreted (possibly stimulated by hPL). After birth, oestrogen levels fall and lactation is stimulated by prolactin and oxytocin. By days 2–3 postpartum, colostrum is replaced by milk. The breasts become swollen and engorged with milk and are tender.

Prolactin

Prolactin stimulates milk production.

Secretion of prolactin—a peptide hormone synthesized by lactotrophic cells in the anterior pituitary gland—increases during pregnancy and lactation. Circulating levels of prolactin are very high during pregnancy, stimulating breast growth and development. After birth the decline in oestrogens allows prolactin to *initiate* the production of milk in acinous cells. Suckling stimulates further prolactin secretion, resulting in more milk production; hence the production of milk is maintained by frequent suckling via a positive feedback loop mechanism (Fig. 11.12).

Once lactation has been initiated, it can continue for months. Basal levels of prolactin decrease but continue to be raised in response to suckling. If breastfeeding is stopped (e.g. at weaning or owing to painful breasts), nipple stimulation diminishes, hence prolactin secretion is reduced and milk production ceases.

The high basal levels of prolactin that occur in lactating women inhibit LH and FSH secretion from the pituitary gland. This means that breastfeeding suppresses ovarian function, i.e. it has a contraceptive effect. However, if suckling is infrequent, the basal levels of prolactin fall and conception is possible. Non-lactating women return to their normal ovarian cycles within 4–5 weeks after birth.

Oxytocin

Oxytocin induces the myoepithelial cells surrounding the acini to contract, resulting in the ejection of milk. Suckling stimulates oxytocin secretion from the posterior pituitary gland; oxytocin stimulates milk ejection required during suckling; hence a positive feedback loop is generated which ensures adequate milk ejection (Fig. 11.12). Oxytocin also elicits maternal behaviour via its action on the brain.

Composition of colostrum and milk

Colostrum is secreted during late pregnancy and early puerperium, until it is replaced by milk. It is a thick yellow fluid that has a high protein, low fat content. It is thought to be important in the protection of the neonate against infection because it is rich in immune antibodies (maternal IgG).

Milk is composed of lipids, milk proteins (casein and whey), lactose, vitamins, minerals, divalent cations, and IgG. The main energy source in the milk is fat. Milk produced by other mammalian females has the same basic composition but the relative quantities of each component differs. This means that human infants cannot be fed with milk from other mammals (e.g. cow's milk). Special formula milks are available to women who choose not to breastfeed.

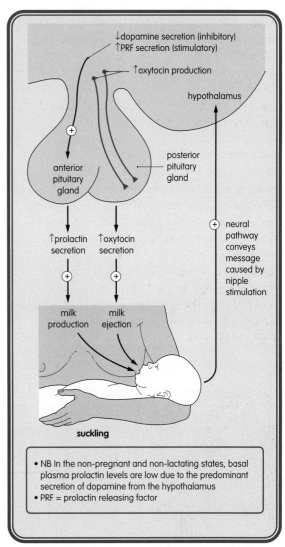

Fig. 11.12 Control of prolactin and oxytocin secretion during lactation and their actions on the breast. Prolactin and oxytocin secretion are both stimulated by suckling (the 'suckling reflex'). It is a positive feedback loop because prolactin and oxytocin increase milk delivery to the suckling infant, which in turn stimulates more prolactin and oxytocin release (as suckling causes nipple stimulation).

- ○ **Describe the anatomy, histology, and development of the breast.**
- ○ **Describe the neuroendocrine control of lactation.**
- ○ **List the components of colostrum and milk.**

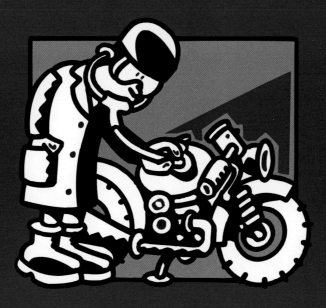

CLINICAL ASSESSMENT

12. Taking a History

INTRODUCTION

The history is the crucial stage in the investigation of a medical problem—it will either lead you directly to the correct diagnosis or suggest a number of differential diagnoses (which can be confirmed or eliminated by appropriate examination and specific investigations).

Patients usually complain of a limited number of symptoms, hence it is important to take a complete history in order to uncover other symptoms that may be connected to the disorder (e.g. increased sweating may not be troublesome to the patient and may not be mentioned unless directly questioned).

Before starting to take a history, there are a number of guidelines to follow:

1. **Present yourself properly**
- Always give your name and status, e.g. medical student.
- Mention the consultant's name—this usually convinces the patient that you are genuine and provides a common link between you and the patient.
- Check that the patient is sitting/lying comfortably.
- Try to put the patient at ease—sit at a comfortable distance from him or her and take the interview at a relaxed pace (do not worry about silences between your questions).
- 'Look the part'—many patients do not feel comfortable giving details of their personal life to young people, especially if they look dishevelled; you will obtain better histories if you are suitably dressed.

2. **Notice the patient's surroundings**
- Try to see the patient walk into the room before the interview (e.g. in outpatient clinics) because any disabilities present can be seen more easily when the patient is moving.
- Note what the patient brings to outpatients with him or her, e.g. inhalers, oxygen, walking sticks/frames, sputum pots, reading material, etc.; on the ward look around the bedside for clues.

3. **Regard the patient's appearance and behaviour**
- Try to be aware of the patient's physical features and clothing.
- Watch the patient's behaviour for clues while taking the history—is he or she agitated or distressed, can you see any tremors, abnormal behaviour, or abnormal eye and body movements?

THE STRUCTURE OF A HISTORY

A history should include the following information:

1. **Patient's details**
Always record:
- the patient's name, age, sex, ethnic group, marital status, occupation, and address;
- the date and time of the interview and how the patient presented, e.g. via ambulance, GP referral, brought in by workmates, follow-up appointment, etc.

2. **Presenting complaint**
Ask the patient what is troubling them and list the complaints in order of severity/importance. Patients often reply with a diagnosis either they or another doctor have come up with (e.g. 'I think I've got diabetes, doctor'). This can be noted in this section but is not the presenting complaint. Therefore ask, 'Why do you think that, then?' This will hopefully elicit the symptoms (e.g. 'Well, I feel tired and thirsty all the time and I seem to be passing water more than I used to')—these are the presenting complaints and it is these that should be recorded, not diagnoses!

It is often useful to write down the complaints in the patient's own words, e.g. a patient may complain of waking up in the night feeling breathless, not of orthopnoea.

3. **History of presenting complaint**
Record the nature of the complaint and the order of events leading to the patient seeking medical attention ('When did it start?; What did you notice first?'), and ask about the following features of the pain and/or symptoms:
- Site.
- Radiation—does the pain move?
- Time and mode of onset (gradual or sudden?) and progression.
- Severity.

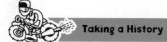

- Character—is the pain sharp, dull, knife-like, colicky?
- Duration and pattern—constant/intermittent; frequency of symptoms?
- Associated features, e.g. nausea, vomiting, weight, appetite.
- Precipitating/relieving factors—does anything seem to make it better/worse?
- Any prior treatment or investigations for this complaint—if so, find out about these episodes.

4. Past medical history

Ask the patient if they have ever been in hospital before and if they have had any illnesses or operations in the past. Record any past medical problems—both chronic (e.g. diabetes mellitus) and acute (e.g. road-traffic accident)—and when they happened.

Ask specifically about diabetes, asthma/bronchitis, TB, jaundice, rheumatic fever, hypertension, heart attacks/angina, strokes, epilepsy, and allergies. These are noted even if they are all negative (often written shorthand as ^{0}DM/Asm/TB/J/RhF/HT/MI/CVA/Ep/Al).

Record the obstetric history in women, i.e. previous pregnancies and their outcomes.

5. Drug history

Ask the patient if they take any tablets or injections regularly or from time to time. Record any medication being taken, either on prescription or over-the-counter (OTC).

Ask women about the contraceptive pill specifically.

Record any exposure to toxins such as alcohol, tobacco, illicit drugs, industrial toxins, etc.

6. Family history

Ask the patient if anyone else in their family has had similar problems, and ask about TB, diabetes, heart disease and any other relevant diseases in the family. Record the age, health, and cause of death (if known) of parents, sibs, and children. It is often useful to sketch the family tree.

7. Review of systems (Fig. 12.1)

Investigate all the body systems when taking a history in case you have missed anything or there is some secondary problem. Use simple language that the patient will understand, but record it in technical terms. Explain to the patient that while much of it will not be relevant, it is necessary to review routinely the body systems (this prevents the patient from thinking that you have 'lost the plot'). Not all the questions will need to be asked—some

will not be appropriate (e.g. it is not always appropriate to enquire about sexual function or contraception).

8. Social history

Try to inquire about a patient's social history without making them feel you are prying. Ask about:

- Children (at home/left home).
- Occupational history.
- Housing (heating, stairs, distance from shops, adequacy).
- Finance (including financial problems caused by illness).
- Diet/exercise/leisure activities.
- Risk behaviours (smoking, alcohol, drug abuse, sexual practices).
- Travel abroad.

9. Summary

'So what you have been telling me is . . .'—always summarize the history back to the patient to check you have not misunderstood anything.

When presenting the case, always give a summary at the end, which should include:

- The patient's name and age.
- The presenting complaint, its duration, and the effect it is having on the patient's life.
- The differential diagnosis.

Accurate history taking is learnt by experience, therefore try to clerk as many patients as possible. Try to present as many patients as possible to house officers/consultants. Compare the history you have taken with that in the patient's notes—this will expose any areas you have not explored sufficiently. Try not to look in the patient's notes before you see the patient as this will not help you learn how to elicit the appropriate information.

Review of systems

General health
- weight loss, appetite, night sweats, fevers, any lumps, itch, fatigue, apathy

Cardiovascular system
- chest pain
- palpitations (awareness of the heart beating)
- exertional dyspnoea (quantify exercise tolerance, e.g. number of flights of stairs that can be managed)
- orthopnoea (breathlessness on lying flat—symptom of left ventricular failure)
- paroxysmal nocturnal dyspnoea (repeated bouts of breathlessness at night)
- claudication (calf pain on walking)
- ankle oedema (sign of right-sided heart failure)
- skin sores/ulcers

Respiratory system
- cough
- sputum (amount, colour)
- haemoptysis (coughing up blood)
- shortness of breath
- wheeze

Gastrointestinal system
- appetite, weight, diet, taste
- nausea, vomiting
- difficulty swallowing
- haematemesis (vomiting blood)
- heartburn
- indigestion
- abdominal pain (site, severity, character, relationship to eating, previous episodes, etc)
- bowel habit (frequency, change, difficulties)
- rectal bleeding

Urinary system ('How are the waterworks?')
- frequency
- nocturia (needing to pass urine in the night)
- urine stream (hesitancy, dribbling)
- dysuria (pain on passing urine)
- haematuria (blood in the urine)
- incontinence

Nervous system
- headaches, fits, faints, loss of consciousness
- changes in vision, hearing, speech, memory
- anxiety, depression, sleep disturbances
- paraesthesiae (pins and needles)
- sensory disturbances (numbness)
- weakness

Reproductive system (female)
- periods (length, cycle, menarche, menopause)
- first day of last menstrual period (LMP)
- contraception
- post-menstrual/intermenstrual bleeding
- vaginal discharge
- dyspareunia (pain on intercourse)
- pregnancies, terminations, births
- problems in pregnancy
- breast symptoms

Reproductive system (male)
- impotence/loss of libido
- scrotal swelling

Musculoskeletal system
- aches or pains in muscles, bones, or joints
- swelling of joints
- limitation of joint movements
- weakness of muscles

Skin
- rashes

Risk factors
- smoking, alcohol consumption, drug abuse
- allergies, foreign travel

Fig. 12.1 Review of systems.

COMMON PRESENTING COMPLAINTS

This section gives examples of the presenting complaints associated with endocrine dysfunction and reproductive disorders. The important aspects of the history that need to be focused on for each presenting complaint are outlined.

Amenorrhoea (Fig. 12.2)
The presenting complaint is a failure to begin menstrual bleeding by the age of 16 years (primary amenorrhoea) or 'missed menstrual periods' (secondary amenorrhoea).

The important questions to be asked and the most common causes are shown in Fig. 12.2. Hyperprolactinaemia is the commonest cause and should be considered in any young woman with amenorrhoea.

Galactorrhoea (Fig. 12.3)
The presenting complaint is the inappropriate production of milk from the mammary glands, i.e. lactation outside the peripartum period. It can occur in males but is extremely rare.

Hyperprolactinaemia is the commonest cause, but often no cause is found (idiopathic galactorrhoea).

Gynaecomastia (Fig. 12.4)

The presenting complaint is the presence of an increased amount of breast tissue in men. Most cases are caused by drugs, e.g. spironolactone, cimetidine, digoxin, cannabis.

Hirsutism (Fig. 12.5)

This presents as increased body and facial hair in women, resembling the male distribution. Polycystic ovary disease is the commonest cause, but in most cases a cause is never found (idiopathic hirsutism).

Obesity (Fig. 12.6)

Obesity describes the condition of excessive fat accumulation whereby the person is 20% above the recommended weight for his or her height, or has a body mass index (BMI; = weight in kilograms/square of height in metres) of 30.0–39.9. The normal BMI is 18.5–24.9. A BMI of 40 constitutes morbid obesity. Endocrine disorders are only very rarely the cause of obesity.

Amenorrhoea		
Find out	**Findings**	**Differential diagnosis**
age of patient	> 50 years	menopause
menstrual history—date of last menstrual period (LMP), normal cycle, length, regular/irregular?	no established menstrual pattern and > 16 years of age	delayed puberty or Turner's syndrome
sexual history— recent intercourse? method of contraception (if any)?	high chance of pregnancy	pregnancy !
associated symptoms/factors	• galactorrhoea, hirsutism, headaches, and/or severe weight loss, stress • weight gain, hirsutism • weight loss, heat intolerance, irritability	• hyperprolactinaemia (due to hypothalamic or pituitary dysfunction) • polycystic ovary disease • hyperthyroidism
obstetric history— previous pregnancies? miscarriages? terminations?	recent pregnancy with postpartum shock and failure to lactate	Sheehan's syndrome (very rare)

Fig. 12.2 Some important questions to be asked when investigating amenorrhoea and the most common causes.

Galactorrhoea		
Find out	**Findings**	**Differential diagnosis**
sexual history—recent intercourse? method of contraception (if any)?	high chance of pregnancy	pregnancy
associated symptoms/factors	• amenorrhoea (in female), impotence (in male), hirsutism, headaches, and/or severe weight loss, stress • weight gain, cold intolerance, lethargy	• hyperprolactinaemia (due to hypothalamic or pituitary dysfunction) • hypothyroidism (rare cause)
drug history	dopamine-receptor antagonists (metoclopramide, haloperidol)	drug-induced galactorrhoea
obstetric history—previous pregnancies? miscarriages? terminations?	recent termination	hyperprolactinaemia

Fig. 12.3 Some important questions to be asked when investigating galactorrhoea and the most common causes.

Gynaecomastia		
Find out	**Findings**	**Differential diagnosis**
age of patient	10–15 years	transient breast enlargement due to puberty
associated symptoms/factors	• recent weight gain • tall stature, scanty body hair, small penis • weight loss, heat intolerance, irritability • high alcohol consumption • symptoms of testicular disease	• obesity • Kleinfelter's syndrome (rare) • hyperthyroidism (rare cause) • liver disease (rare cause) • infection, trauma or tumour of the testis (rare cause)
drug history	spironolactone, cimetidine, digoxin, cannabis	drug-induced gynaecomastia
family history	breast cancer in first-degree relative	breast cancer (rare in men)

Fig. 12.4 Some important questions to be asked when investigating gynaecomastia and the most common causes.

Hirsutism		
Find out	**Findings**	**Differential diagnosis**
age of patient	> 50 years	menopause
associated symptoms/factors	• amenorrhoea, weight gain • cushingoid appearance, easy bruising, myopathy • deep voice, male body form	• polycystic ovary disease • Cushing's syndrome • congenital adrenal hyperplasia
history	exogenous androgens and very high doses of steroids	drug-induced hirsutism
family history	other closely related females have similar hair distribution with unknown cause	constitutional hirsutism

Fig. 12.5 Some important questions to be asked when investigating hirsutism and the most common causes.

Obesity		
Find out	**Findings**	**Differential diagnosis**
patient's view of cause, quantify daily food intake and exercise	excessive food intake and lack of exercise	sedentary lifestyle in combination with an excessive food intake and a genetic predisposition towards obesity
associated symptoms/factors	• overeating/binge eating in response to stress or depression • cold intolerance, lethargy, gynaecomastia (rare) • cushingoid appearance, easy bruising, myopathy	• psychological cause • hypothyroidism • Cushing's syndrome
drug	any drugs that stimulate the appetite or eating behaviour (e.g. steroids, antidepressants), nicotine withdrawal	drug-induced obesity
family history	other family members are obese	environmental or genetic cause (i.e. learnt eating habits or genetic predisposition)

Fig. 12.6 Some important questions to be asked when investigating obesity and the most common causes.

Symptoms of thyroid dysfunction and goitre (Fig. 12.7)

Patients with hyperthyroidism commonly present with heat intolerance, sweating, weight loss despite a good appetite, tremor, fatigue, and mood changes. Rarer symptoms include palpitations, pruritus, amenorrhoea, and thirst.

Patients with hypothyroidism commonly present with no symptoms (disorder only discovered by chance), tiredness (elderly patients often put this down to their age, but hypothyroidism is worth investigating), or symptoms of energy loss, constipation, anorexia, cold intolerance, loss of hair, flaking dry skin, weight gain, hoarseness of the voice, menorrhagia, and occasionally carpal tunnel syndrome.

Goitre commonly presents as a neck lump the patient has found, or as symptoms associated with thyroid disorders.

Symptoms of adrenocortical disorder

(Fig. 12.8)

Patients with cortisol hypersecretion (Cushing's syndrome) commonly present complaining of a change of appearance ('moon-face', hirsutism, acne, increased pigmentation, temporal hair loss, truncal obesity, abdominal striae), proximal-muscle wasting and weakness, unexplained bruising of the skin, ankle oedema, and curving of the spine (due to osteoporosis). Less commonly they present with back and bone pain, polydipsia, nocturia, headache, hypertension, psychotic behaviour, and menstrual disturbances.

Patients with aldosterone hypersecretion (hyperaldosteronism) commonly present with polyuria, polydipsia, hypertension, muscle weakness, cramps and spasms, especially of the hands (carpopedal spasm).

Adrenal androgen hypersecretion commonly presents as virilization of females (temporal balding, a male body form, muscle bulk, deepening of the voice, clitoral enlargement, and hirsutism) and precocious puberty in males.

Patients with adrenal insufficiency commonly present with tiredness, dizziness (postural hypotension), depression, skin pigmentation, anorexia, nausea, vomiting, abdominal cramps, weight loss, and amenorrhoea. Severe cases present acutely with circulatory collapse or coma (addisonian crisis).

Patients usually complain of a limited number of symptoms and it is important to take a complete history in order to uncover other symptoms that may be connected to the disorder.

Symptoms of disordered glucose homoeostasis (Fig. 12.9)

Poorly managed diabetes mellitus may cause episodes of hyperglycaemia and hypoglycaemia. Type 1 diabetes mellitus is due to insulin deficiency resulting from autoimmune disease of the pancreas; type 2 is due to insulin resistance by the tissues.

Approximately 30% of diabetic patients are asymptomatic (diagnosed by routine testing).

Patients with hyperglycaemia commonly present with thirst, polyuria, lethargy, weight loss, and recurrent skin infections. Rarely, severe cases may present with nausea, vomiting, hyperventilation, dehydration, and confusion (all caused by ketoacidosis).

Patients with hypoglycaemia commonly present complaining of nausea, sweating, tremor, a fast and pounding heart beat (palpitations), hunger, drowsiness, and headaches. These symptoms may have disappeared spontaneously or the patient may complain of prolonged episodes. Symptoms are caused by the release of adrenaline (which is a counter-regulatory hormone that mobilizes sufficient glucose into the blood). By far the most common cause of hypoglycaemia is excessive treatment (e.g. relative insulin overdose compared with carbohydrate intake) for diabetes mellitus. Reactive (postprandial) hypoglycaemia occurs in patients who rapidly release excess insulin in response to a meal.

Symptoms of disordered calcium homoeostasis (Fig. 12.10)

Disordered calcium homoeostasis can have variable symptoms (see Figs 15.8 and 15.9) or may be asymptomatic (even at significantly abnormal calcium levels) if calcium levels have changed very gradually (giving the body time to adapt).

Patients with chronic hypercalcaemia commonly present with renal stones and bone aches/fractures. However, many cases are discovered only when the plasma calcium is checked as part of a biochemical screen, and symptoms, if any, are correctly identified only in retrospect. Severe hypercalcaemia of rapid onset commonly presents as abdominal pain, anorexia, nausea, thirst, polyuria, and muscle weakness. Hyperparathyroidism and malignancy are the commonest causes.

Patients with hypoglycaemia commonly present with numbness/'pins and needles' in their hands and feet, and muscle cramps. Rarely, chronic cases present with cataracts. Severe hypocalcaemia of rapid onset commonly presents as carpopedal spasm and

convulsions. Hypoparathyroidism and chronic renal failure are the most common causes.

Symptoms of thyroid dysfunction and goitre		
Find out	**Findings**	**Differential diagnosis**
age of patient	10–15 years (adolescence)	a neck lump may be a transient physiological goitre
medical history	recent thyroid surgery to correct hyperthyroidism, may — hypothyroidism	iatrogenic hypothyroidism
drug history	lithium can cause hypothyroidism; amiodarone can cause hyper- or hypothyroidism	drug-induced thyroid dysfunction
family history	other close relatives have thyroid disease	autoimmune thyroid disease (e.g. Grave's disease, Hashimoto's thyroiditis)

Fig. 12.7 Some important questions to be asked when thyroid dysfunction is suspected and the most common causes.

Symptoms of adrenocortical dysfunction		
Find out	**Findings**	**Differential diagnosis**
medical history	recent TB, sarcoidosis, amyloidosis, meningococcal septicaemia	adrenal insufficiency
associated symptoms/factors	cough, loss of appetite and weight, general tiredness	ACTH-secreting bronchial carcinoma (rare)
drug history	corticosteroids used in many disorders (e.g. asthma, rheumatoid arthritis, dermatitis, organ transplantation)	iatrogenic Cushing's syndrome

Fig. 12.8 Some important questions to be asked when adrenocortical dysfunction is suspected (its causes are usually not evident from the history—further investigations are required).

Symtoms of disordered glucose homoeostasis		
Find out	**Findings**	**Differential diagnosis**
age of patient	• children and young adults • middle and old age	• type 1 DM • type 2 DM
medical history	alcohol abuse	alcohol-induced DM
associated symptoms/factors	• obesity • pregnancy • acute pancreatitis • cushingoid appearance, easy bruising, myopathy	• type 2 DM • gestational DM • transient DM • Cushing's syndrome (rare cause)
drug history	• steroids and thiazides can raise blood glucose levels and predispose to DM • relative insulin or sulphonylurea overdose may cause hypoglycaemia	• drug-induced DM • drug-induced hypoglycaemia
family history	other close relatives have DM	genetic predisposition to DM

Fig. 12.9 Some important questions to be asked when investigating diabetes mellitus (DM).

Vaginal inflammation and abnormal bleeding (Fig. 12.11)

Patients with vaginal inflammation commonly present with an unusual vaginal discharge or genital pruritis. They report a change in the amount or colour of their vaginal discharge; a vaginal odour; and itching, discomfort, or burning of the vulvovaginal tissue.

Other frequently reported symptoms include cystitis, vulvovaginal redness and swelling, and pain on intercourse; rarely, vaginal bleeding. Vaginal inflammation may be caused by infectious agents, chemical agents, mechanical agents, or neoplasms.

Patients with abnormal vaginal bleeding commonly present with heavy or prolonged menstrual periods (menorrhagia) or lack of them (amenorrhoea), intermenstrual bleeding, or unexpected bleeding (e.g. postmenopausal, or during pregnancy). Abnormal ovulatory vaginal bleeding (i.e. abnormal bleeding that is related to ovulatory cycles) is usually associated with crampy abdominal pain and premenstrual symptoms (e.g. nausea, bloating, emotional instability and is normally caused by a disorder in the pelvic organs. Anovulatory vaginal bleeding (i.e. abnormal bleeding that is unrelated to the ovulatory cycle) occurs irregularly and is usually caused by a disorder in the endocrine organs involved in the ovulatory cycle (the hypothalamus, pituitary, ovaries, or adrenal cortex).

Pelvic masses (Fig. 12.12)

These are often asymptomatic and are usually found on pelvic examination or ultrasound, during investigations of other symptoms. They may be caused by infection, cysts, or neoplasia of the reproductive organs (ovaries, fallopian tubes, and uterus) or of the colon and bladder.

Disorders of the breast (Fig. 12.13)

Patients with breast disorders present with breast pain, breast lump, and/or nipple discharge. These symptoms may present individually or together, and can be unilateral or bilateral. They can be caused by physiological cyclic changes, inflammatory conditions, fibrocystic changes, trauma, or neoplasia.

Ask patients presenting with breast pain to describe the pain (site, onset, duration, character, intensity, radiation, any relieving or exacerbating factors) and the patient's opinion of its cause. Distinguish it from chest pain (i.e. musculoskeletal, cardiac, and epigastric pain). Inquire about possible trauma or sexual abuse. Note, pregnancy can cause pricking sensations in the breast.

Ask patients presenting with breast lumps to describe the lump (how and when it was first discovered; its position, size, shape, consistency, tenderness, mobility; skin changes, e.g. redness, dimpling; nipple changes, e.g. discharge or retraction; any changes since it was first noticed) and the patient's

Symptoms of disordered calcium homoeostasis		
Find out	**Findings**	**Differential diagnosis**
presence of physical disability	immobilization	immobilization is a contributing factor to hypercalcaemia (increases bone turnover)
medical history	recent thyroid surgery to correct hyperthyroidism may lead to hypoparathyroidism	iatrogenic hypoparathyroidism
associated symptoms/factors	• malaise, recent weight loss, localized pain • symptoms of hyperthyroidism, sarcoidosis, adrenal insufficiency, or acromegaly • symptoms of chronic renal failure (oedema, lethargy)	• malignancy (bone metastases; breast, bronchial, or prostate cancer; myeloma) • one of these disorders may be the cause of suspected hypercalcaemia • renal failure may be the cause of suspected hypocalcaemia
drug history	thiazide diuretics, antacids, and vitamin A and D intoxication may lead to hypercalcaemia	drug-induced hypercalcaemia

Fig. 12.10 Some important questions to be asked when abnormal plasma calcium levels are suspected and the most common causes.

opinion of its cause. Inquire if any other lumps or general lumpiness is present. Investigate risk factors for breast cancer (increasing age, positive family history, previous breast cancer/atypical biopsy, aged >35 years at first birth, early menarche, early menopause, history of other cancers).

Ask patients presenting with nipple discharge to describe the character, frequency, and colour of the discharge. Serous or bloody discharge tends to indicate more serious pathologies of the breast (e.g. breast cancer), but also is often found in patients with ductal ectasia, papilloma, and fibrocystic disease. Milky or watery discharge is usually caused by galactorrhoea, the early stages pregnancy, or infection.

Vaginal inflammation and abnormal bleeding	
Find out	**Findings**
age of patient	aetiologies are often age dependent
medical history	any previous episodes of similar symptoms and how they were treated?
menstrual history	date of the first day of the last menstrual period (LMP)? normal cycle? length? regular/irregular? possibility of pregnancy?
sexual history	sexual activity? method of contraception? any similar symptoms in sexual partner (penile discharge or discomfort)?
drug history	antibiotics and the oral contraceptive pill can upset the normal vaginal flora, resulting in infection
hygiene	change in soap may result in allergy or predispose to infection
family history	if other family members have had similar problems, there may be an inheritable condition that predisposes to vaginal inflammation or abnormal bleeding, e.g. the patient may have undiagnosed diabetes, making him or her prone to recurrent vaginal infections, or a blood clotting disorder (often familial)

Fig. 12.11 A breakdown of the questions to be asked when investigating vaginal discharge, discomfort, or abnormal bleeding.

Pelvic masses	
Find out	**Findings**
age of patient	different diagnoses are more common in different age groups, e.g.: in women of reproductive age, ovarian cysts are the most common cause; in postmenopausal women, a pelvic mass must be considered a malignancy until proven otherwise
medical history	find out if a similar mass has been found before and if so what was the diagnosis and treatment, e.g. previous surgery for ovarian cancer may signify local recurrence of the tumour
menstrual history	note date of the first day of the last menstrual period (LMP), the possibility of pregnancy (i.e. could mass = pregnant uterus?), and menstrual bleeding (if excessive, suggestive of fibroids)
obstetric history	involuntary infertility suggests the diagnosis of endometriosis or ovarian carcinoma
associated symptoms/factors	urinary frequency may result from uterine fibroids pressing on the bladder or from bladder pathology; gastrointestinal symptoms may suggest the mass is caused by pathology of the colon
family history	gynaecological problems in other family members may be relevant

Fig. 12.12 A breakdown of the history to be asked when investigating pelvic masses.

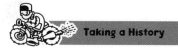

Scrotal masses (Fig. 12.14)

The presenting complaint is a lump in the scrotum. Scrotal masses usually arise in the structures within the scrotal contents but may arise from the intra-abdominal cavity or the retroperitoneum, e.g. inguinoscrotal hernias often allow parts of the small bowel, colon, or even bladder into the scrotum. The underlying cause of a scrotal mass may be structural, infectious, neoplastic, vascular, traumatic, or the result of obstruction of the spermatic cord.

Disorders of the breast	
Find out	**Findings**
medical history	find out if a similar lump, pain, or discharge has occurred before and if so what was the diagnosis and treatment, e.g. previous benign breast lump removed
menstrual history	note the date of the first day of the last menstrual period (premenstrual breast pain may be due to cyclic changes, and infection or tumour are less likely) and the possibility of pregnancy
obstetric history	breast symptoms associated with current or recent lactation could be caused by inflammatory conditions
associated symptoms/factors	night sweats, flushes, and rigors may result from breast infections; obesity can predispose to fat necrosis of the breast; general malaise, loss of weight, and backache may accompany breast cancer
family history	prevalence of breast cancer in the family is very relevant

Fig. 12.13 A breakdown of the history to be asked when investigating disorders of the breast. Breast cancer can present with variable symptoms, therefore a complete history-taking and examination must be carried out (plus investigations) until a carcinoma has been definitively diagnosed or excluded. If symptoms are bilateral, they are less likely to have been caused by a carcinoma (but one must investigate further until carcinoma can be disqualified).

Scrotal masses	
Question	**Comment**
age of patient	congenital masses found in neonates are usually hydrocoeles or inguinoscrotal hernias; in patients aged 10–15 years, torsion is commonest; in patients aged 20–40 years, solid masses are usually testicular tumours; in the elderly, chronic epididymitis is a common cause
history of presenting complaint	ask the patient to describe the mass (how and when it was first discovered, its position, size, shape, consistency, tenderness, mobility, any scrotal skin changes, any changes since it was first noticed) and ask the patient's opinion of its cause; note recent infections or trauma; bilateral masses are usually caused by hydrocoeles
medical history	note previous operations, e.g. a mass in the spermatic cord in vasectomized patients is most likely to be a sperm granuloma (foreign-body immune reaction to the leakage of sperm at this site)
associated symptoms/factors	a reducible lump may suggest an inguinoscrotal hernia or a scrotal varicocoele; a dull ache or insidious pain may suggest a testicular tumour; an acute onset of severe scrotal pain usually signifies torsion of the testicle or acute epididymitis; malaise, fever, acute parotitis, and testicular swelling signifies mumps orchitis; general malaise and loss of weight may suggest testicular cancer with distant metastases

Fig. 12.14 A breakdown of the history to be asked when investigating scrotal masses.

Sexual dysfunction (Fig. 12.15)

In men, the presenting complaints are decreased libido and impotence (failure to maintain an erection suitable for vaginal penetration or the inability to ejaculate). Drugs and alcohol are the most common causes, followed by psychological and then organic factors.

In women, the presenting complaints are decreased libido, pain on intercourse (vaginismus or dyspareunia), and failure to reach orgasm (anorgasmia). Decreased libido often stems from psychological causes (e.g. confidence, trust, anxiety, depression, altered body image), but can be caused by vaginal infection, general illness, medications, and drugs. Neurological and vascular disorders are rare.

Sexual dysfunction	
Question	**Comment**
history of presenting complaint	determine the time of onset, severity, frequency, and other attributes of the patient's sexual dysfunction (e.g. if anorgasmia/impotence is associated with decreased libido) and the patient's opinion of its cause; inquire whether the patient masturbates and whether he or she experiences the same problems during masturbation; inquire about the patient's partner and their relationship
medical history	relevant findings include: history of sexual abuse; diabetes mellitus (can cause autonomic neuropathy — impotence); recent illnesses or operations that may have increased sexual anxiety or decreased libido (e.g. sexually transmitted diseases, gynaecological operations, testicular disorders)
associated symptoms/factors	in men, decreased need to shave and loss of pubic hair suggests testosterone deficiency
drug history	inquire about the use of alcohol, narcotics, prescription drugs, and over-the-counter preparations, and about industrial toxin exposure, e.g. antidepressants may relieve the loss of libido associated with depression but cause anorgasmia/impotence

Fig. 12.15 A breakdown of the history to be asked when investigating sexual dysfunction.

- List the common presenting symptoms for each of the disorders covered in this chapter.
- Outline the important facts from the history that should be sought when investigating each of these disorders.

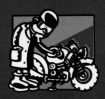

13. Examination of the Patient

GENERAL INSPECTION

First impressions are important—assess if the patient is physically stable and gauge how sick the patient seems to be from his general appearance and behaviour. Whilst taking the history be aware of the patient's demeanour, mental state, and speech, and pay particular attention to:

- Facial features and obvious eye signs (Fig. 13.1).
- Skin complexion (Fig. 13.2).
- Body physique and posture (Fig. 13.3).

Examination of the face	
Finding	**Diagnostic inference**
harsh facial features and abnormal body structure, i.e. 'Punch and Judy' appearance due to large nose, protuberant jaw, and large hands	acromegaly
infant with a broad flat face, widely spaced eyes, and a protruding tongue	cretinism (resulting from hypothyroidism)
eyes that appear to be bulging out of their sockets, i.e. exophthalmos	Graves' disease (not in other forms of thyrotoxicosis)

Fig. 13.1 Examination of the face. Some facial characteristics are so typical of certain diseases that they immediately suggest the diagnosis (although other physical signs must be found and further investigations made to confirm the diagnosis).

Examination of the skin	
Finding	**Diagnostic inference**
generalized pigmentation of the skin	Addison's disease, Cushing's disease (not in Cushing's syndrome)
pale complexion	hypopituitarism
flushed, red skin with excessive sweating	thyrotoxicosis, phaeochromocytoma
boils/skin infections	undiagnosed or poorly controlled diabetes mellitus

Fig. 13.2 Examination of the skin. Depending on the extent to which the patient is clothed and the quality of light in the room, it may be possible to notice features of endocrine disorders in the skin. NB Artificial light does affect the appreciation of colour.

Fig. 13.3 Examination of the body physique and posture. Look specifically for obesity, weight distribution, proximal muscle wasting, height (ask the patient to stand), and limb deformity.

Examination of the body and its posture	
Finding	**Diagnostic inference**
a patient who appears overweight may be carrying excess fat or a foetus, or may be oedematous—look at the distribution of the weight on the face, abdomen, limbs, and shoulders	Cushing's syndrome (abnormal fat distribution in face, shoulders, and trunk, but thin wasted limbs) hypothyroidism (may be overweight and have non-pitting oedema of the legs), pregnancy
short stature	hypopituitarism (GH deficiency), hypothyroidism in infants (cretinism)
short stature with bone deformities ('knock-knees' or 'bow-legs')	rickets (vitamin D deficiency; very rare in UK)
female with short stature but with a masculine body shape (wide shoulders, narrow pelvis, underdeveloped breasts) and webbed shoulders	Turner's syndrome (chromosome configuration 45, XO)
male with tall stature and normal male hair growth but with a female distribution of fat around the breasts and pelvis	Kleinfelter's syndrome (chromosome configuration 47, XXY)

EXAMINATION OF THE HANDS, NAILS, LIMBS, AND FEET

Signs found in the hands, nails, limbs and feet which may suggest endocrine disorders include:

- Structural abnormalities (e.g. bone and muscle changes).
- Skin changes.
- Neurological disorders (e.g. paraesthesia, anaesthesia).

- Cardiovascular disorders (e.g. perfusion deficits, abnormal pulses, hypertension).

All formal examination begins with the hands. As well as providing a wealth of information (Fig. 13.4), inspecting the hands is not intrusive and allows the patient to get used to your physical contact before you progress to more personal areas. The specific features to look for in the nails, limbs and feet are outlined in Figs 13.5, 13.6, and 13.7, respectively.

Examination of the hands	
Finding	**Diagnostic inference**
hands are enlarged, greasy, spade-like, with thickened skin	acromegaly
fingers are short (especially the 4th and 5th) owing to short metacarpals	pseudohypoparathyroidism
palms are warm and moist	thyrotoxicosis
palms are cold and dry	hypothyroidism
palmar creases are pigmented—caused by excess plasma adrenocorticotrophic hormone (ACTH)	Addison's disease, ectopic ACTH syndrome
note the extent of the areas where the patient complains of 'pins and needles' (paraesthesia) or numbness (anaesthesia) in the fingers and hands	diabetes mellitus, hypocalcaemia
Trousseau's sign, showing neuromuscular irritability—test by occluding the blood flow to the hands, using an inflated blood pressure cuff around the upper arm, which causes a typical contraction of the hand (thumb adducts, fingers extend) within 2 minutes	hypocalcaemia
Tinel's sign, showing carpal tunnel thickening (i.e. carpal tunnel syndrome)—diagnose by tapping over the flexor retinaculum and causing paraesthesia in the medial fingers	hypothyroidism, acromegaly
decreased skin turgor, signifying dehydration—present if skin on the back of the hand does not return to normal immediately after being pinched	uncontrolled diabetes mellitus, diabetes insipidus, hypercalcaemia

Fig. 13.4 Examination of the hands. When examining the hands, you should:
- Observe specifically the size and shape of the hands and fingers, their temperature, skin colour.
- Look for tremors and signs of dehydration.
- Demarcate any areas of anaesthesia or paraesthesia.
- Test for Trousseau's sign and Tinel's sign if the history suggests this is appropriate.

Examination of the nails	
Finding	**Diagnostic inference**
separation of the nail from its bed (onycholysis) and nail tips appear white	thyrotoxicosis
clubbing of the fingertips (acropachy), caused by swelling of the soft tissue at the base of the nail	Graves' disease (not in other forms of thyrotoxicosis)
nails look broken and weak (fragile nails)	hypocalcaemia
deformed nails with inflammation of the surrounding skin is a sign of infection (often caused by *Candida albicans*)	uncontrolled diabetes mellitus

Fig. 13.5 Examination of the nails. Nail features are not always present—they tend to more obvious in severe disorders.

Examination of the limbs		
Feature	Finding	Diagnostic inference
pulse rate and rhythm	rapid pulse rate of >100 beats per minute (tachycardia)	thyrotoxicosis, phaeochromocytoma
	slow pulse rate of < 60 beats per minute (bradycardia)	hypothyroidism
	irregular pulse rhythm (signifying cardiac arrhythmias)	thyrotoxicosis
	reduced or absent pulses in the feet and legs (caused by peripheral vascular disease)	diabetes mellitus
skin, muscle, and bone structure of the limbs	infected or ulcerated skin (look especially on the lower leg and ankles)	diabetes mellitus, Cushing's syndrome (both cause poor wound healing)
	multiple bruising over the skin, with no history of trauma	Cushing's syndrome
	thickened skin over the tibia, with elevated dermal nodules and plaques (pretibial myxoedema)	Graves' disease (not in other forms of thyrotoxicosis)
	proximal muscle wasting (observe and feel the biceps and quadriceps muscles)	Cushing's syndrome, hypothyroidism, thyrotoxicosis
	bone deformity, e.g. 'bow-legs' or 'knock-knees' (observe when the patient is standing)	rickets (vitamin D deficiency; rare in UK)
	pitting oedema at the ankles (caused by salt and water retention)	Cushing's syndrome (SIADH does not cause oedema)
blood pressure	high blood pressure (hypertension)	Cushing's syndrome, diabetes mellitus, acromegaly
	low blood pressure whilst moving from lying to standing position (postural hypotension)	Addison's disease, diabetic autonomic neuropathy

Fig. 13.6 Examination of the limbs. When examining the limbs, you should:
- Palpate the radial pulse at the wrist to determine the rate and rhythm of the heart beat.
- Palpate all the pulses in the lower limb (i.e. in the groin, knee, ankle and foot) to check that perfusion of the limb is adequate.
- Inspect the skin, musculature, bone structure and joints of the arms and legs and check ankles for the presence of oedema.
- Measure the blood pressure.

Examination of the feet	
Finding	Diagnostic inference
feet are large and wide and patient's shoe size has recently increased	acromegaly
skin ulcers and/or gangrene	diabetes mellitus
dry, cold, hairless skin of the feet, and weak or absent foot pulses— may signify ischaemia caused by peripheral vascular disease (check by testing capillary refill)	diabetes mellitus
note the extent of the areas where the patient complains of 'pins and needles' (paraesthesia) or numbness (anaesthesia) in the feet and lower legs	diabetes mellitus, hypocalcaemia

Fig. 13.7 Examination of the feet. When examining the feet, you should:
- Observe specifically the size and shape of the feet, their temperature, skin colour.
- Palpate the foot pulses
- Demarcate any areas of anaesthesia or paraesthesia.

Being the most peripheral region of the body, the feet show the first signs of peripheral disease, i.e. peripheral vascular disease and peripheral neuropathy.

Symmetrical numbness of both feet signifies loss of sensory innervation that can be caused by peripheral neuropathy and it may extend up into the legs in a 'stocking pattern' distribution.

This chapter can be used to test your knowledge of the physical effects caused by endocrine and reproductive disorders—e.g. cover up one of the columns and try to remember the associated feature or disorder.

EXAMINATION OF THE HEAD AND NECK

Signs found in the head and neck which may suggest endocrine disorders are numerous and include:

- Structural abnormalities and changes in the hair, skin and buccal mucosa. (Fig. 13.8).
- Eye signs (Figs 13.9 and 13.10).
- Signs of thyroid disease in the neck (Fig. 13.11).

Examination of the head		
Feature	Finding	Diagnostic inference
bone structure, facial features and complexion	increased head circumference, protuberant jaw, coarse facial features, nose and jaw enlarged, malaligned teeth with spaces between them in the lower jaw, thickened facial skin folds	acromegaly
	protuberant forehead	rickets (vitamin D deficiency; rare in UK)
	pale, puffy face with coarse features	hypothyroidism
	round 'moon-face'	Cushing's syndrome
	acne on face, neck, and chest	Cushing's syndrome, acromegaly
	Chvostek's sign, showing neuromuscular irritability—diagnose by gently tapping the facial nerve where it passes through the parotid gland and causing the facial muscles to twitch briskly on the same side of the face	hypocalcaemia
Hair distribution	lack of normal beard growth in postpubescent males	delayed puberty, hypopituitarism causing gonadotrophin deficiency
	excessive facial hair (hirsutism) in females	polycystic ovary disease
Mouth	hyperpigmented buccal mucosa	Addison's disease, Cushing's disease (not in Cushing's syndrome)
	malaligned teeth, enlarged tongue (possibly causing dysarthria, i.e. difficulty in pronunciation)	acromegaly
	swollen tongue and a hoarse, croaky voice	hypothyroidism

Fig. 13.8 Examination of the head. When examining the head, you should:
- Inspect the bone structure, facial features and complexion (e.g. size and shape of the head, face, eyes, nose, jaw and tongue).
- Observe the hair distribution and texture.
- Examine the mouth.

Examination of the eyes

Finding	Diagnostic inference
lid lag—descent of the upper lid lags behind descent of the eyeball	hyperthyroidism
lid retraction—at rest, the superior limbus of the iris and possibly even some sclera above it (white of the eye) is visible (see Fig. 13.10)	hyperthyroidism
exophthalmos—the eye appears to bulge out of its socket and it is possible to see the whole of the iris and sometimes even sclera surrounding its circumference (see Fig. 13.10)	Graves' disease (not in other forms of thyrotoxicosis)
anaemia—the inner surface of the lower lid looks pale if anaemia is present	menorrhagia
retinal disease—look for ischaemic change and neovascularisation using an ophthalmoscope (appearance of 'dots' and 'blots' signify presence of microaneurysms and microhaemorrhages, respectively)	diabetes mellitus
papilloedema (caused by raised intracranial pressure)—both optic discs appear convex and their margins appear blurred	pituitary tumour
impaired visual acuity—test the visual acuity in both eyes separately using an eye chart	diabetes mellitus
bitemporal hemianopia visual field deficits—test the visual fields in each eye separately	pituitary tumour

Fig. 13.9 Examination of the eyes. When examining the eyes, you should:
- Observe the appearance of the eyes and their movements.
- Examine the cornea, lens, retina and the optic disc using an ophthalmoscope.
- Test visual acuity and visual fields.

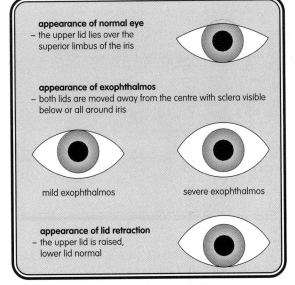

appearance of normal eye
– the upper lid lies over the superior limbus of the iris

appearance of exophthalmos
– both lids are moved away from the centre with sclera visible below or all around iris

mild exophthalmos   severe exophthalmos

appearance of lid retraction
– the upper lid is raised, lower lid normal

Fig. 13.10 Eye signs found in hyperthyroidism

Examination of the neck

Finding	Diagnostic inference
anterior neck swelling in the thyroid position which ascends during swallowing	goitre
swelling in the neck (0.5–5 cm diameter) between the chin and the 2nd tracheal ring which moves with swallowing	congenital thyroglossal cyst

Fig. 13.11 Examination of the neck. When examining the neck, you should:
- Observe changes in the skin such as scars (e.g. from previous thyroidectomy), unusual pigmentation, hair growth and acne.
- Describe the characteristics of any swellings in the neck—i.e. determine its site, size, shape, symmetry, movement with swallowing (all thyroid swellings ascend during swallowing), surface, consistency and tenderness.

EXAMINATION OF THE THORAX AND THE BREAST

Signs found in the thorax and breast which may suggest endocrine disorders and breast pathology include:

- Structural abnormalities (e.g. size and shape of breast and ribs, fat deposition).
- Skin and nipple changes (e.g. complexion and hair distribution).
- Respiratory disorders (e.g. respiratory distress).

A complete examination of the thorax and breast (Figs 13.12, 13.13, and 13.14) should involve:

- Observation (looking) of the structure, skin and respiratory rate.
- Palpation (feeling) of the breasts, axillary lymph nodes and heart beat.
- Percussion (tapping) to demarcate the heart and areas of lung disease.
- Auscultation (listening) of the heart and breath sounds.

Only the observable and palpable signs are included in this text because other signs (i.e. of heart and lung disease) are usually not useful in the diagnosis of endocrine disorders. However the cardiovascular and respiratory systems should be always be examined to check for co-existing heart and lung disease.

A reasonably accurate clinical diagnosis can be made from breast examination, but usually it is followed by further investigations (e.g. mammogram, fine needle aspiration, biopsy) to confirm the diagnosis, as numerous breast disorders can resemble carcinoma. A complete examination of the breast includes:

- Observation (Fig. 13.14).
- Palpation (Fig. 13.13).

Palpation of the breast	
Finding	**Diagnostic inference**
a solitary, stony-hard, painless lump with an irregular surface and an indistinct edge, which may or may not involve the skin, underlying muscle, and regional lymph nodes	breast carcinoma
a solitary, firm, painless lump with a spherical (or knobbly) surface, which tends to be highly mobile, and no lymphadenopathy	fibroadenoma—nevertheless, further investigations must be performed
a lump or diffuse swelling that is tender, soft/solid, and spherical, with hot overlying skin and lymphadenopathy	breast abscess
palpable regional lymph nodes	breast infection, breast carcinoma

Fig. 13.13 Palpation of the breast. When palpating the breasts, you should:
- Feel the normal breast first in order to determine what is normal for the patient because breast texture varies from individual to individual.
- If a mass is noted or suspected it should be described in terms of its position, size, shape, consistency, surface texture, edge, mobility, tenderness and any attachment to surrounding muscle or skin.
- Palpate the regional lymph nodes in the axilla and in the supraclavicular and infraclavicular regions for lymphadenopathy—record the number, size, consistency and fixity of any palpable glands.
- Feel the abdomen and lumbar spine for signs of metastases (e.g. hepatomegaly, ascites, spinal pain, limitation of spinal movement).

Examination of the thorax	
Finding	**Diagnostic inference**
a 'pigeon chest' or 'rickety rosary' (outward bowing and thickening of the costochondral junctions)	rickets (vitamin D deficiency; rare in UK)
decreased chest hair in men	hypopituitarism
truncal obesity (abnormal fat distribution) and increased chest hair in men and women	Cushing's syndrome
respiratory distress—deep, rapid hyperventilation ('air-hunger'), called Kussmaul's breathing	diabetic ketoacidosis

Fig. 13.12 Examination of the thorax. When examining the thorax, you should:
- Inspect the chest wall for abnormalities in bone structure, skin, hair distribution, fat deposition, breast size, and nipple pigmentation.
- Note the presence of respiratory distress.

Observation of the breast	
Finding	**Diagnostic inference**
scar due to mastectomy (removal of breast)	previous breast carcinoma
breast size decreased bilaterally in women	hypopituitarism
enlargement of the female breast (unilateral or bilateral)	benign hyperplasia of the breast, breast infection/ inflammation, breast neoplasm
enlargement of the male breast (unilateral or bilateral)	gynaecomastia (see Fig. 12.3), breast carcinoma
skin appears pulled in and puckered	underlying breast carcinoma
skin has an 'orange peel' appearance (peau d'orange) because of oedema-induced widening of the orifices of sweat glands and hair follicles	breast carcinoma that is blocking the lymphatic drainage and causing oedema
skin nodules, abnormal skin texture and colour	skin infiltrated with tumour cells from a breast carcinoma
skin is erythematous (reddened)	infection of the breast or the overlying skin
skin ulceration (determine its position, size, shape, colour, edge, and base)	breast carcinoma
nipple and surrounding skin is thickened, red, encrusted, and oozy, with an underlying breast lump	Paget's disease of the nipple
nipple pigmentation decreased	hypopituitarism
nipple pigmentation increased	Addison's disease (pregnancy)
nipple asymmetry and/or retraction	underlying breast carcinoma
nipple discharge	infection, benign or malignant breast tumours, lactation
nipple duplication—can occur anywhere along the 'milk line', which runs from the axilla to the groin	supernumerary nipples (rare)
redness and swelling of the axilla and arm (caused by lymphadenopathy and oedema)	metastases in the axillary lymph nodes from a breast carcinoma

Fig. 13.14 Observation of the breast. When examining the breasts, you should:
- Assess their size, shape and symmetry.
- Inspect for changes in the skin and in the nipple, and the presence of any localised swelling.
- Look for redness or swelling of the axillae and arms, and distended veins.

EXAMINATION OF THE ABDOMEN

Signs found in the abdomen which may suggest endocrine and reproductive disorders include:
- Structural abnormalities (e.g. fat deposition, enlarged organs, pelvic masses, vertebral collapse).
- Skin changes (e.g. colour, scars, purple striae, hair distribution).

A complete examination of the abdomen involves:
- Observation (looking)—see Fig. 13.15.
- Palpation (feeling)—see Fig. 13.16.
- Percussion (tapping)—see fig 13.17.
- Auscultation (listening) of bowel sounds and the foetal heart.

Diarrhoea and constipation can be associated with endocrine disorders but do not attempt to diagnose them by listening to the bowel sounds—bowel sounds do vary depending upon the rate of intestinal motility, but the terms 'increased' or 'decreased' are meaningless because motility varies normally, depending upon when a meal was last eaten. Foetal heart sounds can be heard over a pregnant uterus using a handheld doppler ultrasound at 10 weeks gestation and a stethoscope at 25 weeks.

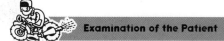

Observation of the abdomen	
Finding	**Diagnostic inference**
scars (e.g. from previous adrenalectomy, hysterectomy, or other gynaecological surgery)	previous surgery to treat endocrine or reproductive system disorder
wide purple striae (linear wrinkled 'stretch' marks) and increased abdominal hair (hirsutism) in women	Cushing's syndrome
abdominal distension (can be caused by fat, fluid, foetus, flatus, faeces, or large solid tumours)	Cushing's syndrome (fat), hypothyroidism (fat), pelvic mass (e.g. fibroids, ovarian disease, or pregnancy)
excessive outward curvature of the spine (kyphosis) or excessive inward curvature of the spine (lordosis)—both can be caused by vertebral collapse due to crush fractures (back pain may be present or may have subsided)	osteoporosis (secondary to menopausal hormone failure, Cushing's syndrome, or thyrotoxicosis)

Fig. 13.15 Observation of the abdomen. When examining the abdomen, you should:
- Inspect for asymmetry, abnormalities in skin, hair distribution, abdominal distension and any obvious masses.
- Note the shape and mobility of the spine.

Palpation of the abdomen	
Finding	**Diagnostic inference**
enlarged liver, spleen, and kidneys (organomegaly)	acromegaly
mass found and its lower edge cannot be palpated	pelvic mass (e.g. fibroids, ovarian disease, or pregnancy)
bony tenderness of the vertebral column (caused by crush fractures)	osteoporosis (secondary to menopausal hormone failure, Cushing's syndrome, or thyrotoxicosis)

Fig. 13.16 Palpation of the abdomen. When palpating the abdomen, you should:
- Feel for enlarged organs (liver, spleen, kidney), abdominal and pelvic masses.
- Feel the spine to detect tenderness or vertebral collapse.
- Describe the physical signs of any masses—position, size, shape, consistency, surface, edge, mobility, tenderness, fluctuation, fluid thrill, resonance and pulsitility.

The pregnant uterus is regularly assessed by palpation to make sure that the foetus is growing at a normal rate.

Percussion of the abdomen	
Finding	**Diagnostic inference**
pelvic mass is dull to percussion (i.e. not gas filled) and has a fluid thrill	cystic mass (e.g. ovarian cyst)
pelvic mass is dull to percussion and does not have a fluid thrill	solid mass (e.g. ovarian tumour)

Fig. 13.17 Percussion of the abdomen. Percuss over the whole abdomen, the liver and over any masses (to deduce their size and tenderness).

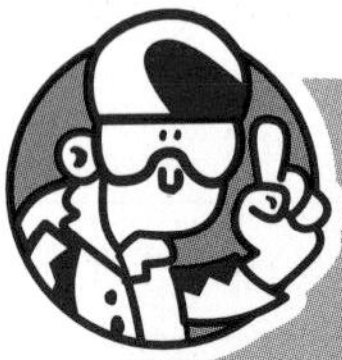

Not all signs of a particular endocrine disorder have to be present in order to make the diagnosis (presence and severity of specific signs depend on the duration and severity of the disorder).

EXAMINATION OF THE FEMALE REPRODUCTIVE SYSTEM

Examination of the vulva (external genitalia)

When examining the vulva (Fig. 13.18), you should:
- Inspect the skin and mucous membranes for rashes, ulceration, warts, scars, sinus openings or the presence of lumps.
- Note any anatomical abnormalities (e.g. vaginal prolapse), the size and shape of the clitoris, and any vaginal discharge.
- Swab any non-bloody discharge from the urethra or vagina should be swabbed and send samples off to the microbiology and histology laboratories for culture and microscopical examination.

Digital examination of the vagina and cervix

When examining the vagina and cervix, you should:
- Locate the cervix and note its position, size, shape, consistency, tenderness and mobility.

- Palpate the cervix and vagina for softening, tears, polyps or foreign bodies (e.g. retained tampon).
- Note the characteristics and location of any palpable masses.

Bimanual examination of the uterus, ovaries and tubes

Palpate the uterus bimanually. Position the index and middle fingers of the right hand in the anterior vaginal fornix and with the left hand placed just below the umbilicus, gently press down and backwards, and:
- Note whether the uterus is anterior (anteverted) or posterior (retroverted) in its position.
- Estimate its size, shape, consistency, mobility and attachments.
- Check for the presence of tumours or tenderness.

A large nodular mobile uterus suggests fibroids, while smooth enlargement suggests pregnancy or cancer. The ovaries and fallopian tubes are not usually palpable, but they can be felt if they are enlarged or tender.

Further investigations are required to confirm the cause of uterine, ovarian or tubular abnormalities (e.g. pelvic ultrasound, CT scan, laparoscopy, biopsy).

Male students and doctors should always be accompanied by a chaperone during a gynaecological examination, primarily to reassure the patient but also for medico-legal reasons.
Before any examination (and especially before gynaecological examination), always explain the procedures fully and obtain the patient's consent.

Internal examination using a speculum

Examine the vagina and cervix using a well-lubricated bivalve speculum. The following specimens can be taken:
- A smear for cervical cytology to detect cervical dysplasia or cancer.

Fig. 13.18 Examination of the vulva (female external genitalia).

Examination of the vulva	
Finding	**Diagnostic inference**
rashes (redness, swelling, or white thickened areas of leucoplakia)	often caused by infections (e.g. thrush or trichomoniasis), dermatological conditions (e.g. lichen sclerosus), chemical irritants, or allergies to soap, contraceptive creams, etc.
injury or scars	can be due to trauma (e.g. childbirth, female circumcision, or sexual abuse)
enlarged clitoris (clitoromegaly)	congenital adrenal hyperplasia (excessive androgen secretion)
red painful cystic lump beneath the posterior part of the labium majora	Bartholin's cyst or abscess (acute bartholinitis)
bloody vaginal discharge	menstruation, miscarriage, cancer, cervical polyp, or erosion
purulent vaginal discharge	vaginitis, cervicitis, endometritis (e.g. caused by gonorrhoea)
frothy, watery, pale, yellow-white or purulent discharge and pruritus	infection caused by *Trichomonas vaginalis*
thick, white, cottage-cheese-like discharge and inflammation of the skin and mucous membranes	infection caused by *Candida albicans*

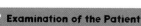

- Swabs for wet slides to detect trichomonas or thrush (if indicated).
- Cultures to detect gonorrhoea and chlamydia (if indicated).

EXAMINATION OF THE MALE GENITALIA

Examination of the external Genitalia
A full examination comprises the following:
- Observation (Fig. 13.19).
- Palpation (Fig. 13.20).

Examination of a scrotal mass
The possible causes of swellings in the scrotum are illustrated in Fig. 13.21. If a scrotal mass is found, describe its:
- Position—i.e. is it a testicular mass, an epididymal mass, or does it arise from the abdomen?
- Size.
- Shape.
- Surface—smooth, rough, regular, irregular or bosselated?
- Edge—clearly defined or indistinct?
- Consistency—soft, spongy, rubbery, firm, hard or stony hard?
- Mobility—attachment to surrounding structures?
- Tenderness—pain on palpation?
- Translucency—cystic masses transmit light.
- Reducibility—can it be compressed so that it disappears temporarily?
- Groin lymph nodes—size, tenderness, consistency.

Examination of the prostate gland
A rectal examination is required to examine the prostate gland and the seminal vesicles. The normal prostate is firm, bilobed and 2–3 cm across with a smooth surface and a shallow central sulcus.

An enlarged, lobulated, mobile prostate with no involvement of the rectal mucosa is caused by benign hypertrophy.

An irregular, hard enlargement of the prostate with an indistinct edge, distorted central sulcus and fixed rectal mucosa is caused by prostatic carcinoma

Observation of the male external genitalia	
Finding	Diagnostic inference
skin/mucosal rashes or ulceration (a swab or biopsy of the lesion, together with a complete history, is required to determine the cause)	infection (e.g. STD, scabies), inflammation (e.g. allergic dermatitis, chemical irritants), connective tissue disease, squamous cell carcinoma
decreased pubic hair	hypogonadism, hypopituitarism
small penis	hypogonadism
abnormal position of the external urethral meatus	hypospadias

Fig. 13.19 Observation of the male external genitalia.
- Inspect the skin on and around the genitals and on the scrotum for rashes, ulceration, oedema, sebaceous cysts and observe the pubic hair distribution.
- Observe the size and shape of the penis, the skin colour and condition, and note the presence or absence of the foreskin.

Palpation of the male external genitalia	
Finding	Diagnostic inference
urethral discharge	infection or inflammation (e.g. caused by Chlamydia trachomatis)
empty scrotum (unilateral or bilateral)	undescended or retractile testis, previous excision
small firm testes (bilateral)	hypogonadism, testicular atrophy due to alcohol or drugs
small firm testis (other testis normal)	mumps orchitis
exquisitely tender testis with oedematous swelling of the entire scrotal contents	torsion of the testis (twisting within the scrotal sac)

Fig. 13.20 Palpation of the male external genitalia.
- Palpate the groin lymph nodes first—enlargement of these is lymph nodes is most commonly caused by sexually transmitted disease, but can be caused by metastatic spread from testicular tumours.
- Retract the foreskin to expose the glans penis and the external urethral meatus—look for urethral discharge; if present, collect a specimen using a swab.
- Feel for the testes, epididymides, and the cords—the testes are normally equal in size, smooth and relatively firm.
- In the absence of one or both testes, search for incompletely descended or retracted testes in the inguinal canal or for ectopic testes in sites such as the groin.

Normal testis

• testes are equal in size, smooth and relatively firm

Inguinoscrotal hernia

• a mass that arises in the abdomen (cannot feel above it in the scrotum) and may be reducible and/or tender

Testicular tumour

• a mass which is part of the testis and solid (non-translucent) is likely to be a tumour

Hydrocoele (a collection in the tunica vaginalis of the testis)

• a cystic (translucent) mass which surrounds the testis

Epididymal cyst

• a small, firm mass which is cystic (translucent) and is located within the epididymis (appears separate from the testis)

Epididymitis

• a mass that is not cystic, appears to be separate from the testis, and may be tender is probably caused by chronic epididymitis (acute epididymitis is exquisitely tender)

Varicocoele (bunch of dilated, tortuous veins in the pampiniform plexus)

• a mass above the testis that feels like a 'bag of worms' and is reducible when the patient lies flat

Spermatocoele (cystic swelling that contains sperm)

• a small, non-tender, translucent mass that arises out of the epididymis

Fig. 13.21 The possible causes of masses in the scrotum

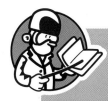

○ **List examples of the features of each endocrine and reproductive disorder that can be found on examination.**
○ **What are the important features to describe when examining the breasts in order to diagnose breast pathology?**
○ **Describe the procedures for examining the male and female reproductive systems.**

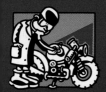

14. Further Investigations

INVESTIGATION OF ENDOCRINE FUNCTION

This section outlines the tests used to assess endocrine function. If an excess or deficiency of a hormone is suspected from the history and examination, such tests can be performed to confirm the diagnosis and investigate its cause.

Endocrine function is investigated by:
- Measuring the hormone level directly. The plasma and urine hormone levels using radioimmunoassay (RIA) or enzyme-linked immunosorbent assay (ELISA; see Fig. 1.13).
- Measuring the hormone level indirectly. Some hormones produce metabolic changes and their levels can be evaluated by measuring the plasma and urine solute concentrations and osmolality—e.g. osmolality is measured to determine plasma antidiuretic hormone (ADH) levels; plasma glucose levels are measured to evaluate plasma insulin levels.
- Testing the endocrine gland secretory function using stimulation or suppression tests—these tests involve administering a substance into the body that affects the secretion of a specific hormone, and comparing the resultant plasma hormone levels with the expected levels.

Anterior pituitary function
Hormone assays
To investigate pituitary function, the plasma levels of the pituitary hormones and the hormones that are released in response to them must be measured, e.g. the pituitary hormone thyroid-stimulating hormone (TSH) stimulates the thyroid gland to release thyroxine and tri-iodothyronine (T_4 and T_3), and T_4 and T_3 act back on the pituitary to inhibit TSH secretion.

However, it is not always useful to measure basal plasma hormone levels to diagnose endocrine dysfunction. Stimulation and suppression tests are used to diagnose abnormal secretion of hormones that:
- Have a short half life (e.g. adrenocorticotrophic hormone, ACTH).
- Are secreted in quantities that are too small to be measured accurately (e.g. hypothalmic hormones).

- Are normally secreted episodically causing their plasma levels to fluctuate (e.g. growth hormone, GH).

The combined pituitary test
When secretion of one anterior pituitary hormone is suspected to be abnormal, secretion of all the anterior pituitary hormones is tested to make sure that they are not abnormal as well.

The combined pituitary test (CPT) stimulates the anterior pituitary gland to increase hormone secretion in response to provocation by the intravenous injection of:
- Insulin (which induces hypoglycaemia) to stimulate ACTH, GH, and prolactin secretion (Fig. 14.1).
- Thyrotrophin-releasing hormone (TRH) to stimulate TSH and prolactin secretion.
- Gonadotrophin-releasing hormone (GnRH) to stimulate luteinizing hormone (LH) and follicle-stimulating hormone (FSH) secretion.

The resultant plasma hormone levels are measured using RIA and compared with the levels expected; hence, abnormal secretion of specific hormones can be observed.

Further tests for anterior pituitary hormone secretion
Further tests used to evaluate ACTH, TSH, and LH and FSH secretion are described in the sections on adrenal, thyroid, and gonadal function, respectively.

Plasma levels of prolactin can be measured directly and accurately using RIA (provocative tests are not required to diagnose abnormal prolactin secretion, although its levels are measured after the CPT test to compare its secretion with the other anterior pituitary hormones).

Plasma levels of GH can not be accurately assessed by RIA alone because it is secreted episodically and normal levels are usually too low to be detectable.

GH deficiency is diagnosed using provocation tests, such as: insulin-induced hypoglycaemia stress test (see Fig. 14.1); glucagon test (intramuscular injection of glucagon stimulates GH secretion); clonidine test (oral clonidine stimulates GH secretion).

GH excess (causing acromegaly or gigantism) is diagnosed using suppression tests, such as the oral

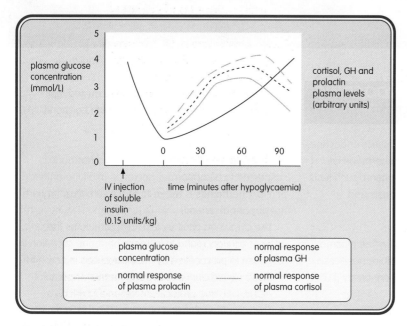

Fig. 14.1 Normal response of cortisol, growth hormone, and prolactin to the insulin-induced hypoglycaemia stress test (part of the CPT). NB hypoglycaemia stimulates ACTH secretion but cortisol plasma levels are usually measured instead of ACTH (increased ACTH secretion results in increased cortisol secretion). (Adapted from *Lecture Notes on Endocrinology 5e*, by WJ Jeffcoate. Courtesy of Blackwell Science, 1993.)

glucose tolerance test. In this, 75 g oral glucose is given and the plasma levels of GH are measured every 30 minutes for 2 hours. Increased blood glucose normally suppresses GH secretion, but in acromegaly or gigantism GH levels fail to decrease.

Posterior pituitary function

Hormone assays

ADH secretion is assessed by measuring the urine and plasma osmolality—if the urine is dilute and the plasma concentrated, and there is no other cause of solute diuresis, then ADH secretion must be deficient; conversely, if the urine is concentrated and the plasma dilute, then ADH secretion must be excessive.

Plasma levels of ADH can be measured accurately using RIA. However, because ADH levels vary depending on the plasma osmolality, random plasma samples are of little value and levels should be measured only in combination with provocation tests (see below).

Oxytocin secretion is not tested because abnormal plasma levels do not cause any recognized pathology.

The water deprivation test

This is used to check for ADH deficiency—diabetes insipidus (DI)—by testing the body's ability to concentrate water, i.e. it does not measure ADH directly.

The procedure is to deprive the patient of food and

water for 6 hours after an overnight fast and—at 60-minute intervals—to measure the urine volume and osmolality, and the plasma osmolality, and weigh the patient (abandon the test if the patient loses >5% body weight).

Normally, water deprivation causes ADH levels to rise in order to reduce water excretion—this maintains the normal plasma osmolality (280–295 mOsmol/kg) and results in an increased urine osmolality (>750 mOsmol/kg) and a decreased urine volume. If the peak plasma osmolality increases out of the normal range (i.e. >295 mOsmol/kg) and the peak urine osmolality remains low (<300 mOsmol/kg), then DI is diagnosed.

The desmopressin test

This is used to test whether DI is caused by deficient ADH secretion by the pituitary (cranial DI) or by the failure of the kidney to respond to ADH (nephrogenic DI).

It is used in conjunction with the water deprivation test. After the 6 hours of water deprivation, 2 mg desmopressin (an ADH analogue) is given intramuscularly and the patient is allowed to drink. Plasma and urine osmolality are measured at 1 hour and 2 hours after the desmopressin.

If the peak urine osmolality remains low (<300 mOsmol/kg) after desmopressin, the patient has nephrogenic DI; if it increases to >750 mOsmol/kg, the patient has cranial DI.

Thyroid function
Hormone assays
Plasma T$_4$, T$_3$, and TSH levels should be measured to determine thyroid function.

Both free and plasma-protein-bound levels of T$_4$ and T$_3$ are measured by RIA because levels of thyroxine binding globulin (TBG) can vary (e.g. during pregnancy and with the oral contraceptive pill) and give erroneous results.

Low plasma levels of T$_4$ and T$_3$ indicate hypothyroidism; high levels indicate hyperthyroidism.

TRH stimulation test
This test can be used to investigate TSH deficiency, but is not often applied now that immunoassays are sensitive enough to measure basal TSH levels.

TRH—the hypothalamic thyrotrophin-releasing hormone that stimulates TSH secretion from the anterior pituitary gland—is administered intravenously in a dose of 200–500 mg. Plasma TSH levels are measured 0, 20, and 60 minutes later, and compared with the expected TSH response (Fig. 14.2).

Thyroid autoantibody assays
ELISA and RIA can be used to detect thyroid autoantibodies (present in autoimmune thyroid diseases):
- The presence of thyroid-stimulating antibodies (TsAb) indicates Graves' disease.
- The presence of anti-thyroid-peroxidase (anti-TPO) antibodies and anti-thyroglobulin antibodies (anti-TgAb) indicates Hashimoto's thyroiditis.

Adrenal function
Hormone assays
If a disorder of the adrenal cortex is suspected from the history and examination, the plasma or urine levels of the hormone thought to be causing the disorder can be measured using RIA.
- Urinary levels of free cortisol measured over a 24-hour period are used to estimate the output of cortisol by the adrenal cortex—most cortisol is excreted in a metabolized form, but the free (i.e. unmetabolized) cortisol can be measured using RIA (normal is <700 nmol/24 hours).
- Basal plasma cortisol and ACTH are measured at

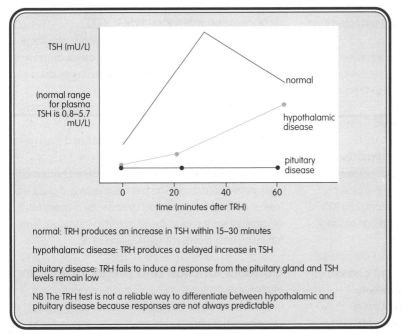

Fig. 14.2 Response of TSH plasma levels to the TRH stimulation test. (Adapted from *Lecture Notes on Endocrinology 5e,* by WJ Jeffcoate. Courtesy of Blackwell Science, 1993.)

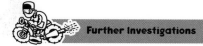

9 a.m. because they vary diurnally (but they are not as reliable as the urinary levels of free cortisol and they can be affected by abnormal levels of plasma protein).

- Random plasma or urinary levels of aldosterone and renin, together with plasma potassium levels, are measured to assess aldosterone secretion from the adrenal cortex (e.g. in Conn's syndrome, aldosterone is high, renin and potassium low).
- Plasma or urinary levels of the catecholamines and their metabolites (e.g. vanillylmandelic acid—VMA) are measured to assess adrenal medulla function (e.g. in phaeochromocytoma, VMA levels are raised).

Dexamethasone suppression test

Dexamethasone is a synthetic steroid that normally suppresses ACTH and corticotrophin-releasing hormone (CRH) secretion, hence also cortisol secretion.

The low-dose (overnight) dexamethasone suppression test is used to investigate Cushing's syndrome (cortisol hypersecretion). It involves the oral administration of 2 mg dexamethasone at 11 p.m., with measurement of plasma cortisol at 9 a.m. the next morning (normal is <170 nmol/L). If the test fails to suppress cortisol, the patient has Cushing's syndrome.

The high-dose dexamethasone suppression test is used to diagnose Cushing's disease (pituitary hypersecretion of ACTH) and to rule out adrenal disease and ACTH-secreting tumours. In this test, 2 mg dexamethasone is administered orally every 6 hours for 48 hours, and plasma cortisol is measured at 9 a.m. when the test is completed (cortisol is suppressed in Cushing's disease).

Synacthen stimulation test

This test is used to investigate cortisol hyposecretion, i.e. adrenal insufficiency.

Synacthen, a synthetic analogue of ACTH, normally stimulates cortisol secretion.

In the short Synacthen test, 0.25 mg Synacthen is injected intramuscularly and plasma cortisol levels are measured at 0 and 30 minutes. If the initial plasma cortisol level is >140 nmol/L and the second is >500 nmol/L (or >200 nmol/L above the initial cortisol level), adrenal insufficiency can be ruled out.

If the short Synacthen test does not exclude adrenal insufficiency, the prolonged Synacthen test is performed. This involves the injection of 1.0 mg Synacthen intramuscularly daily for 3 successive days and measurement of the plasma cortisol levels at 0 and 6

hours after the third injection. Adrenal insufficiency is diagnosed if plasma cortisol is <690 nmol/L at 6 hours after the third injection, whereas pituitary ACTH deficiency is diagnosed if plasma cortisol is >690 nmol/L at this time.

CRH stimulation test

This test is not often used, but it is useful to investigate cortisol and ACTH deficiency that is caused by hypothalamic CRH deficiency.

Exogenous CRH (100 mg) is administered intravenously. The resultant plasma cortisol levels are measured every 15 minutes for 2 hours and compared with the expected cortisol response. If the response to a CRH test is normal but the response to an insulin stress test is insufficient, this suggests that hypothalamic CRH is deficient.

Pancreatic function
Random and fasting blood glucose assays

These are used to diagnose diabetes mellitus (caused by insulin deficiency or insensitivity). Insulin causes the plasma glucose levels to decrease, therefore lack of insulin results in abnormally high plasma glucose levels.

If pancreatic dysfunction is suspected from the history and examination, a blood sample can be taken, either at random or after a 6-hour fast, and its glucose level measured. Diabetes mellitus is indicated by:

- A random blood glucose level of >11.1 mmol/L.
- A fasting blood glucose level of >7.8 mmol/L.

Oral glucose tolerance test (OGTT)

If the results from a fasting blood glucose assay show that the patient has impaired glucose tolerance, an OGTT is indicated. This test is used to evaluate the patient's response to a glucose load to see whether they are diabetic rather than merely having impaired glucose intolerance.

To test, the patient is fasted overnight and then given 75 g glucose in water to drink.

The venous plasma glucose is measured before and 2 hours after the drink. The first measurement gives the lowest (fasting) level of blood glucose; by 2 hours after glucose intake it should be returning to this basal level, following an initial rise (Figs 14.3 and 14.4).

Gonadal function and pregnancy testing
Hormone assays

In the male, if gonadal failure is suspected (e.g. from two abnormally low sperm counts), plasma levels of

FSH, LH, testosterone, and prolactin should be measured using RIA. For testosterone, three blood samples need to be taken in the morning at 20-minute intervals and the mean plasma testosterone level calculated, because testosterone levels are higher in the morning and it is secreted in a pulsatile fashion (normal range for plasma testosterone is 10–35 nmol/L).

In the female, if gonadal failure is suspected (e.g. from amenorrhoea or failure to conceive), plasma levels of FSH, LH, oestradiol-17β, progesterone, and prolactin should be measured using RIA. The normal levels of FSH, LH, oestradiol-17β, and progesterone vary during the menstrual cycle, so it is important to calculate the day of the cycle on which the blood sample was taken (although an oestradiol of <110 pmol/L at any time of the cycle indicates gonadal failure).

Plasma prolactin levels are measured because hyperprolactinaemia inhibits the action of LH and FSH.

Low levels of gonadal hormones with high levels of LH and FSH indicate primary gonadal failure.

Low levels of gonadal hormones with low or normal levels of LH and FSH indicate hypothalamic–pituitary dysfunction.

Clomiphene stimulation test

This test can be used to investigate gonadal failure in both men and women.

Clomiphene is a weak antioestrogen that blocks oestrogen receptors in the hypothalamus, causing a functional oestrogen deficiency; this leads to the increased secretion of GnRH from the hypothalamus, which in turn stimulates the pituitary to secrete LH and FSH.

Clomiphene (100 mg) is taken orally twice daily for 10 days and the plasma hormone levels measured on day 0 and 10 of the test (plasma hormone levels before and after the test are compared).

- In men, the normal response is an increase in LH, FSH, and testosterone.
- In women, LH and FSH are increased, followed by an

Fig. 14.3 OGTT diagnostic criteria.

OGTT diagnostic criteria			
Blood glucose level (mmol/L)	Normal	IGT	Diabetes mellitus
after a 6-hour fast	6.0	>6.0 but <7.8	>7.8
2 hours after glucose intake	<7.8	7.8–11.1	>11.1

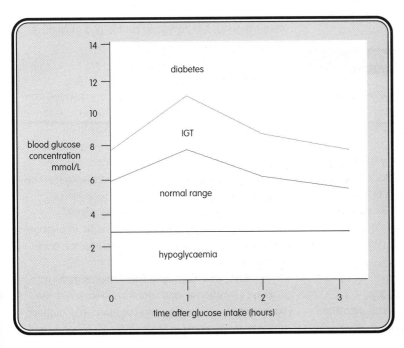

Fig. 14.4 The OGTT blood glucose ranges diagnostic of normal, impaired glucose tolerance (IGT), and diabetes mellitus (DM). IGT signifies that glucose levels are abnormal but not enough to be classed as DM. NB IGT does not produce symptoms of DM but patients may be prone to macrovascular disease and to acquiring type 2 DM. (From *Fundamentals of Obstetrics and Gynaecology 6E,* by D Llewellyn-Jones, Mosby, 1994.)

increase in oestradiol and progesterone, and ovulation is induced.

Failure of LH and FSH levels to rise after this test shows hypothalamic–pituitary dysfunction. NB Clomiphene is also used to induce superovulation—this is used in assisted conception techniques.

Pregnancy test

The early test used to diagnose pregnancy involves the detection of human chorionic gonadotrophin (hCG) in the urine, i.e. if hCG is present, the test is positive. This test is highly sensitive and specific—hCG (produced by the developing placenta) can be detected in the maternal urine approximately 10 days after conception.

- Describe the stimulation and suppression tests that are used to investigate endocrine function.
- How are the levels of hormone in the blood measured directly and indirectly.

ROUTINE INVESTIGATIONS

This section outlines the investigations that would be used to assess the endocrine and reproductive systems in a patient who presents to an Accident and Emergency department or an outpatients' clinic.

Blood samples are always taken, for evaluation of the full blood count and levels of urea and electrolytes (U&Es).

Biopsies and samples for cytological or microbiological examination are taken if appropriate (i.e. if the history and examination indicate a cellular abnormality or infective aetiology).

Clinical chemistry

The concentrations of the ionic and organic components of the blood and urine can be measured by the chemistry laboratory.

The individual components of the blood are considered separately in Fig. 14.5, however, in practice, the overall blood concentrations must be examined together. This is because concentrations of the ionic and organic components are interrelated, e.g. Addison's disease causes the plasma concentrations of calcium and potassium to be elevated and the plasma concentrations of sodium and bicarbonate to be low, because of the effect of aldosterone deficiency in the kidney.

Chemical analysis of random urinary samples is useful only in combination with the blood results because concentrations are so variable in the urine.

Inappropriate excretion of electrolytes can be observed by testing the urine (e.g. if the history is appropriate, a dilute urine together with an abnormally concentrated plasma is suggestive of diabetes insipidus).

Haematology

Changes in the blood cell indices can be caused by endocrine and reproductive disorders, e.g. erythropoeitin deficiency causes a decrease in the haemoglobin concentration.

The percentage of haemoglobin that is glycosylated gives a measure of the average control of blood glucose in a diabetic patient over the preceding 6–8 weeks (glucose non-enzymatically attaches itself to the β chains of the haemoglobin molecule). If the percentage of glycosylated haemoglobin is high then the patient has not had good control and must have had periods of hyperglycaemia.

Microbiology and virology

If a differential diagnosis of infection is suspected from the history and examination, an appropriate specimen is sent off to the microbiology laboratory to be examined and tested for specific microorganisms.

Acute infections of the endocrine glands are uncommon. Idiopathic endocrine disorders may have an infective aetiology but the organisms are no longer detectable by the time the endocrine disorder is diagnosed; e.g. it is suspected that some cases of diabetes mellitus may result from a previous viral infection of the endocrine pancreas.

Endocrine disorders including diabetes mellitus, Cushing's syndrome, and hypothyroidism make the body more prone to acquiring infections; e.g. diabetic patients are susceptible to staphylococcal and fungal

Do not interpret laboratory reports except in the light of clinical assessment, i.e. provisional or differential diagnoses are made from the patient's history and examination and clarified by the blood/urine chemistry, not vice versa.

Normal concentration ranges for ionic and organic components of the blood and endocrine causes of abnormally high or low concentrations		
Component and its normal range	Endocrine causes of abnormally high concentration	Endocrine causes of abnormally low concentration
plasma sodium: 135–145 mmol/L	diabetes insipidus, Cushing's syndrome (rarely), Conn's syndrome (rarely)	syndrome of inappropriate antidiuretic hormone secretion (SIADH), Addison's disease, diabetes mellitus
plasma potassium: 3.5–5.0 mmol/L	Addison's disease, diabetes insipidus, diabetes mellitus	Cushing's syndrome, hyperaldosteronism, SIADH, hyperthyroidism
plasma urea: 2.5–7.5 mmol/L; plasma creatinine: <120 mmol/L	diabetes insipidus, diabetes mellitus, Addison's disease	SIADH
plasma osmolality: 270–300 mOsmol/kg	diabetes insipidus, diabetes mellitus (NB abnormal aldosterone levels do not affect osmolality)	SIADH
pH: 7.35–7.45; bicarbonate: 24–30 mmol/L	Cushing's syndrome, Conn's syndrome	Addison's syndrome, diabetic ketoacidosis, hyperparathyroidism (mild)
plasma calcium: 2.25–2.55 mmol/L	hyperparathyroidism, vitamin D toxicity, hyperthyroidism, acromegaly, Addison's disease (NB abnormal calcitonin levels do not affect plasma calcium levels)	hypoparathyroidism, vitamin D deficiency, Cushing's syndrome
plasma phosphate: 0.8–1.5 mmol/L	hypoparathyroidism, hyperthyroidism, acromegaly	hyperparathyroidism, vitamin D deficiency, diabetes mellitus
fasting blood glucose: 3.5–6.0 mmol/L	diabetes mellitus, Cushing's syndrome, acromegaly, hyperthyroidism, phaeochromocytoma	exogenous insulin overdose, Addison's disease, pituitary insufficiency
fasting plasma triglycerides: 0.55–1.90 mmol/L	diabetes mellitus	
plasma ketone bodies: not normally present in the blood	diabetes mellitus	

Fig. 14.5 Normal concentration ranges for ionic and organic components of the blood and endocrine causes of abnormally high or low concentrations.

infections of the skin (boils and carbuncles), candidal infections (thrush), and TB.

The reproductive system can acquire numerous infections, the most common being the sexually transmitted diseases (STDs). Specimens for investigations are taken by swabbing, scraping, or aspirating the infected region.

Opportunistic infections (e.g. secondary to AIDS or immunosuppression) can infect the endocrine glands and reproductive organs.

Histopathology and cytology

Biopsies of the thyroid, parathyroid, and adrenal glands, and of the breast, cervix, uterus, ovaries, and testes, can be taken if a mass or abnormality is detected. Biopsied material is sectioned using a microtome, stained, and examined under a microscope for abnormal cells and abnormal tissue structure.

Cell samples from cervical smears and from fine-needle aspiration of cystic lesions in the breast are stained and examined under a microscope to detect the presence of abnormal cells (dyskaryosis).

The specimens are examined for evidence of:

- Inflammatory cells, showing presence of inflammation of infection.
- Tissue structure changes, e.g. necrosis, hyperplasia, dysplasia. NB In biopsied material only—cytological examination does not show tissue structure.
- Abnormal cells, e.g. changes in cell shape, colour, polarity, nucleus:cytoplasm ratio, and the presence of mitotic figures.

○ **What tests are routinely used to investigate endocrine and reproductive disorders.**

IMAGING OF THE ENDOCRINE AND REPRODUCTIVE SYSTEMS

Plain X-rays

Plain X-rays are useful to demonstrate bony structures and calcified areas within organs because bone and calcified tissues are radio-opaque compared with the surrounding soft tissues of the body. They are used, therefore, to investigate endocrine disorders that cause bone abnormalities (e.g. acromegaly, hyperparathyroidism, rickets, Cushing's syndrome, thyrotoxicosis—see Figs 14.6 and 14.7) and to observe endocrine glands that are either encased by bone (e.g. pituitary) or may have become calcified in association with the disorder (e.g. adrenal glands, pancreas).

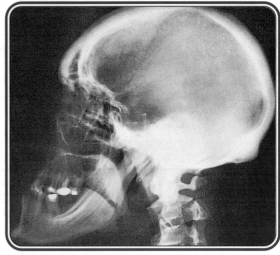

Fig. 14.6 Plain lateral X-ray of the skull of a patient with acromegaly, showing the characteristic enlarged jaw (prognathism), enlarged pituitary fossa, and thickened skull vault. (From *Atlas of Endocrine Imaging* by M Besser and M Thorner, Mosby Europe Ltd, 1993.)

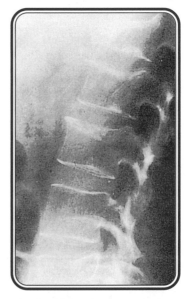

Fig. 14.7 Plain lateral X-ray of the lumbar vertebrae of a patient with osteoporosis, showing reduced bone density, thin cortex, and vertebral collapse (endocrine causes of osteoporosis include Cushing's syndrome and thyrotoxicosis). (From *Atlas of Endocrine Imaging* by M Besser and M Thorner, Mosby Europe Ltd, 1993.)

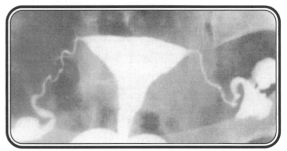

Fig. 14.8 Hysterosalpingogram showing a normal uterus and Fallopian tubes. (From *Fundamentals of Obstetrics and Gynaecology 6E*, by D Llewellyn-Jones, Mosby, 1994.)

Contrast medium and dyes

The soft tissues can be examined on plain X-rays using radio-opaque contrast medium (inert substances that have an absorptive capacity for X-rays that differs from that of the body tissues).

The contrast material can be ingested, or injected into a specific body compartment to allow this compartment to be examined using X-rays. For example:

- In angiography, contrast medium is injected intravenously, permitting the blood vessels, and consequently the organ that the blood vessels supply (e.g. adrenals, pancreas), to be visualized.
- In hysterosalpingography, contrast medium is injected into the cervix and its progression along the tubes is monitored using image-intensified television (Fig. 14.8). The X-ray can be repeated a few hours later to confirm the tubes are patent (in which case there would be contrast medium in the peritoneal cavity).
- In fluorescein angiography, fluorescein dye is injected intravenously and the retina photographed using ultraviolet light while the blood containing the fluorescein is passing through the eye. This technique is used to gain a detailed image of the retinal vessels and is useful in the investigation of diabetic retinopathy (Fig. 14.9).

Mammography

Mammography—in combination with a comprehensive

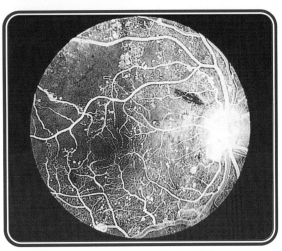

Fig. 14.9 Fluorescein angiogram showing diabetic retinopathy [lesions include capillary closure (C), microaneurysms (M), and neovascularization.] (L, leakage.) (From *A Colour Atlas of the Eye and Systemic Disease,* by EE Kritziner and BE Wright, Wolfe Medical Publications Ltd, 1994.)

history, physical examination, and ultrasonography—can be used to investigate breast lumps (be they due to normal lumpiness, or cystic, benign, or malignant) and has a pivotal role in the early detection of breast cancer.

Mammograms showing the architecture of a normal breast and a breast containing a breast carcinoma are presented in Figs 14.10 and 14.11, respectively. Most patients with breast lumps present before they have progressed to the stage shown in Fig. 14.11.

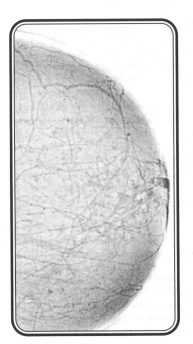

Fig. 14.10 Mammogram showing the architecture of the normal breast—the blood vessels are outlined and the breast has a trabeculated appearance with no areas of increased density that would be suggestive of a mass. (From *Fundamentals of Obstetrics and Gynaecology 6E,* by D Llewellyn-Jones, Mosby, 1994.)

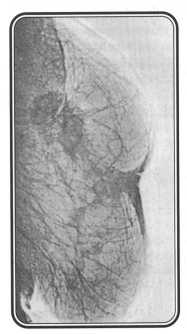

Fig. 14.11 Mammogram of a breast containing a breast carcinoma (which is also causing the skin to thicken and the nipple to retract). (From *Fundamentals of Obstetrics and Gynaecology 6E,* by D Llewellyn-Jones, Mosby, 1994.)

Ultrasonography

Ultrasonography uses mechanical pressure waves (like audible sound waves, but of much higher frequency). These are reflected differently by various tissues in the body according to their composition. An image of the reflected waves can be formed—fluid appears black; denser structures that attenuate the ultrasound reflect brightly.

Ultrasonography is used to investigate the size of a 'lump' and whether it is cystic or solid. 'Lumps' examined using ultrasound include breast, ovarian, testicular, thyroid, and adrenal masses (Figs 14.12 and 14.13)

Ultrasound imaging is also used to examine the foetus routinely (Figs 14.14 and 14.15) and to investigate any abnormalities that may be suspected clinically.

CT and MRI scans
CT scans

Computerized tomography (CT) involves the detection of X-rays from a source that is rotated around the region of the body under investigation and the formation of a computerized image—bone appears dense (white) and other tissues less dense (dark).

CT scanning is used to visualize numerous disease processes, including enlargement of organs and neoplasms, and can be used to locate tumours during biopsy (CT-guided biopsy) and prior to surgery (e.g. adrenal tumours).

Intravenous injection of contrast medium is often utilized to allow better visualization of blood vessels and

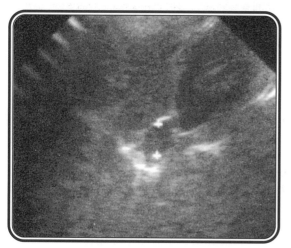

Fig. 14.12 Transverse ultrasound scan showing a 2 cm adrenal mass in the left adrenal gland. (From *Atlas of Endocrine Imaging* by M Besser and M Thorner, Mosby Europe Ltd, 1993.

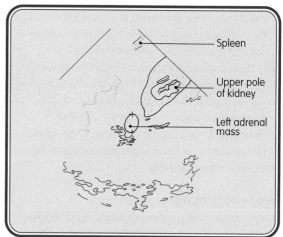

Fig. 14.13 Line drawing showing the main features of the adrenal scan in Fig. 14.12. (From *Atlas of Endocrine Imaging* by M Besser and M Thorner, Mosby Europe Ltd, 1993.)

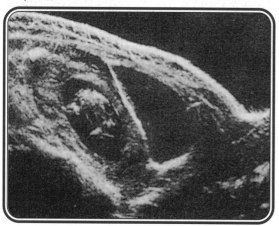

Fig. 14.14 Sagittal ultrasound scan showing the appearance of a normal foetus at week 12 of gestation. (From *Fundamentals of Obstetrics and Gynaecology 6E,* by D Llewellyn-Jones, Mosby, 1994.)

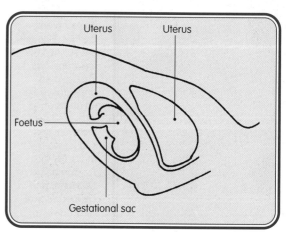

Fig. 14.15 Line drawing showing the main features of the scan in Fig. 14.14. (From *Fundamentals of Obstetrics and Gynaecology 6E,* by D Llewellyn-Jones, Mosby, 1994.)

to improve the density differences between tumours and adjacent tissues.

A transverse CT scan of the head of a patient with Graves' disease is shown in Fig. 14.16.

MRI scans

Magnetic resonance imaging (MRI) uses strong magnetic fields and radiofrequency energy to detect the density and behaviour of protons within the tissues. The radiofrequency causes the protons in the tissues to align within the magnetic field. Removal of the radiofrequency allows the protons to 'relax' back—as they do so, they release energy that can be detected as a radio signal. Air, bone, and fast-flowing blood appear black; other tissues appear as different shades of grey, depending on their density and the character of the protons within them.

MRI scans can be T1 or T2 weighted, depending on the proton relaxation times measured (different tissues can be visualized better under T1 or under T2).

MRI scans have advantages over CT scans in that they do not involve potentially harmful X-rays, they do not require contrast media, and they have a better resolution.

MRI is used to detect tumours and to ascertain the size and nature of the tumour (Fig. 14.17).

Radioisotope scans

Radioisotope scans involve the ingestion or injection of isotopes that accumulate in specific tissues (e.g. radioactive iodine accumulates in the thyroid gland) and the detection of their radioactive emission by a gamma camera. This allows specific endocrine glands (e.g. thyroid, parathyroid, adrenal) to be visualized, and the pattern of radioisotope uptake within the gland exposes any abnormal areas.

Thyroid scanning is used to determine the activity of the gland (e.g. the thyroid is hyperactive in Graves' disease) and to evaluate palpable nodules (e.g. benign or malignant). Oral radioactive iodine (^{123}I) is ingested and the thyroid scanned 5 and 24 hours later. In this way, the thyroid can be imaged (shows abnormal anatomy, and the size and location of nodules) and its function tested—increased radioactive iodine uptake (RAIU), measured by a gamma detector, indicates hyperactivity (normal uptake is 5–15% of the oral dose at 5 hours and 10–30% at 24 h).

Intravenous technetium-99m pertechnetate is a less toxic alternative that is also used to image the thyroid—the thyroid is scanned 20 minutes after injection, and the resolution is better than that with [123]I (Figs 14.18–14.21).

Parathyroid scanning—using the radiotracer technetium-99m Sestamibi—is used to detect and localize parathyroid adenomas.

Adrenal imaging is used to localize adrenal tumours:
- ^{131}I-iodonorcholesterol (NP-59) is used to examine the adrenal cortical structure and function.

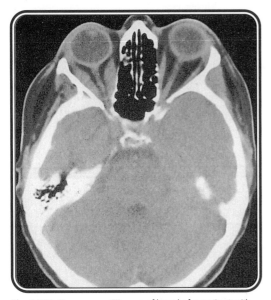

Fig. 14.16 Transverse CT scan of head of a patient with Graves' disease, showing exophthalmos of the left eye caused by thyroid peroxidase autoantibodies (orbital rectus muscles hypertrophy and cause the eye to protrude). (From *A Colour Atlas of Endocrinology 2e*, by R Hall and D Evered, Wolfe Medical Publications Ltd, 1990.)

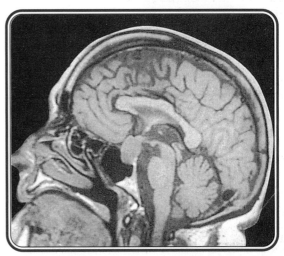

Fig. 14.17 Sagittal T1-weighted MRI scan of the head of a patient with hyperprolactinaemia, showing a large homogeneous pituitary adenoma. (From *Atlas of Endocrine Imaging* by M Besser and M Thorner, Mosby Europe Ltd, 1993.)

- ^{131}I- meta-iodo-benzyl-guaindine (mIBG) is used to label the medulla—it selectively collects in tissues that store catecholamines, especially in tumours of the adrenal medulla (e.g. phaeochromocytoma).

These radiotracers contain radioactive iodine, which is potentially harmful to the thyroid, so Lugol's solution is given both the day before and on the test day to reduce its uptake by the thyroid.

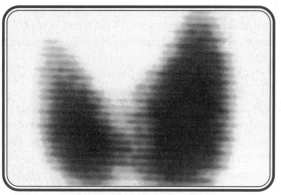

Fig. 14.18 Thyroid image (using technetium-99m pertechnetate) from a patient with Graves' disease, showing abnormally increased uptake throughout the enlarged gland. (From *Atlas of Endocrine Imaging* by M Besser and M Thorner, Mosby Europe Ltd, 1993.)

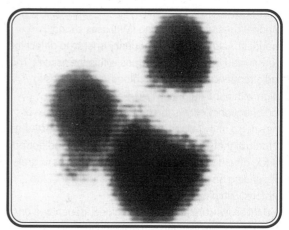

Fig. 14.19 Thyroid image (using technetium-99m pertechnetate) from a patient with a toxic multinodular goitre, showing nodules with increased uptake separated by areas of normal tissue whose function has been suppressed. (From *Atlas of Endocrine Imaging* by M Besser and M Thorner, Mosby Europe Ltd, 1993.)

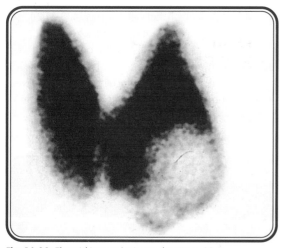

Fig. 14.20 Thyroid image (using technetium-99m pertechnetate) from a patient with a solitary palpable lump in the thyroid gland, showing a 'cold' nodule (i.e. area of thyroid with reduced radiotracer uptake)—the 'cold' nodule could be caused by a haemorrhage, a cyst, or follicular thyroid cancer (ultrasound is used to investigate the nodule further). (From *Atlas of Endocrine Imaging* by M Besser and M Thorner, Mosby Europe Ltd, 1993.)

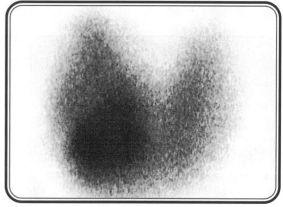

Fig. 14.21 Thyroid image (using technetium-99m pertechnetate) from a patient with a solitary palpable lump in the thyroid gland, showing a 'hot' nodule (i.e. area of thyroid with increased radiotracer uptake) surrounded by normal thyroid tissue—'hot' nodules are usually caused by benign thyroid tumours. (From *Atlas of Endocrine Imaging* by M Besser and M Thorner, Mosby Europe Ltd, 1993.)

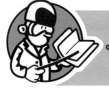 ○ **Outline the imaging techniques used to investigate endocrine disorders and abnormalities in the breast and reproductive systems.**

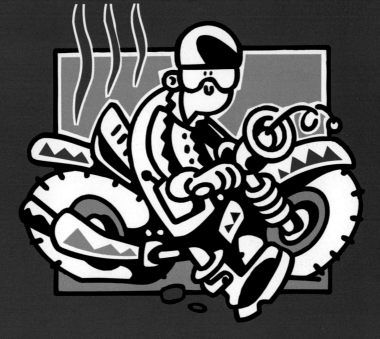

BASIC PATHOLOGY

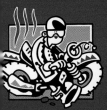

15. Pathology of the Endocrine Glands

DISORDERS OF THE PITUITARY GLAND AND HYPOTHALAMUS

Disorders of the pituitary gland include:

- Hyperpituitarism—excessive secretion of a pituitary hormone.
- Hypopituitarism—insufficient secretion of a pituitary hormone.
- Panhypopituitarism—insufficient secretion of more than one pituitary hormone.

Aetiology of pituitary gland and hypothalamic disorders

Possible causes of disorders of the pituitary gland and hypothalamus include:

- Invasion—tumours in or surrounding the hypothalamus and pituitary, e.g. large pituitary tumours, primary CNS tumours, craniopharyngiomas (these are cysts derived from the remnants of Rathke's pouch which increase in size owing to accumulation of fluid, not cell division).

  Tumours are by far the commonest cause of disorders of these organs. They can cause: compression of the pituitary gland, leading to panhypopituitarism; compression of the hypothalamus and/or the portal vessels (and hence block the delivery of hypothalamic releasing hormones), leading to panhypopituitarism and excess prolactin secretion. (Prolactin secretion is unusual in that it is normally inhibited by the hypothalamic hormone dopamine.)

  Pituitary adenomas commonly cause a combined deficiency/excess syndrome in which one pituitary hormone (depending on the cell type that the tumour arises from) is secreted in excess and the other pituitary hormones are deficient (owing to compression of their secretory cells).

- Infarction—ischaemic damage to the pituitary can lead to panhypopituitarism, e.g.:
  (A) Sheehan's syndrome—postpartum pituitary necrosis, which can occur after massive postpartum haemorrhage (→ systemic hypotension and hypoxia) because the pituitary is enlarged and very vascular at the time of delivery and therefore is susceptible to total infarction. Women with this rare condition will not lactate, develop amenorrhoea, and suffer loss of body hair. It may lead to death if untreated. (It is the only pituitary disorder in which the prolactin levels are low.)
  (B) Pituitary apoplexy—spontaneous haemorrhagic infarction, causing sudden severe headache or collapse. It is a neurosurgical emergency.

- Idiopathic (i.e. no underlying cause is found)—e.g. idiopathic diabetes insipidus (acquired ADH deficiency); idiopathic hypopituitarism of the elderly—normal hypothalamic function declines with age (degenerative process) and can lead to hypopituitarism.

- Iatrogenic—e.g. surgery or irradiation therapy for previously overactive pituitary can cause hypopituitarism.

- Injury—e.g. severe head trauma.

- Infiltration—e.g. sarcoidosis, haemochromatosis, histiocytosis X.

- Infection—e.g. tuberculosis, syphilis, abscesses (now very rare causes).

- Immunologic—autoimmune processes, e.g. lymphocytic hypophysitis (very rare).

- Inherited—congenital deficiency of an individual hypothalamic or pituitary hormone is very rare.

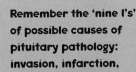

Remember the 'nine I's' of possible causes of pituitary pathology: invasion, infarction, injury, infiltration, infection, immunologic, iatrogenic, idiopathic, and inherited.

Empty sella syndrome

This describes the condition where the sella turcica partially fills with cerebrospinal fluid, causing it to enlarge, and the pituitary gland is compressed within it. It is not always pathological (some cerebrospinal fluid is found within the sella in at least 50% of normal individuals). Causes include congenital incompetence of the diaphragma sellae, pituitary surgery or irradiation, postpartum pituitary infarction (Sheehan's syndrome), and coexisting pituitary tumour.

It is diagnosed using magnetic resonance imaging (MRI—demonstrates presence of fluid) and the combined pituitary test (checks for hormone insufficiency by stimulating the release of each of the pituitary hormones).

It does not have to be treated unless an endocrine disturbance is associated with it.

Effects of pituitary gland and hypothalamic disorders
Local effects
These are commonly due to tumour growth causing compression of surrounding structures. They usually occur in advanced cases only, and include the following symptoms:

- Headaches (not related to tumour size).
- Loss of peripheral vision owing to compression of the optic nerve (bitemporal hemianopia with macular sparing).
- Cranial nerve palsy (with fast-growing tumours only).
- Raised intracranial pressure and occasionally hydrocephalus.

Pituitary tumour can grow down into the nasopharynx and present as a 'nasal polyp'.

Systemic effects
Pituitary gland and hypothalamic disorders result in the abnormal secretion of hormones that have systemic effects.

Effects of abnormal secretion of hypothalamic hormones
Deficiency of the hypothalamic releasing hormones will result in insufficient secretion of the corresponding anterior pituitary hormones (hypopituitarism):

- Growth-hormone-releasing hormone (GHRH) deficiency leads to reduced growth hormone (GH) secretion from the pituitary.
- Gonadotrophin-releasing hormone (GnRH) deficiency leads to reduced luteinizing hormone (LH) and follicle-stimulating hormone (FSH) secretion from the pituitary.

Idiopathic GnRH deficiency in children, associated with congenital anosmia or colour blindness is known as Kallman's syndrome.

- Thyrotrophin-releasing hormone (TRH) deficiency leads to reduced thyroid-stimulating hormone (TSH) secretion (extremely rare).
- Corticotrophin-releasing hormone (CRH) deficiency leads to reduced adrenocorticotrophic hormone (ACTH) secretion (extremely rare).

Deficiency of the hypothalamic inhibiting hormone dopamine will, however, lead to hyperprolactinaemia (prolactin secretion is unusual in that it is normally under dominant negative control by dopamine).

Excessive secretion of hypothalamic hormones does not tend to occur.

Effects of abnormal secretion of anterior pituitary hormones
Deficiency of the anterior pituitary hormones will result in insufficient secretion of hormones from other endocrine glands (see Fig. 15.1).

In panhypopituitarism, GH, LH, and FSH are usually lowered/lost first, followed by ACTH and then TSH (prolactin deficiency is rare except after pituitary necrosis).

The pituitary has a great secretory reserve—more than 75% of it must be destroyed before clinical manifestations are evident.

Symptoms of anterior pituitary disorders depend on the specific hormone that is secreted abnormally, and on the severity and duration of the abnormal secretion.

Excess of the anterior pituitary hormones (hyperpituitarism) will result in excessive secretion of

Deficiencies of the anterior pituitary hormones (in order of prevalence) and their effects	
Deficiency	**Effect**
GH	dwarfism in children, adult GH deficiency syndrome (abnormal body composition, weight loss, lethargy, and impaired physical performance) in adults
LH and FSH (usually occur together)	failure to enter puberty, low levels of sex hormones hypogonadism, infertility, reduced libido, and hair loss in males, and amenorrhoea in females
ACTH (rare)	reduced cortisol secretion by the adrenals (adrenal insufficiency)
TSH (rare)	reduced thyroid hormone secretion (hypothyroidism)
prolactin (very rare)	failure of postpartum lactation (only occurs with panhypopituitarism)

Fig. 15.1 Deficiencies of the anterior pituitary hormones (in order of prevalence) and their effects.

Excesses of the anterior pituitary hormones (in order of prevalence), tumours responsible, and their effects		
Excess	**Tumour**	**Effect**
prolactin	prolactinomas (≈ 50% of all pituitary tumours), non-functioning adenomas (≈ 20% of all pituitary tumours)	hyperprolactinaemia—commoner in females, where it causes galactorrhoea, menstrual disturbance, infertility, hirsutism; in males, there may be galactorrhoea, impotence, loss of libido (does not cause gynaecomastia)
GH	somatotrophic cell adenomas (≈ 20% of all pituitary tumours)	gigantism in children (generalized increase in body size and stature), acromegaly in adults (excessive growth confined to soft tissues and bones of the hands, feet, and jaw—see Fig. 15.3)
ACTH	corticotrophic cell adenomas (≈ 5% of all pituitary tumours; very rare, <5 cases/million/year)	Cushing's disease → symptoms of Cushing's syndrome (owing to cortisol and androgen hypersecretion), adrenal hyperplasia, pigmentation of the skin and mucous membranes
LH and FSH	gonadotrophic cell adenomas (very rare)	infertility, visual impairment (because tumours often large when patient presents)
TSH	thyrotrophic cell adenomas (very rare)	hyperthyroidism, visual impairment (because tumours often large when patient presents)

Fig. 15.2 Excesses of the anterior pituitary hormones (in order of prevalence), tumours responsible, and their effects.

hormones from other endocrine glands (see Fig. 15.2).

The hormone most commonly secreted in excess is prolactin. This is because prolactinomas are the commonest pituitary tumours and because non-secreting pituitary tumours can upset the delivery of dopamine (inhibiting factor) to the prolactin-secreting cells, causing excessive prolactin secretion.

The signs and symptoms of excessive GH secretion in adults (acromegaly) are shown in Fig. 15.3.

Effects of abnormal secretion of posterior pituitary hormones

A deficiency of oxytocin can lead to difficulty with breastfeeding, whereas an excess of oxytocin has no ill effects.

Factors associated with abnormal secretion of antidiuretic hormone (ADH) are listed in Fig. 15.4—ADH deficiency causes cranial diabetes insipidus; ADH excess causes SIADH (syndrome of inappropriate secretion of ADH).

Other effects of hypothalamic dysfunction

Lesions in the hypothalamus can cause many other abnormalities, including disorders of consciousness, behaviour, thirst, satiety, and temperature regulation. These disorders usually occur together with hypopituitarism and diabetes insipidus.

The biblical giant Goliath may have suffered from pituitary disease—he was very big (possibly due to excessive GH secretion) and perhaps had impaired peripheral vision because he failed to see David's stone coming (possibly due to a somatotrophic pituitary tumour)

Diagnosis of pituitary gland and hypothalamic disorders

Pituitary and hypothalamic disorders are diagnosed from:
- Symptoms—e.g. symptoms of Cushing's disease lead to suspicion of ACTH excess.
- Abnormal basal hormone levels in the blood—e.g. hyperprolactinaemia.
- Provocation tests—these involve the administration of hormone analogues that stimulate hormone secretion and are used when hormone secretion is believed to be deficient, to see if the pituitary is able to respond normally (basal hormone levels are too

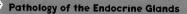

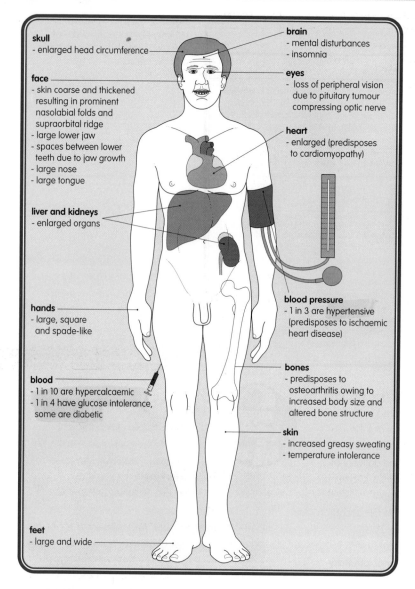

skull
- enlarged head circumference

face
- skin coarse and thickened resulting in prominent nasolabial folds and supraorbital ridge
- large lower jaw
- spaces between lower teeth due to jaw growth
- large nose
- large tongue

liver and kidneys
- enlarged organs

hands
- large, square and spade-like

blood
- 1 in 10 are hypercalcaemic
- 1 in 4 have glucose intolerance, some are diabetic

feet
- large and wide

brain
- mental disturbances
- insomnia

eyes
- loss of peripheral vision due to pituitary tumour compressing optic nerve

heart
- enlarged (predisposes to cardiomyopathy)

blood pressure
- 1 in 3 are hypertensive (predisposes to ischaemic heart disease)

bones
- predisposes to osteoarthritis owing to increased body size and altered bone structure

skin
- increased greasy sweating
- temperature intolerance

Fig. 15.3 Signs and symptoms of acromegaly (caused by excessive growth hormone secretion in adults). Usually occurs in 3rd–4th decade and is usually caused by pituitary adenomas of the somatotroph cells, but ectopic GH-producing tumours do occur.

low to test directly); e.g. the water deprivation test and the desmopressin test are used to check for ADH deficiency (see Chapter 14).
- Visual field assessment—to detect a possible pituitary tumour.
- MRI scan—to detect abnormal anatomy, e.g. a pituitary tumour (see Fig. 14.17).

Clinical manifestations take time to appear, therefore if one anterior pituitary hormone is found to be abnormally secreted, the other pituitary hormones are tested (by the combined pituitary test—see Chapter 14) to make sure that they are not insufficient or excessive.

Treatment and management of pituitary gland and hypothalamic disorders
The causes of pituitary and hypothalamic disorders are treated by:
- Surgery—e.g. surgical removal of pituitary adenoma; aspiration and excision of craniopharyngioma cyst capsule.
- Irradiation—e.g. postoperative irradiation of pituitary adenoma to prevent recurrence.
- Drug therapy—to treat infection, inhibit hormone secretion, and to shrink tumours; e.g. bromocriptine (dopamine agonist) inhibits prolactin secretion and shrinks prolactinomas.

Causes, effects, and symptoms and signs of diabetes insipidus and SIADH		
	Cranial diabetes insipidus	**SIADH**
causes	• commonest cause = idiopathic (20%) • other causes = traumatic, autoimmune, hypothalamic tumours (cf. nephrogenic diabetes insipidus—caused by the failure of the kidneys to respond to ADH)	• excessive secretion of ADH by the posterior pituitary due to drugs that stimulate ADH release, trauma, infections, and other endocrine disorders, e.g. adrenal insufficiency; • ectopic secretion of ADH, e.g. by bronchial carcinomas
effect	the body is unable to conserve body water because insufficient water is reabsorbed from the kidney tubule	retention of body water because excessive water is reabsorbed from the kidney tubule
symptoms and signs	thirst, polyuria, nocturia, weakness, apathy, postural hypotension, syncope, confusion, raised pulse	asymptomatic when mild but may cause headaches, apathy, vomiting, and may lead to coma and death; does not cause oedema

Fig. 15.4 Causes, effects, and symptoms and signs of cranial diabetes insipidus and SIADH.

Hormone abnormalities caused by pituitary and hypothalamic disorders are treated by:

- Hormone replacement (either of the deficient pituitary hormone or of the hormone that it normally stimulates)—e.g. GH deficiency is treated using GH replacement therapy (GH is now made using recombinant DNA techniques); ADH deficiency is treated using desmopressin (ADH analogue); ACTH deficiency is treated by administering hydrocortisone.
- Hormone suppression—e.g. GH excess is treated temporarily using octreotide (synthetic somatostatin) to reduce GH secretion.

- **Discuss the aetiology of pituitary and hypothalamus disorders.**
- **Describe the local and systemic effects caused by pituitary and hypothalamic hormone abnormalities.**
- **List the signs and symptoms of acromegaly.**
- **Review the diagnosis and treatment of pituitary and hypothalamus disorders.**

THYROID DISORDERS

Hyperthyroidism

Hyperthyroidism is the excessive secretion of thyroid hormones (T_3 and T_4) resulting from an overactive thyroid gland.

Aetiology of hyperthyroidism

The causes of hyperthyroidism are (in approximate order of frequency):

- Graves' disease—autoimmune disease of unknown cause. Autoantibodies of the IgG class are produced, and these bind to the thyroid epithelial cells and mimic the stimulatory action of TSH. These autoantibodies are known as long-acting thyroid stimulators (LATS) or as thyroid-stimulating antibodies (TsAb) and their effect on the thyroid can be described as a form of hypersensitivity reaction. LATS stimulate the activity and growth of the thyroid follicular epithelium, resulting in increased T_3 and T_4 release. This disease may occur at any age and is more common in women.
- Toxic multinodular goitre— small benign nodules within the thyroid gland. The cells within the nodules are unresponsive to secretory control mechanisms and secrete excess T_3 and T_4.
- Functioning adenoma—small, benign tumours of the thyroid gland. The tumour cells are unresponsive to secretory control mechanisms and secrete excess T_3

and T_4. However, not all adenomas (only 1%) secrete sufficient T_3 and T_4 to cause thyrotoxicosis.

- Thyrotoxicosis factitia—exogenous T_4 intake. This is caused by self-treatment with levothyroxine, e.g. for weight reduction.
- Other causes (rare)—include the toxic phase of subacute thyroiditis (symptoms subside spontaneously); TSH-secreting pituitary tumour; some cases of thyroid follicular carcinoma; certain drugs (e.g. amiodarone—an antiarrhythmic drug that contains 35% iodine).

Effects of hyperthyroidism

Hyperthyroidism causes the clinical syndrome thyrotoxicosis, the clinical symptoms and signs of which are listed in Fig. 4.10 and shown in Fig. 15.5.

Graves' disease causes the usual features of thyrotoxicosis plus the following:

- Exophthalmos (thyroid eye disease)—caused by specific autoantibodies that affect both the thyroid and the retro-orbital tissues, leading to infiltration of the orbital tissues by lymphocytic cells, which in turn causes protruding eyes (can lead to exposure keratitis and, less commonly now, blindness due to optic nerve compression, see Fig. 14.16).
- Diffuse goitre (enlarged thyroid gland).
- Pretibial myxoedema (thickening of the skin over the shins).
- Acropachy (similar to finger clubbing).

Thyrotoxic crisis ('thyroid storm') is the acute exacerbation of all the symptoms of thyrotoxicosis. This is a medical emergency and should be managed by administration of fluids, propranolol, carbimazole, Lugol's solution, and treatment of the underlying cause. It can occur after an acute infection or trauma, or after thyroid surgery (if the patient is not properly controlled preoperatively).

Diagnosis of hyperthyroidism

Thyroid function tests are used to demonstrate the presence and/or cause of thyroid overactivity. The excessive secretion of T_3 and T_4 is demonstrated by the measurement of serum TSH, free T_3, and free T_4 by radioimmunoassay (RIA). A suppressed TSH and elevated free T_3 and free T_4 establish the diagnosis of hyperthyroidism.

Radioisotope scanning (using easily measurable and non-thyrotoxic isotopes) is used to demonstrate the size of the thyroid gland and to visualize any abnormal

areas within it. The isotopes normally accumulate in the thyroid, but their distribution in an abnormal thyroid gland can aid diagnosis, e.g. in toxic multinodular goitre, the areas of hyperactivity accumulate more isotope and appear denser on the scan (so-called hot nodules). See Fig. 14.21.

Enzyme-linked immunosorbent assay (ELISA) or RIA is used in Graves' disease to demonstrate the presence of thyroid autoantibodies (LATS) in the serum.

Treatment and management of hyperthyroidism

Three effective methods of treatment are available:

- Surgery (partial thyroidectomy)—the majority of the gland is removed, leaving the parathyroids behind. Patients must be made euthyroid (normal blood levels of thyroid hormones) using Lugol's solution before surgery, as this reduces postoperative shock. Lugol's solution contains iodine in excess (5% I_2 + 10% KI), which inhibits T_3 and T_4 secretion and decreases the size and vascularity of the gland. More often than not, too much of the gland is removed and hormone replacement therapy with oral thyroxine daily is required for life to achieve normal levels of T_3 and T_4.
- Radioactive iodine therapy (using ^{131}I)—^{131}I is selectively taken up by the thyroid tissue (via the 'iodine-trap' mechanism) and damages the cells, leading to reduced T_3 and T_4 synthesis. The response is slow and supplementary antithyroid drugs may be required.
- Antithyroid drug therapy (e.g. thiouracil, carbimazole, methimazole)—these accumulate in the thyroid gland and reduce T_3 and T_4 secretion by inhibiting the peroxidase reactions of T_3 and T_4 synthesis (propylthiouracil also inhibits the peripheral deiodination of T_4 into its active form, T_3). The onset of action is delayed (3–4 weeks) until the preformed hormones are depleted (propranolol is administered to reduce the symptoms of thyrotoxicosis until hormone stores become depleted). These drugs may cause allergic reactions.

The choice of therapy varies according to the nature and severity of the illness, the response to previous therapies, and the preference of the hospital, e.g. in the USA radioactive iodine tends to be used; in Europe there is a preference for antithyroid drug therapy or surgery.

The prognosis depends on the aetiology of the thyrotoxicosis, e.g. Graves's disease—like many

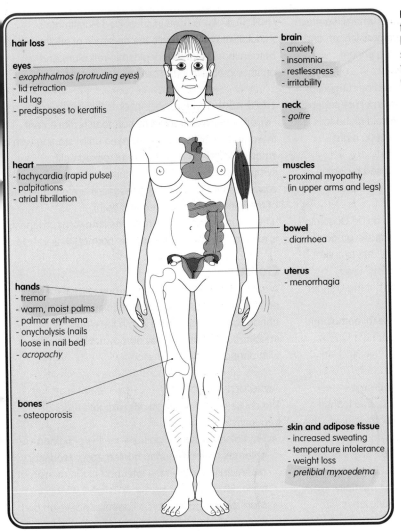

hair loss

eyes
- *exophthalmos (protruding eyes)*
- lid retraction
- lid lag
- predisposes to keratitis

heart
- tachycardia (rapid pulse)
- palpitations
- atrial fibrillation

hands
- tremor
- warm, moist palms
- palmar erythema
- onycholysis (nails
  loose in nail bed)
- *acropachy*

bones
- osteoporosis

brain
- anxiety
- insomnia
- restlessness
- irritability

neck
- *goitre*

muscles
- proximal myopathy
  (in upper arms and legs)

bowel
- diarrhoea

uterus
- menorrhagia

skin and adipose tissue
- increased sweating
- temperature intolerance
- weight loss
- *pretibial myxoedema*

Fig. 15.5 Symptoms and signs of thyrotoxicosis (caused by hyperthyroidism). The features shown in italics are exclusive to thyrotoxicosis that is caused by Graves' disease.

autoimmune diseases—remits and relapses and therefore patients require surveillance.

Hypothyroidism

Hypothyroidism is the insufficient secretion of T_3 and T_4 resulting from underactivity of the thyroid gland.

Aetiology of hypothyroidism

The causes of hypothyroidism are (in approximate order of frequency):

- Primary atrophic hypothyroidism and Hashimoto's thyroiditis—autoimmune diseases of unknown cause. The autoimmune reactions cause the gland to be infiltrated by lymphocytes and plasma cells, and colloid content is reduced. Initially, the autoimmune damage to the thyroid follicles may

cause the release of excessive T_3 and T_4, resulting in a transient phase of thyrotoxicosis (which is rarely recognized clinically), followed by a period of normal thyroid function (euthyroid), but later the thyroid gland becomes atrophic and fibroses, leading to hypothyroidism.

Hashimoto's thyroiditis causes a goitre, primary atrophic hypothroidism does not. Two autoimmune antibodies can be detected in most patients with Hashimoto's thyroiditis: one reacts with the endoplasmic reticulum of thyroid epithelial cells, the other with thyroglobulin.

These autoimmune diseases may occur at any age, but are more common in women aged 60–70 years.

- Iatrogenic hypothyroidism may result from previous treatment for thyrotoxicosis (e.g. partial

157

thyroidectomy or radioactive iodine) where too much thyroid tissue was removed/damaged; lithium and antithyroid drugs may also render a patient hypothyroid.

- Congenital hypothyroidism is caused by congenital agenesis of the thyroid gland (very rare) or congenital dyshormonogenesis where the thyroid gland fails to synthesise T_3 and T_4 (occurs in 1 in 4000 births).
- Other causes are rare but include:
  (A) dietary hypothyroidism (e.g. caused by iodine deficiency or the ingestion of goitrogens that suppress thyroid function);
  (B) subacute thyroiditis (also known as De Quervain's thyroiditis or granulomatous thyroiditis)—an acute inflammatory disorder of the thyroid due to a viral infection (initially causes thyrotoxicosis, fever, malaise, and soreness in the neck, but may render the patient hypothyroid);
  (C) hypothalamic or pituitary disease (hypothalamic TRH and/or pituitary TSH deficiency).

Effects of hypothyroidism
Hypothyroidism causes the clinical syndrome myxoedema, but this is rarely seen now due to the early recognition and treatment of hypothyroidism. The clinical symptoms and signs of hypothyroidism are listed in Fig. 4.10 and shown in Fig. 15.6.

Congenital hypothyroidism may result in defective brain development and the child will be mentally subnormal (cretinous), hence thyroid function is routinely screened a week after birth.

Many patients with hypothyroidism have minimal signs and are diagnosed only by chance, or because they feel generally unwell or they have noticed unexplained weight gain.

Severe hypothyroidism may cause myxoedema coma. This is a medical emergency and is managed by warming the patient, giving fluids, and intravenous injections of T_3 and hydrocortisone.

Diagnosis of hypothyroidism
Thyroid function tests are used to demonstrate the presence and/or cause of thyroid underactivity. The insufficient secretion of T_3 and T_4 is demonstrated by the measurement of serum TSH, free T_3, and free T_4 by RIA. An elevated TSH and low free T_3 and free T_4 establish the diagnosis of hypothyroidism (TSH may be low if hypothyroidism is caused by a pituitary disorder, but this is very rare).

ELISA or RIA is used in suspected Hashimoto's thyroiditis to demonstrate the presence of antithyroid autoantibodies (anti-endoplasmic-reticulum and antithyroglobulin) in the serum.

Treatment and management of hypothyroidism
Hypothyroidism is treated by hormone replacement therapy—levothyroxine (T_4) is taken daily, starting with a small dose, which is gradually increased until symptoms subside and TSH returns to normal. T_4 is converted into T_3 in the body tissues, therefore only one of the hormones is required (not both).

With appropriate treatment, the long-term prognosis is excellent and life expectancy is normal.

Goitre
A goitre is a swelling of the neck due to generalized enlargement of the thyroid gland (diffuse goitre) or an abnormally enlarged area within the gland (multinodular goitre). It may or may not be associated with abnormal thyroid function.

Aetiology of goitre
The causes of goitre are (in approximate order of frequency):
- Physiological (simple goitre)—the thyroid gland enlarges normally during adolescence, pregnancy, and lactation, and in the later part of the menstrual cycle.
- Multinodular goitre—cysts commonly develop and may distend so that they become palpable lumps within the thyroid gland. Cysts are not painful but are often removed for cosmetic reasons or to ensure they are not due to tumour growth.
- Dietary (rare)—the thyroid gland enlarges during iodine deficiency and after ingestion of goitrogens in the diet (e.g. cabbage, cassava, and cow's milk). Early this century, goitre caused by iodine deficiency was endemic in Derbyshire ('Derbyshire neck') due to the population living off food grown in iodine-depleted soils. Lack of iodine and/or suppression of thyroid function by goitrogens causes a decrease in T_3 and T_4 synthesis and hence a decrease in their secretion. The pituitary responds to the low circulating T_3 and T_4 levels by releasing increased amounts of TSH (TSH causes thyroid hyperplasia).
- Other causes include:
  (A) congenital dyshormonogenesis (thyroid gland fails to synthesize T_3 and T_4);

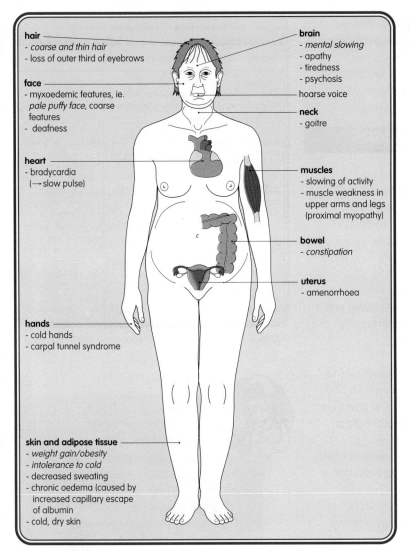

Fig. 15.6 Symptoms and signs of hypothyroidism. The most common symptoms are shown in italics.

hair
- *coarse and thin hair*
- loss of outer third of eyebrows

face
- myxoedemic features, ie.
  pale puffy face, coarse
  features
- deafness

heart
- bradycardia
  (→ slow pulse)

hands
- cold hands
- carpal tunnel syndrome

skin and adipose tissue
- *weight gain/obesity*
- *intolerance to cold*
- decreased sweating
- chronic oedema (caused by
  increased capillary escape
  of albumin
- cold, dry skin

brain
- *mental slowing*
- apathy
- tiredness
- psychosis

hoarse voice

neck
- goitre

muscles
- slowing of activity
- muscle weakness in
  upper arms and legs
  (proximal myopathy)

bowel
- *constipation*

uterus
- amenorrhoea

(B) autoimmune diseases (e.g. Graves' disease and Hashimoto's thyroiditis)—often cause goitres due to inflammation, lymphocytic infiltration, and hyperplasia of thyroid gland;

(C) viral infection (e.g. De Quervain's thyroiditis)—causes the thyroid gland to enlarge and become hard and painful;

(D) TSH-secreting pituitary tumour (very rare);

(E) neoplasms (benign or malignant tumours)—often present as solitary thyroid masses.

Treatment and management of goitre
It is important to treat both the cause and any associated symptoms (e.g. hyperthyroidism or hypothyroidism).

Treatment may involve the surgical removal of the thyroid gland for cosmetic reasons or, to remove neoplastic tissue, or to prevent compression of adjacent structures (e.g. with a retrosternal goitre).

Neoplasia of the thyroid
Tumours in the thyroid are usually benign follicular adenomas, which present as a solitary thyroid nodule that only very rarely causes thyrotoxicosis (if they do synthesize excess T_3 and T_4, they appear as 'hot' nodules on radioisotope scans).

Primary malignant thyroid tumours (carcinomas) and tumours of lymphoid tissue within the thyroid gland (lymphomas) are very rare and are usually associated with radiation exposure (secondary metastatic carcinomas occur in the thyroid because of its high blood supply). The different types of primary malignant thyroid tumours are listed in Fig. 15.7.

Treatment for tumours comprises surgical removal and/or radioactive iodine therapy.

PARATHYROID DISORDERS

Hyperparathyroidism

Hyperparathyroidism is the excessive secretion of parathyroid hormone (PTH) from the parathyroid gland(s), and usually results in hypercalcaemia.

Aetiology of hyperparathyroidism

Primary hyperparathyroidism

This is the inappropriate hypersecretion of PTH (in relation to the prevailing plasma calcium levels) and is one of the most common endocrine disorders (incidence is approximately 1 in 1000).

The commonest cause of primary hyperparathyroidism is parathyroid adenoma (80%); other causes comprise parathyroid hyperplasia (20%) and carcinoma (<1%). Approximately 5% of cases are inherited, including those associated with multiple endocrine neoplasia (MEN) syndromes.

It occurs more commonly after the age of 45 years and in postmenopausal women (female:male ratio = 2:1).

It may remain asymptomatic for many years, but usually presents with symptoms of hypercalcaemia.

Secondary hyperparathyroidism

This is the appropriate hypersecretion of PTH in response to persistent hypocalcaemia.

Persistent hypocalcaemia can be caused by calcium malabsorption (due to a deficiency of vitamin D) or by renal failure (due to the failure of vitamin D hydroxylation by the kidney).

Secondary hyperparathyroidism caused by renal failure is also known as renal osteodystrophy.

Secondary hyperparathyroidism does not cause hypercalcaemia.

Tertiary hyperparathyroidism

This is the continued hypersecretion of PTH after hypocalcaemia has been corrected.

The parathyroid glands may become autonomous after longstanding secondary hyperparathyroidism, and

Four types of primary malignant thyroid tumours		
Tumour	**Behaviour**	**Prognosis**
papillary adenocarcinoma (most common type)	slow-growing, well-differentiated tumour; often curable	excellent—5-year survival rate is 95%
follicular adenocarcinoma	often metastasize to lung and bone	poor—5-year survival rate is 70%
anaplastic carcinoma (rare, occur more often in the elderly and in females)	aggressive, undifferentiated tumour that spreads locally; effectively incurable	very poor—5-year survival is 10% (often invades trachea ⟶ respiratory obstruction)
medullary carcinoma (rare tumours of the parafollicular C cells) —can arise as part of familial MEN II syndrome	very slow-growing, locally invasive tumours that secrete excess calcitonin (may also secrete ACTH and serotonin)	variable, tend to recur—5-year survival is 80% (familial cases tend to be more aggressive)

Fig. 15.7 Four types of primary malignant thyroid tumours.

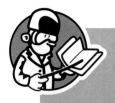

- **Summarize the causes, effects, diagnostic methods, and treatment of hyperthyroidism and hypothyroidism.**
- **Discuss the aetiology and treatment of goitres.**
- **Describe the types of benign and malignant thyroid neoplasias.**

even when calcium levels have returned to normal, they continue to secrete high levels of PTH, resulting in hypercalcaemia.

Effects of hyperparathyroidism

Excessive PTH secretion may remain asymptomatic for many years, but it tends to cause characteristic bone features—seen on X-ray—due to bone resorption (bone features are not always present and probably reflect disease duration and severity).

Primary and tertiary hyperparathyroidism cause hypercalcaemia, but the disease is slowly progressive, hence relatively high levels of plasma calcium can be tolerated with few symptoms.

The symptoms and signs of hypercalcaemia are listed in Chapter 8 and shown in Fig. 15.8.

Diagnosis of hyperparathyroidism
Primary hyperparathyroidism is diagnosed from:
- The presence of symptoms of hypercalcaemia.
- Abnormally high plasma calcium levels and low plasma phosphate levels.
- Abnormally high plasma PTH levels (measured by RIA).
- The abnormal appearance of the bones on chest, skull, and pelvic X-rays (rarely seen now due to the earlier detection of hyperparathyroidism).

- Isotope scans of the parathyroid glands (may be useful in localizing tumours).

Treatment and management of hyperparathyroidism
Primary and tertiary hyperparathyroidism are treated surgically (parathyroidectomy), medically (with drugs, e.g. calcitonin, bisphophonates), or managed conservatively (i.e. patients are advised to restrict their calcium intake and increase oral fluids), depending on the cause and extent of the disorder.

After surgery, calcium supplements may be required, and the underlying cause of tertiary hyperparathyroidism needs to be treated in order to prevent recurrence.

Secondary hyperparathyroidism is corrected by

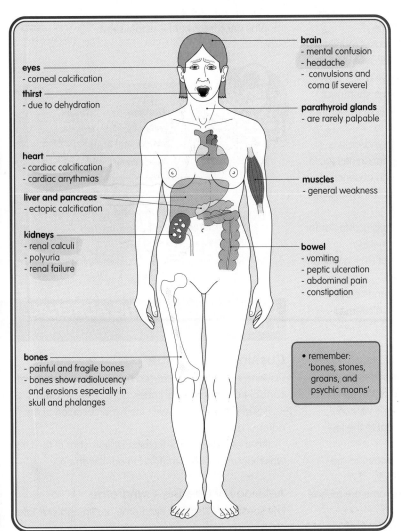

Fig. 15.8 Symptoms and signs of hypercalcaemia.

brain
- mental confusion
- headache
- convulsions and coma (if severe)

eyes
- corneal calcification

thirst
- due to dehydration

parathyroid glands
- are rarely palpable

heart
- cardiac calcification
- cardiac arrythmias

muscles
- general weakness

liver and pancreas
- ectopic calcification

kidneys
- renal calculi
- polyuria
- renal failure

bowel
- vomiting
- peptic ulceration
- abdominal pain
- constipation

bones
- painful and fragile bones
- bones show radiolucency and erosions especially in skull and phalanges

- remember: 'bones, stones, groans, and psychic moans'

treating the underlying cause, e.g. giving vitamin D supplements such as Alfacalcidol.

Hypoparathyroidism

Hypoparathyroidism is the insufficient secretion of PTH from the parathyroid gland(s), resulting in hypocalcaemia.

Aetiology of hypoparathyroidism

The causes of hypoparathyroidism are (in approximate order of frequency).

- Iatrogenic—caused by surgical removal/damage to the parathyroid glands during thyroidectomy or during surgery to correct hyperparathyroidism.
- Idiopathic—autoimmune disease of unknown cause produced by the destruction of the parathyroid cells by an autoantibody. It is associated with other organ-specific autoimmune diseases, e.g. 50% of cases form part of the HAM syndrome (hypoparathyroidism, Addison's disease, moniliasis).
- Inherited (pseudoparathyroidism)—tissues do not respond to PTH. Affected people have a characteristic short, round face, with a short neck and short metacarpals. They have hypocalcaemia but levels of PTH are high.
- Congenital deficiency—DiGeorge's syndrome is where the third and fourth pharyngeal arches fail to develop in the embryo, resulting in an absence of the thymus and parathyroid glands. The syndrome arises sporadically and is very rare.
- Magnesium depletion—magnesium is a cofactor for some actions of PTH, therefore magnesium depletion causes decreased action of PTH, although levels of PTH are normal or elevated.
- Neonatal—the foetal parathyroid glands can be suppressed if the mother has hypercalcaemia.

Effects of hypoparathyroidism

Insufficient PTH secretion causes symptoms of hypocalcaemia. However, these are surprisingly few, considering the levels of hypocalcaemia that can be reached, because the condition develops very gradually, so the body has time to adapt to the low levels of calcium.

The symptoms and signs of hypocalcaemia are listed in Chapter 8 and shown in Fig. 15.9.

The most commonly reported symptoms are muscle cramps, paraesthesia, and tetany.

Diagnosis of hypoparathyroidism

Hypoparathyroidism is diagnosed from:

- Symptoms of hypocalcaemia (suggest hypoparathyroidism as a differential diagnosis).
- Abnormally low plasma calcium levels and high plasma phosphate levels.
- Inappropriately low or absent plasma PTH levels (measured by RIA).

Treatment and management of hypoparathyroidism

Hormone replacement therapy is not available.

The aim of the treatment is to compensate for the lack of PTH by giving calcium and vitamin D supplements (e.g. Alfacalcidol) to increase calcium absorption from the gut and combat the hypocalcaemia.

Plasma calcium levels should be monitored every 6 months once treatment is established.

- **Discuss the causes, effects, diagnostic methods, and treatment of hyperparathyroidism and hypoparathyroidism.**
- **List the signs and symptoms of hypercalcaemia and hypocalcaemia.**

DISORDERS OF THE ADRENAL CORTEX

Cushing's syndrome

Cushing's syndrome is caused by the hypersecretion of cortisol from the adrenal cortex.

It is often associated with the hypersecretion of the adrenal androgens.

It is a rare disorder (<5 cases/million/year in the UK) which occurs more commonly in adult women.

Aetiology of Cushing's syndrome

The causes of Cushing's syndrome are (in approximate order of frequency):

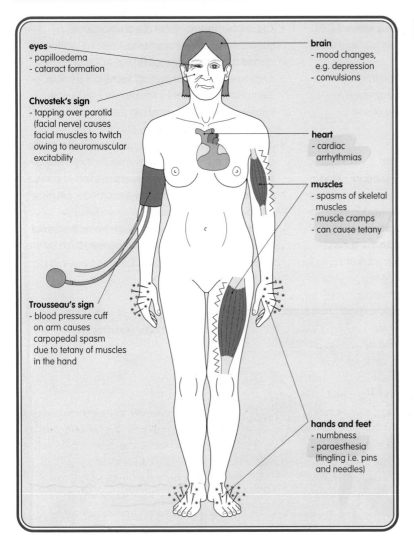

Fig. 15.9 Symptoms and signs of hypocalcaemia.

eyes
- papilloedema
- cataract formation

Chvostek's sign
- tapping over parotid (facial nerve) causes facial muscles to twitch owing to neuromuscular excitability

Trousseau's sign
- blood pressure cuff on arm causes carpopedal spasm due to tetany of muscles in the hand

brain
- mood changes, e.g. depression
- convulsions

heart
- cardiac arrhythmias

muscles
- spasms of skeletal muscles
- muscle cramps
- can cause tetany

hands and feet
- numbness
- paraesthesia (tingling i.e. pins and needles)

- Hypersecretion of ACTH from the anterior pituitary gland (Cushing's disease)—ACTH stimulates the adrenal cortex to secrete cortisol, therefore excess ACTH leads to bilateral adrenal cortical hyperplasia and excessive secretion of cortisol. This is the commonest cause in adults (75% of cases of Cushing's; see Fig. 15.2).
- Adrenal cortical tumour—tumour (adenoma or carcinoma) secretes excess cortisol inappropriately. This is the commonest cause in children and the cause in 10% of adults.
- Iatrogenic—excessive administration of exogenous ACTH or cortisol, given for medical reasons, causes Cushing's syndrome. Corticosteroids are used in the long-term treatment of many chronic diseases (e.g. inflammatory bowel disease, rheumatoid arthritis)—

doses must be monitored to prevent the occurence of cushingoid symptoms.
- Hypersecretion of ACTH from non-pituitary tissue (very rare)—e.g. from some oat cell bronchial carcinomas or from some tumours of the thymus, pancreas, or ovary. These types are called ectopic ACTH syndromes and involve the secretion of very high levels of ACTH.

Effects of Cushing's syndrome

The effects of excess cortisol are listed in Fig. 5.10 and shown in Fig. 15.10.

The main features include obesity, hirsuitism, hypertension, diabetes, and osteoporosis.

In children, excess cortisol also causes growth retardation.

If Cushing's syndrome is caused by excessive ACTH secretion, then there is also hyperpigmentation of the skin and mucous membranes.

The increased secretion of adrenal androgens associated with Cushing's syndrome may result in hirsutism or male pattern baldness, and cause menstrual irregularities.

Diagnosis of Cushing's syndrome

Laboratory tests are used to determine adrenal gland function, including:

- Measurement of cortisol levels in the blood and urine—levels are inappropriately high in Cushing's syndrome and diurnal variation in plasma cortisol levels is lost. The 24-hour urinary excretion of cortisol is measured (normal is <700 nmol/24 h).

- The overnight (low-dose) dexamethasone suppression test—dexamethasone is a synthetic steroid that normally suppresses ACTH and CRH secretion, and hence cortisol secretion. If it fails to suppress cortisol levels, the patient has Cushing's syndrome (does not ascertain the cause of excess cortisol secretion).

- Measurement of ACTH—required to determine the cause of the Cushing's syndrome. It differentiates between primary adrenal hypersecretion of cortisol and ACTH hypersecretion (by the anterior pituitary gland or ectopic tumours).

  ACTH is low/undetectable in patients with adrenal cortical tumours, as excess cortisol secretion by the adrenal tumours feeds back on the pituitary to decrease ACTH release.

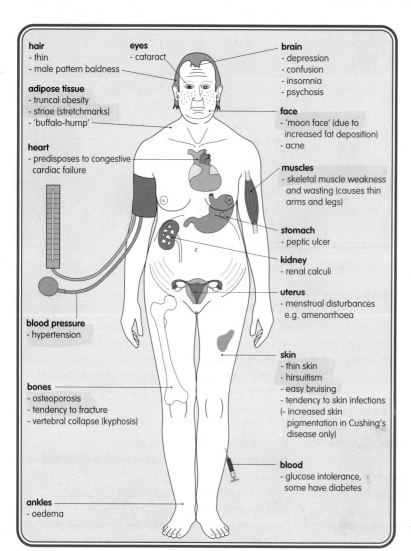

Fig. 15.10 Symptoms and signs of Cushing's syndrome.

hair
- thin
- male pattern baldness

eyes
- cataract

adipose tissue
- truncal obesity
- striae (stretchmarks)
- 'buffalo-hump'

heart
- predisposes to congestive cardiac failure

blood pressure
- hypertension

bones
- osteoporosis
- tendency to fracture
- vertebral collapse (kyphosis)

ankles
- oedema

brain
- depression
- confusion
- insomnia
- psychosis

face
- 'moon face' (due to increased fat deposition)
- acne

muscles
- skeletal muscle weakness and wasting (causes thin arms and legs)

stomach
- peptic ulcer

kidney
- renal calculi

uterus
- menstrual disturbances e.g. amenorrhoea

skin
- thin skin
- hirsuitism
- easy bruising
- tendency to skin infections
(- increased skin pigmentation in Cushing's disease only)

blood
- glucose intolerance, some have diabetes

ACTH is high in patients with ACTH-secreting pituitary tumours, and ACTH hypersecretion causes the adrenal glands to secrete excess cortisol. ACTH is very high in patients with ectopic ACTH-secreting tumours.

- The high-dose dexamethasone suppression test— required to differentiate between pituitary disease and ectopic tumours. If high-dose dexamethasone suppresses cortisol, the patient has pituitary disease.

Treatment and management of Cushing's syndrome

If the disorder is due to a primary change in the adrenals, the treatment is removal of the abnormal adrenal tissue. After bilateral adrenalectomy, patients will require exogenous cortisol replacement.

If the disorder is due to overstimulation of the adrenals by excess ACTH secreted by a pituitary tumour, the treatment is surgical removal or irradiation of the pituitary.

Treatment of Cushing's syndrome caused by an ectopic ACTH-secreting tumour, such as some bronchial carcinomas, involves the surgical removal or irradiation of the tumour.

Patients with inoperable malignant disease causing Cushing's syndrome or those with residual cortisol excess after an operation can be treated with metyrapone, a drug that interferes with the biosynthesis of steroid hormones.

Prognosis depends on the aetiology of the Cushing's syndrome. For untreated Cushing's syndrome, the 5-year survival is 50%.

Hyperaldosteronism

Hyperaldosteronism is caused by the hypersecretion of aldosterone from the adrenal cortex.

Aetiology of hyperaldosteronism

Primary hyperaldosteronism (Conn's syndrome)
In primary hyperaldosteronism, aldosterone is high and renin is low.

It is caused by generalized hyperplasia or adenoma of the zona glomerulosa which secrete excess aldosterone inappropriately, i.e, control of secretion is lost.

Carcinoma of the zona glomerulosa is extremely rare.

Secondary hyperaldosteronism
In secondary hyperaldosteronism, both aldosterone and renin are high.

This is the most common cause of hyperaldosteronism. It is caused by excess renin secretion by the kidney (primary hyperreninaemia):

- The renin–angiotensin system is stimulated owing to reduced glomerular perfusion (e.g. due to narrowing of the renal arteries or due to reduced blood volume).
- Renin stimulates aldosterone secretion from the zona glomerulosa in an attempt to correct this reduced perfusion.
- Aldosterone secretion is raised but appropriate in relation to the renin levels.

Effects of hyperaldosteronism
The effects of excess aldosterone are listed in Fig. 5.12.

It results in systemic hypertension associated with potassium depletion and alkalosis.

The patient often complains of polyuria and muscle weakness, and might have cramps and spasms, especially of the hands (carpopedal spasm).

There is no oedema.

Diagnosis of hyperaldosteronism
Conn's syndrome is suspected from the symptoms and from hypokalaemia. It is confirmed by demonstrating a high plasma or urinary aldosterone in association with suppressed renin.

Secondary hyperaldosteronism is demonstrated by raised aldosterone and renin levels.

Treatment and management of hyperaldosteronism
Spironolactone, an aldosterone antagonist, is used to treat hyperaldosteronism where there is bilateral zona glomerulosa hyperplasia.

Unilateral adrenalectomy is the choice treatment for adrenal adenoma (or rarely carcinoma).

Hyperandrogenism

Hyperandrogenism is caused by the hypersecretion of adrenal androgens from the adrenal cortex.

Aetiology of hyperandrogenism
The causes of hyperandrogenism are:

- Adrenal cortical tumours—some adrenal cortical tumours secrete excess adrenal androgens, e.g. in Cushing's syndrome both cortisol and adrenal androgens are usually secreted in excess.
- Congenital adrenal hyperplasia—inherited defect of steroid synthesis in the adrenal glands. This is

usually due to a deficiency of 21-hydroxylase, which results in the failure to make cortisol and aldosterone. The adrenals cannot synthesize cortisol and aldosterone, but in their attempt to do so they make excess androgens. Failure of cortisol production leads to increased ACTH secretion, resulting in hyperplasia of the adrenal cortex and pigmentation of the skin.

Effects of hyperandrogenism
Hyperandrogenism causes virilization/masculinization of females and precocious puberty in males.

Virilization is characterized by temporal balding, a male body form, muscle bulk, deepening of the voice, enlargement of the clitoris, and hirsutism.

Congenital adrenal hyperplasia also causes symptoms of cortisol and aldosterone deficiency (see Figs. 5.10, 5.12 and 15.11).

Deficiency of 21-hydroxylase is dangerous because aldosterone deficiency causes life-threatening salt loss unless replacement therapy is given.

Diagnosis of hyperandrogenism
Laboratory findings include elevation of plasma ACTH, androgens, and excretory products of adrenal androgens (pregananetriol) in the urine.

Treatment and management of hyperandrogenism
Oestrogen therapy reduces the effects of the circulating androgens by increasing serum sex-hormone-binding globulins.

Cosmetic treatment (depilation or bleaching of the hair) can reduce signs of hirsutism.

In 21-hydroxylase deficiency, corticosteroid (e.g. hydrocortisone) and mineralocorticoid (e.g. fludrocortisone) treatments are required.

Adrenal insufficiency
Adrenal insufficiency results in the hyposecretion of cortisol, aldosterone, and adrenal androgens from the adrenal cortex.

Aetiology of adrenal insufficiency
Adrenal insufficiency can be due to:
- Addison's disease—chronic insufficiency of the adrenal cortex, which can be caused by autoimmune disease, tuberculosis infection, secondary tumours of the cortex, sarcoidosis, and amyloidosis. Autoimmune destruction of the cortex is associated with other 'organ-specific' autoimmune diseases, e.g. pernicious anaemia, Hashimoto's thyroiditis, insulin-dependent diabetes mellitus, and hypoparathyroidism. The adrenal cortex becomes infiltrated by lymphocytes and atrophies. It causes a combined lack of cortisol and aldosterone.
- Waterhouse–Friderichsen syndrome—acute insufficiency of the adrenal cortex caused by acute haemorrhagic necrosis of the adrenals due to meningococcal septicaemia. It causes a combined lack of cortisol and aldosterone.
- Pituitary ACTH deficiency—lack of ACTH leads to decreased secretion of cortisol but normal aldosterone.
- Iatrogenic—treatment for Cushing's syndrome (e.g. bilateral adrenalectomy or excessive metyrapone therapy) may cause adrenal insufficiency. Prolonged steroid therapy can also lead to adrenal atrophy and adrenal insufficiency once treatment is stopped.
- Congenital adrenal hyperplasia (see under 'Hyperandrogenism').

Effects of adrenal insufficiency
The clinical effects of adrenal insufficiency are due to the lack of cortisol and aldosterone. The effects of cortisol and aldosterone deficiency are listed in Figs 5.10 and 5.12 and shown in Fig. 5.11.

The main features include weight loss, lethargy, abdominal pain, postural hypotension, pigmentation, hyperkalaemia, and hyponatraemia.

Symptoms of adrenal insufficiency tend to be insidious in onset, but patients can present in an acute Addisonian crisis.

An Addisonian crisis is precipitated by minor illnesses, trauma, and surgery, and causes vomiting, fluid loss, electrolyte disturbances, and circulatory collapse (shock).

Emergency treatment of an Addisonian crisis consists of giving intravenous saline (to replace salt deficiency) and hydrocortisone.

Diagnosis of adrenal insufficiency
Adrenal insufficiency can be diagnosed by the following:
- Blood chemistry—shows hyperkalaemia, hyponatraemia, uraemia, and mild acidosis (hypercalcaemia and eosinophilia are rare).
- Measurement of ACTH, cortisol, and aldosterone—plasma cortisol and aldosterone are low; plasma ACTH is raised in primary adrenal insufficiency.
- The short Synacthen test—Synacthen is a synthetic analogue of ACTH and hence stimulates cortisol

secretion from a normal adrenal gland. If it fails to stimulate cortisol secretion, the patient has adrenal insufficiency (confirm with the prolonged Synacthen test).

- The prolonged Synacthen test—similar to the short Synacthen test but a higher dose is administered and it is repeated for 3 successive days. Primary adrenal insufficiency is diagnosed if, after the last injection, the plasma cortisol is not increased as much as expected. If the adrenal insufficiency is secondary to pituitary ACTH deficiency, there is an increase in plasma cortisol with prolonged Synacthen stimulation.
- The hypoglycaemia stress test—administration of insulin induces hypoglycaemia, which leads to increased CRH secretion by the hypothalamus (CRH stimulates ACTH and hence cortisol secretion). If the plasma cortisol levels fail to increase, in the presence of a normal response to ACTH (Synacthen) administration, then secondary adrenal insufficiency (pituitary ACTH deficiency) is diagnosed.

Treatment and management of adrenal insufficiency

Long-term management requires hormone replacement therapy, i.e. deficient hormones are replaced by synthetic hormones that have the same actions as cortisol and aldosterone—hydrocortisone (a corticosteroid) and fludrocortisone (a mineralocorticoid) are taken in tablet form daily. Aldosterone is not always deficient in adrenal insufficiency, therefore fludrocortisone does not always have to be administered.

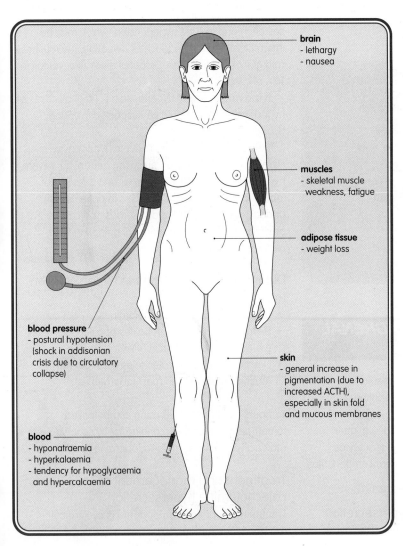

Fig. 15.11 Symptoms and signs of adrenal insufficiency.

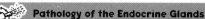
The dose of the hormone is adjusted according to the clinical effects, so the correct amount for the individual patient is achieved.

The patient must be educated about the dangers of abruptly discontinuing hydrocortisone treatment (Addisonian crisis) and how the dose should be increased during intercurrent illness.

Life span is normal if the condition is treated.

Non-functional adrenocortical neoplasias
Non-functional adenomas are found in about 2% of adult autopsies. These tumours do not secrete hormones and therefore do not cause systemic symptoms.

Adrenal cortical carcinoma is a rare tumour that does not tend to be hormone-secreting, although some have been found to secrete adrenal androgens. They are usually large and invasive.

- **List the symptoms and signs of Cushing's syndrome.**
- **How is Cushing's syndrome caused and how should it be managed?**
- **Outline the causes, effects, diagnostic methods and treatment of hyperaldosteronism, hyperandrogenism, and adrenal insufficiency.**

DISORDERS OF THE ADRENAL MEDULLA

Hyperfunction of the adrenal medulla results in hypersecretion of catecholamines (adrenaline, noradrenaline, and dopamine).

Hypofunction of the adrenal medulla (e.g. after adrenal atrophy) causes no clinical consequences because the sympathetic nervous system compensates for catecholamine deficiency.

Aetiology of catecholamine hypersecretion
Catecholamine hypersecretion can be caused by:

- Phaeochromocytomas.
- Neuroblastomas and ganglioneuromas—both very rare.

A phaeochromocytoma is a catecholamine-secreting tumour derived from adrenal medullary chromaffin cells:
- 10% are malignant
- 10% are multiple
- 10% are extra-adrenal.

Phaeochromocytomas are often bilateral (70%) and are found more commonly in middle-aged women. They may be familial and associated with other endocrine tumours [e.g. multiple endocrine neoplasia (MEN) syndrome types II and III].

Effects of catecholamine hypersecretion
Symptoms and signs are due to excess catecholamine secretion and include hypertension (which may be intermittent), pallor, headaches, sweating, nervousness, and glucose intolerance. Diabetes mellitus develops in 10% of cases.

It is a rare cause of hypertension (<1% of all cases of hypertension), but should be suspected in young hypertensive patients.

Patients can present in an acute hypertensive crisis (symptoms include pallor, pulsating headache, severe hypertension of >200/120 mmHg, and a feeling of 'about to die'). Hypertensive crises in patients with phaeochromocytoma are dangerous and can be precipitated by stress, abdominal palpation, and general anaesthesia.

Diagnosis of catecholamine hypersecretion
Laboratory findings include:
- Elevation of urinary catecholamines.
- Elevation of urinary metabolites of catecholamines, e.g. vanillylmandelic acid (VMA).
- Elevation of plasma catecholamines (but not routinely measured in most laboratories).

Tumours can be localized using computerized tomography (CT) or MRI scanning, or by scanning with radioactively labelled meta-iodobenzylguanidine (mIBG).

Treatment and management of catecholamine hypersecretion
Treatment of phaeochromocytoma is by surgical excision of the tumour.

Prior to surgery it is necessary to block the actions of the catecholamines by administering an α-blocker (phenoxybenzamine) and a β-blocker (propranolol) for 3 days.

After surgery, urinary catecholamine levels are measured for 24 hours and blood pressure is monitored (risk of hypotension).

Life span is normal if the condition is treated.

○ **What effects do haeochromocytomas cause and how are they treated?**

DISORDERS OF THE ENDOCRINE PANCREAS

Diabetes mellitus

Diabetes mellitus is a disorder caused by the lack (relative or absolute) or diminished effectiveness of endogenous insulin.

It is characterized by a chronically raised blood glucose level (hyperglycaemia) and abnormalities in fat and protein metabolism.

It is a common disease with a prevalence of about 2% in Europe, 6% in the USA (depends on ethnic groups), and higher in isolated populations (e.g. 35% in the Pima Indians of Arizona).

Aetiology of diabetes mellitus

Type 1 diabetes mellitus (insulin-dependent diabetes mellitus—IDDM)

This usually has a juvenile onset (childhood or early adult life).

Onset is rapid (weeks or days).

It is caused by total or near-total insulin deficiency.

Insulin deficiency results from the destruction of pancreatic β cells, caused by 'organ-specific' autoimmune disease (islet cell antibodies are present in 85% of cases at the time of diagnosis). The cause of the autoimmune disease is usually idiopathic, but can be secondary to viral infections of the pancreas and to toxins (e.g. the rat poison Vacor).

There is a strong genetic link to the human leucocyte antigen (HLA) haplotypes DR3 and DR4—there is a 50% concordance in identical twins and a positive family history in 10% of patients.

It may be associated with other autoimmune diseases (e.g. Hashimoto's thyroiditis, Graves' disease, Addison's disease, pernicious anaemia).

Patients require insulin replacement therapy.

If they are not treated, patients will die from ketoacidosis.

Type 2 diabetes mellitus (non-insulin-dependent diabetes mellitus—NIDDM)

This usually has a late onset (in middle/old age) and is often associated with obesity (70–80% of cases).

Onset is insidious (years).

It is caused by impaired insulin secretion from the pancreas and/or insulin resistance in the tissues, i.e. the body cells fail to respond to insulin.

Impaired insulin secretion from the pancreas may be due to the accumulation of amyloid peptide in the pancreas that is seen in some cases of type 2 diabetes.

Peripheral resistance to insulin is thought to be a post-receptor malfunction, but the mechanism is unknown.

Genetic factors are important, although there is no HLA link—there is almost a 100% concordance in identical twins and a positive family history in 30% of patients.

Patients must lose weight and watch their diet (reduce intake of readily assimilable sugars and saturated fats, and increase intake of fibre).

Patients do not usually require insulin but those not controlled by diet need to take oral hypoglycaemic agents (e.g. sulphonylureas, metformin, acarbose), which increase the secretion of insulin or potentiate its actions.

Patients are not prone to ketoacidosis unless they become very ill from infection or vascular event.

Maturity-onset diabetes of young people (MODY)

This is type 2 diabetes mellitus that occurs in young people.

The family history is often positive and it seems to be inherited as an autosomal dominant condition with incomplete penetrance.

Gestational diabetes mellitus (GDM)

This is diabetes during pregnancy.

There is an increased risk of miscarriage and maternal morbidity, but this is decreased by tight control of blood glucose levels during pregnancy.

Babies born to mothers with GDM tend to be large but developmentally immature.

About 70% of women with GDM will revert back to normal glucose tolerance postpartum; the rest will remain diabetic or have impaired glucose tolerance.

Approximately 75% of women who develop GDM will develop type 2 diabetes as they age, although this risk is also associated with obesity.

Secondary diabetes mellitus

This is diabetes mellitus secondary to conditions that cause insulin resistance (e.g. acromegaly, Cushing's syndrome, phaeochromocytoma).

Malnutrition-related diabetes mellitus (tropical diabetes mellitus)

This usually occurs in adolescents with a history of severe malnutrition and is more common in the developing world.

Other pancreatic diseases causing diabetes mellitus

Diabetes mellitus can also be caused by:
- Acute pancreatitis (may result in diabetes temporarily).
- Pancreatectomy (e.g. to remove pancreatic cancer).
- Haemochromatosis (rare congenital disorder of iron metabolism)—causes iron to be deposited in various organs, including the skin and pancreas. The iron deposits disrupt pancreatic function, leading to diabetes mellitus (called bronze diabetes due to the associated brown pigmentation of the skin).
- Glucagonomas (rare tumour of islet α cells).

Impaired glucose tolerance syndrome

This has a uncertain clinical significance.

Only about 4% of cases per year develop frank diabetes (usually type 2 diabetes).

Patients may have an increased risk of developing chronic complications associated with diabetes (e.g. nephropathy, atherolsclerosis).

Management includes loss of weight and exercise.

Effects of diabetes mellitus

Insulin promotes anabolic processes in the body (i.e. increases cell uptake and storage of nutrients)—this means that in insulin deficiency catabolic processes prevail (i.e. stores are broken down and cells are less able to take up nutrients).

Diabetes mellitus causes:
- A raised blood glucose (hyperglycaemia)—dietary glucose cannot be taken up or utilized by the body cells when insulin is deficient, and the liver responds to low

intracellular glucose levels by producing and releasing more glucose (gluconeogenesis).
- Increased breakdown of protein (proteolysis) and decreased protein synthesis, especially in muscle.
- Increased breakdown of fats (lipolysis) in adipose tissue.

Glucose is needed by the body cells as a fuel, therefore when the cells do not get enough glucose the body responds by increasing the breakdown of energy stores (fats, protein, and glycogen). The liver uses the breakdown products (fatty acids and amino acids) to synthesize glucose and ketones, which can be used by the body cells to provide energy. Hence, energy stores are utilized, resulting in weight loss.

Similar processes occur during starvation, to increase blood glucose and ketones; however, in diabetes, the blood glucose is elevated because the body cells are unable to use glucose in the absence of insulin.

The acute symptoms and signs of diabetes mellitus (types 1 and 2) are shown in Fig. 15.12. The main features are polyuria, polydipsia, tiredness, weakness, and recurrent infections.

Patients may present in a diabetic coma (occurs in less than 50% of diabetic patients). This is caused by dehydration, hyperglycaemia, and ketoacidosis (increased levels of ketones in the blood causes the acidosis). This can occur at any time because of withdrawal of adequate insulin therapy or because of an intercurrent illness.

Treatment of ketoacidosis involves administration of fluids, insulin therapy, and careful monitoring of the plasma potassium levels (plasma potassium falls in response to insulin).

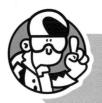

Think of diabetes mellitus as 'starvation in the midst of plenty'.

Chronic complications of diabetes mellitus

The risk of getting chronic complications decreases if the diabetes is well managed (i.e. blood sugar levels are closely monitored and kept as normal as possible with appropriate treatment).

Tissue complications are due to osmotic damage, altered redox state, or glycation of proteins. These are caused by the increased glucose levels in the blood.

Chronic tissue complications include (see Fig. 15.13):

- Microangiopathy (disease of the small blood vessels)—this causes damage especially to the peripheral nerves, retina, and kidneys, leading to neuropathy, retinopathy, and nephropathy, respectively. Patients complain of numbness, tingling, or burning sensations in their feet (bilateral and in a 'stocking pattern' distribution), and impaired vision or blindness.
- Macroangiopathy (disease of the large blood vessels)—this is essentially an accelerated form of atherosclerosis, causing peripheral vascular disease (e.g. claudication and gangrene), strokes, and coronary heart disease. Any evidence of vascular disease (or neuropathy) puts the patient at high risk of foot ulceration, which—once present—is hard to cure and if not rigorously treated may lead to the patient losing the foot because of gangrene.
- Cataracts—caused by osmotic changes or glycation of the lens (both due to hyperglycaemia), making it opaque. Patients complain of impaired vision.
- Chronic infections—high glucose levels in the blood

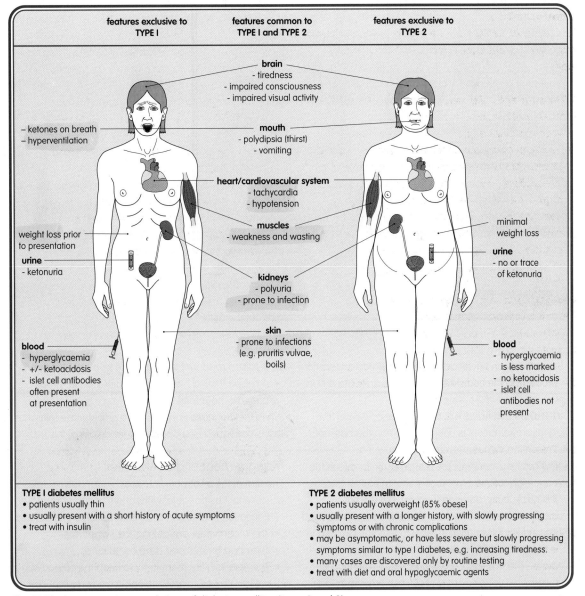

Fig. 15.12 Acute symptoms and signs of diabetes mellitus (types 1 and 2).

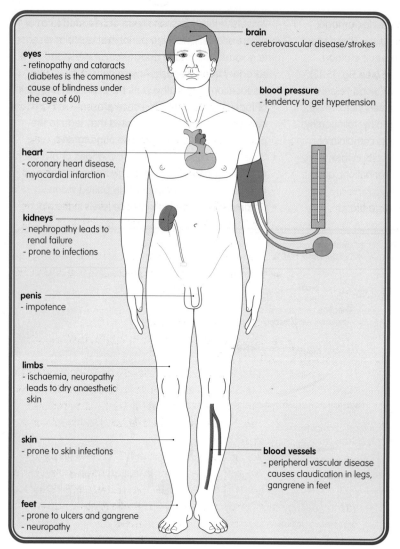

Fig. 15.13 Chronic complications of diabetes mellitus.

brain
- cerebrovascular disease/strokes

eyes
- retinopathy and cataracts (diabetes is the commonest cause of blindness under the age of 60)

blood pressure
- tendency to get hypertension

heart
- coronary heart disease, myocardial infarction

kidneys
- nephropathy leads to renal failure
- prone to infections

penis
- impotence

limbs
- ischaemia, neuropathy leads to dry anaesthetic skin

skin
- prone to skin infections

blood vessels
- peripheral vascular disease causes claudication in legs, gangrene in feet

feet
- prone to ulcers and gangrene
- neuropathy

and effects on bactericidal and immunological function predispose the body to infection, especially of the skin.

Diagnosis of diabetes mellitus

Diagnosis of diabetes is usually made on the basis of:
- Presenting symptoms, e.g. thirst, polyuria.
- Urinanalysis to test for the presence of glucose in the urine—glycosuria is used as a screening test because it is quick, easy, and non-invasive, but it is not diagnostic of diabetes (because of the huge intra- and interindividual variation in renal threshold). Glycosuria is measured using a Diastix, which is dipped into the urine—the test strips are impregnated with glucose oxidase, which oxidizes any glucose present in the urine, causing a colour change.

- A raised random blood glucose level (>11.1 mmol/L).
- A raised fasting blood glucose level (>7.8 mmol/L after a 6-hour fast).

When the diagnosis is in doubt, an oral glucose tolerance test is performed (see Chapter 14 for details of this test).

Management of diabetes mellitus

The aim of the treatment is to reach normoglycaemia, or as close to it as possible, without disrupting normal life.

Education is crucial in order that patients understand:
- The reason they are getting the symptoms.
- The need for diet and drug compliance.
- The necessity for them to try to keep their blood sugar well controlled to prevent long-term complications.
- How to monitor their blood and urine glucose at home.

- The fact that treatment may cause hypoglycaemic episodes ('hypos'), i.e. their blood glucose levels may become low.
- What a 'hypo' feels like and how to abort it with sweets.
- The need to increase the amount of insulin injected during illness.

Treatment for diabetes mellitus may cause hypoglycaemia when the intake of carbohydrates is low or if the patient is taking increased amounts of exercise.

Hypoglycaemia causes unpleasant symptoms, including sweating, palpitations, tachycardia, and aggressive behaviour (due to mental confusion), and can lead to convulsions and coma. These symptoms are due to the increased release of adrenaline in response to low blood glucose levels.

Hypoglycaemic coma is treated by giving 50% dextrose solution intravenously and, when the patient regains consciousness, giving sugary drinks.

Diet and drugs used to treat diabetes mellitus
Diet
Dietary recommendations include:
- Reduced intake of readily assimilable sugars (to reduce hyperglycaemia after eating).
- Eating regularly to avoid hypoglycaemia if on insulin or oral hypoglycaemic agents.
- Weight reduction in the overweight (obesity can induce type 2 diabetes).
- 'Healthy eating'—a diet that is high in fibre and low in saturated fats, and alcohol in moderation only.

Patients may need to snack between meals or take glucose supplements if they feel their blood sugar is low (hypoglycaemic symptoms).

Some milder forms of type 2 diabetes can be treated by diet alone. However, these guidelines should be followed by all diabetic patients.

In reality, more than 50% of patients fail to follow their diet and very few manage to maintain weight loss.

Insulin replacement therapy
This is used to treat type 1 diabetes mellitus (total or near-total loss of pancreatic insulin).

Porcine insulin (used in the past) has been replaced by human insulin, which can be made by recombinant genetic techniques using yeasts and bacteria.

If insulin were administered orally, it would be digested and inactivated; hence it has to be administered by subcutaneous injection (usually into the thigh area).

Administration of insulin needs to be coordinated with meal times—insulin is required for the cells to take up glucose and amino acids, therefore blood levels of insulin need to be high at meal times and lower between them.

The insulin regimen used can be varied depending on:
- The insulin preparation (short, medium or long acting).
- The dose.
- The number and timing of injections given per day.

Examples of different insulin regimens are shown in Fig. 15.14.

The choice of regimen is decided by what suits the patient's lifestyle best and what gives the best control for that patient.

Doses are adjusted according to requirements (more with more food, less if taking more exercise) and to the response of the blood sugar.

Oral hypoglycaemic agents
These are used to treat type 2 diabetes mellitus only and comprise:
- Sulphonylureas (e.g. gliclazide and glibenclamide)—increase insulin release from β cells by inhibiting the ATP-sensitive K$^+$ channel in the β-cell membrane (see Fig. 6.7). Side effects include weight gain and hypoglycaemia.
- Biguanides (e.g. metformin)—act peripherally to increase glucose uptake and reduce hepatic glucose output. Their mechanism of action is not understood but they do not increase insulin release. Side effects include nausea and diarrhoea.
- Acarbose—a new drug that inhibits intestinal α-glucosidase and therefore the digestion of starch, so blood glucose does not shoot up after a meal (useful in combating postprandial hyperglycaemia). Side effects include flatulence and diarrhoea.

Monitoring control of diabetes mellitus
Blood glucose levels are monitored to make sure they are well controlled using the following methods:
- Direct measurement using blood-testing strips (Glucostix strips contain enzymes and reagents that react with glucose and produce a colour change proportional to the amount of glucose present)—measures control of glucose at the time of testing.
- Assessment of the percentage of glycosylated haemoglobin in the blood—measures the average glycaemic control in the preceding 6–8 weeks.
- Evaluation of the serum fructosamine concentration

(represents glycosylated serum protein, mostly albumin)—measures the average glycaemic control in the preceding 2–3 weeks.

Measurement of the amount of ketones in the blood or urine (using Ketostix strips) can also be used to assess diabetic control.

Screening and management of diabetic complications

Complications should be detected before they become symptomatic.

Microalbuminuria should be screened for to detect nephropathy (caused by microangiopathy). If it is present, the patient should be advised to increase the compliance to treatment because of the increased risk of developing hypertension, vascular disease, retinopathy, and renal failure. Angiotensin-converting enzyme (ACE) inhibitors are effective in treating microalbuminuria and hypertension.

Feet should be examined regularly by a chiropodist because they are often affected by peripheral neuropathy and peripheral vascular disease, making them prone to injury, ulceration, and infection, which may lead to gangrene and even necessitate amputation.

Eyes should be tested for changes in visual acuity and for retinopathy. Proliferative retinopathy and maculopathy may be treated effectively by laser photocoagulation.

Any complications detected should be treated as far as possible and closely monitored for any further progression, and the patient should be encouraged to achieve better glucose control.

Islet cell tumours

These are all extremely rare tumours that present with endocrine effects due to excess hormone secretion:

- Insulinoma is a pancreatic β-cell tumour that secretes insulin in excess and causes hypoglycaemia.
- Glucagonoma is a pancreatic α-cell tumour that secretes glucagon in excess and causes secondary diabetes mellitus and a skin rash.
- VIPoma is a pancreatic PP-cell tumour that secretes excess vasoactive intestinal peptide (VIP), which causes watery diarrhoea and flushing of the skin.
- Somatostatinoma is a pancreatic δ-cell tumour that secretes excess somatostatin and causes diabetes mellitus, decreased gastric acid secretion, gall stones, steatorrhoea, and weight loss.

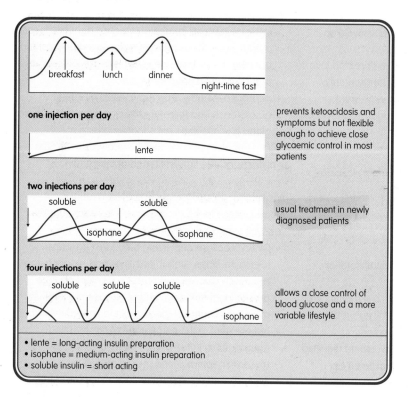

Fig. 15.14 Examples of different insulin regimens.

- Discuss the aetiology of diabetes mellitus, and specify the differences between type 1 and type 2.
- State the symptoms, signs, and chronic complications of diabetes.
- Summarize the diagnosis and management of diabetes.
- Define the four types of islet cell tumours and the endocrine effects that they cause.

MULTIPLE ENDOCRINE NEOPLASIA SYNDROMES

Multiple endocrine neoplasia (MEN) describes disorders resulting from the association of two or more different hormone-secreting tumours in the same person (Fig. 15.15)

MEN is very rare and may be sporadic or familial. Inherited forms are usually autosomal dominant, but with incomplete penetrance (i.e. an individual who inherits the abnormal gene may not necessarily develop MEN).

Treatment is essentially the treatment of each tumour individually.

Classification of MEN syndromes	
Class	Types of tumour present
type I	parathyroid, pancreatic tumours, and pituitary adenomas
type IIa	medullary carcinoma of the thyroid, phaeochromocytoma, parathyroid adenomas
type IIb	medullary carcinoma of the thyroid, phaeochromocytoma, mucosal neurofibromas (nerve cell tumours that distort the lips and jaw)

Fig. 15.15 Classification of MEN syndromes.

Aetiology of MEN syndromes
It is not known why certain tumours commonly occur together in MEN syndromes, but there are three theories that suggest:
- The common origin of the endocrine tissues was abnormal, e.g. abnormal APUD cells (see Chapter 6).
- A circulating growth factor is abnormal and induces mitosis in numerous different endocrine tissues.
- A genetic abnormality is expressed in certain endocrine cells and results in tumour growth.

ECTOPIC HORMONE SYNDROMES

Ectopic hormone syndromes cause endocrine disorders due to the uncontrolled secretion of hormones from tumours in non-endocrine organs (or in endocrine organs that do not normally secrete the hormone in question). Hence, tumours may secrete hormones even though the tissue that they are derived from does not normally do so, e.g. breast cancer cells may secrete a PTH-like peptide that is not normally secreted by the breast tissue.

'Ectopic' means 'out of place', and is possibly a misnomer in that some hormone-secreting tumours in organs regarded as non-endocrine are actually derived from cells that do normally secrete that hormone, e.g. oat cell carcinoma of the lung often secretes ACTH, but it has since been discovered that cells of the bronchial mucosa do normally secrete limited amounts of ACTH.

Examples of syndromes caused by ectopic hormone secretion are listed in Fig. 15.16.

Treatment of the tumours by surgical removal, irradiation, or chemotherapy where possible will correct the endocrine disorder.

Aetiology of ectopic hormone syndromes
It is not known why some tumours secrete specific hormones, but there are three theories:
- There is 'dedepression' of genetic information coding for a hormone that is usually not expressed in an organ (this theory does not readily explain why specific hormones are associated with specific cancers).
- The tumour originates from cells that actually do normally secrete hormone, e.g.cells of the bronchial mucosa normally secrete ACTH, and oat cell carcinoma of the lung secretes ACTH.
- Activation of specific oncogenes in certain tumours causes the activation of hormone production.

Peptide hormones are usually produced by hormone-

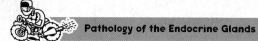

secreting tumours because their synthesis requires expression of only a single gene.

Steroid hormones are not produced by hormone-secreting tumours because steroid synthesis requires the expression of a whole series of enzymes (which requires an unlikely change in gene expression in the tumour cells).

Often tumours secrete hormone analogues rather than the hormones themselves (e.g. breast cancer cells secrete PTH-like peptide).

Examples of syndromes caused by ectopic hormone secretion		
Syndrome	**Hormone secreted by tumour cells**	**Tumour**
hypercalcaemia	parathyroid hormone (PTH) or PTH-like peptide	squamous cell carcinoma of the lung, breast carcinoma
hyponatraemia	ADH	oat cell carcinoma of the bronchus, some intestinal tumours
hypokalaemia (symptoms of Cushing's syndrome caused by ACTH excess have not always developed by the time the patient presents)	ACTH and ACTH-like peptides	oat cell carcinoma of the bronchus, medullary carcinoma of the thyroid, thymic carcinoma, islet cell tumours
gynaecomastia	human placental lactogen	carcinoma of the bronchus, liver, or kidney
galactorrhoea	prolactin	carcinoma of the bronchus, hypernephroma
polycythaemia	erythropoietin	hypernephroma, carcinoma of the uterus
hypoglycaemia (caused by the excessive consumption of glucose by highly active tumours that do not secrete hormones)	insulin (rare)	hepatomas, large mesenchymal tumours
no syndrome	calcitonin	oat cell carcinoma of the lung

Fig. 15.16 Examples of syndromes caused by ectopic hormone secretion.

- List the MEN syndromes.
- Give examples of the syndromes that can be caused by ectopic hormone secretion.

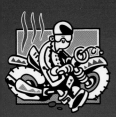

16. Pathology of the Reproductive Function

MENSTRUAL DISORDERS

Amenorrhoea

Amenorrhoea is divided into primary and secondary amenorrhoea. It occurs in 1–2% of women of reproductive age.

Primary amenorrhoea is the failure to start menstruating, and is usually accompanied by growth failure and the absence of secondary sexual characteristics—in most patients, puberty is just late. Rarely it can be caused by vaginal atresia, or ovarian or uterine absence. Ovarian dysgenesis occurs in Turner's syndrome, where the individual lacks an X chromosome (karyotype is 45,XO), and they tend to have other distinguishing characteristics (e.g. short stature, webbed neck).

Primary amenorrhoea also occurs in the rare disorder called testicular feminization—this is where the individual is genetically male (XY chromosomes), but, due to the failure of their tissues to respond to testosterone, their testes do not descend and they have female external genitalia, a short vagina, and are reared as girls. They develop female secondary sexual characteristics at puberty, but do not start menstruating because they do not possess a uterus, or ovaries.

Secondary amenorrhoea is when women who normally have menstrual periods fail to menstruate for 6 months or more. The cause of the lack of cyclical menstruation can be due to a disorder in the hypothalamus, pituitary gland, ovaries, thyroid or adrenal gland, or in the reproductive outflow tract (uterus or cervix). The most common endocrine causes and their relative frequencies are listed in Fig. 16.1.

Amenorrhoea is diagnosed from the history, examination of the reproductive system, investigations of hormone levels—e.g. prolactin, follicle-stimulating

Amenorrhoea after stopping the use of the oral contraceptive pill was once diagnosed as 'post-Pill amenorrhoea', but is now regarded as being due to a disorder in the hypothalamic–pituitary–ovarian axis that was previously masked by the hormonal effect of the Pill.

Most common endocrine causes of amenorrhoea and their approximate relative frequencies		
Disorder	**Cause of disorder**	**Relative frequency**
hypothalamus	GnRH deficiency due to psychological stress, excess physical exercise, weight loss	40%
anterior pituitary gland	hyperprolactinaemia, hypopituitarism (rare)	15%
ovaries	polycystic ovarian disease (excessive androgen production caused by the incomplete maturation of too many follicles in each cycle), ovarian dysgenesis, premature menopause, pelvic radiotherapy	40%
systemic disease	Cushing's syndrome, hypothyroidism, adrenal insufficiency	5%

Fig. 16.1 The most common endocrine causes of secondary amenorrhoea and their approximate relative frequencies.

hormone (FSH), luteinizing hormone (LH), and thyroid function tests—and ultrasound scan of the pelvis.

Treatment depends on the cause of the amenorrhoea. Hyperprolactinaemia is treated using bromocriptine that inhibits prolactin secretion. Polycystic ovarian disease is often associated with other problems (e.g. hirsuitism, insulin resistance, and obesity) that can be improved by dietary advice and anti-androgen treatment. Infertility caused by polycystic ovarian disease is treated with clomiphere (an anti-oestrogen that blocks oestrogen receptors in the hypothalamus, resulting in FSH an LH release that stimulate normal follicular maturation).

Menorrhagia
Menorrhagia is excessive or prolonged menstrual bleeding caused by abnormal shedding of the endometrium. Normal menstrual blood loss is about 30 mL; loss of >80 mL is pathological and can lead to iron-deficiency anaemia. Excess blood loss can be regular or irregular, i.e. menstrual or intermenstrual bleeding.

Regular heavy periods are associated with ovulation and are usually caused by localized disorders of the reproductive tract, including myometrial tumours (e.g. uterine fibroids) and endometriosis.

Irregular bleeding may be associated with anovulatory cycles (e.g. disorders of the hypothalamic–pituitary–ovarian axis). This causes abnormal progesterone and oestrogen levels within the menstrual cycle that lead to irregular endometrial shedding. Alternatively, it may be due to localized pelvic pathology, including:
- Tumours or infection of the endometrium (see Chapter 17).
- Dysfunctional uterine bleeding—this is the most common cause of the menorrhagia that tends to occur as menopause approaches. This diagnosis is given only after other pelvic pathologies have been excluded. It may be caused by abnormal prostaglandin synthesis in the endometrium (PGE2 causes vasodilatation and inhibition of blood clotting).
- Trauma—e.g. caused by an intrauterine contraceptive devices (IUCD)—see Chapter 11.

Hyperthyroidism may also cause menorrhagia.

Treatment is of the cause or in the case of dysfunctional uterine bleeding, a progestogen-containing IUCD may decrease bleeding, or a hysterectomy may be indicated.

Dysmenorrhoea
Dysmenorrhoea is severely painful menstrual periods caused by:
- Excessive uterine contractions—endometrial prostaglandins may be abnormal.
- Infection—e.g. pelvic inflammatory disease.
- Endometriosis.
- Ovarian tumours.
- Psychological disorders—e.g. history of sexual abuse.

It may be associated with menorrhagia, dyspareunia, or infertility.

Treatment is of the cause. If no organic or psychological cause can be found, it is treated symptomatically using nonsteroidal anti-inflammatory agents (which decrease prostaglandin synthesis) or the oral contraceptive pill (anovulatory bleeding is less painful).

Premenstrual syndrome (PMS)
PMS describes the symptoms that may occur 7–10 days prior to the onset of menstruation (Fig. 16.2). The overall incidence of PMS is unknown, but 5–15% of women suffer from severe, life-disrupting PMS. The condition is not related to age, race, or class, and remains poorly understood. It is thought to be caused by an abnormal response to, or metabolism of, progesterone or prostaglandin. It is diagnosed from the history and by using a diary of when symptoms occur (often PMS may be discounted as symptoms do not correlate with the menstrual cycle).

Symptoms can be treated individually (e.g. with analgesics or antidepressants) or by hormonal drugs (e.g. oral contraceptive pill) that inhibit the ovarian cycle.

- Discuss the causes of primary and secondary amenorrhoea.
- What is the commonest cause of menorrhagia and how is it treated?
- List the causes of dysmenorrhoea.
- State the symptoms premenstrual syndrome.

178

Symptoms of premenstrual syndrome		
Psychological	**Behavioural**	**Physical**
anxiety depression increased appetite irritability loss of libido sleep disturbance tension	anger impulsiveness and accident- prone behaviour poor concentration poor tolerance to stress	acne weight gain breast tenderness and swelling abdominal bloating change in bowel habit headache pelvic pain

Fig. 16.2 Symptoms of premenstrual syndrome.

THE MENOPAUSE

The menopause occurs in females at 48–56 years of age (average 51 years) and it marks the end of a woman's reproductive life. Ovulation and menstruation cease completely, caused by the permanent failure of the ovaries. The menopause is preceded by the climacteric (lasts 1–5 years), where there is progressive failure of the ovarian follicles to respond to gonadotrophins (LH and FSH). The failure of the ovarian follicles to develop causes anovulation and a decline in the production of ovarian oestrogens and progesterone. During the climacteric, the fluctuating levels of the gonadotrophins rise acutely in response to oestrogen deficiency, but, as menopause progresses, their levels decline. Oestrogen deficiency is responsible for the majority of the menopausal symptoms and complications. There is, however, a limited amount of oestrogen production during menopause in the peripheral adipose tissue. Here, the weak adrenal androgen androstenedione is aromatized into oestrone. However, oestrone is a weak oestrogen and only protects against oestrogen deficiency when it is produced in sufficient quantities, i.e. in very obese women.

Menopause is a normal event but it does cause acute symptoms and long-term complications (Fig. 16.3). Acute signs and symptoms that may occur include:

- Hot flushes, sweating, and tachycardia—these can be very unpleasant and are caused by vasomotor instability (resulting from fluctuations of excess gonadotrophin secretion). Night sweats can cause sleep disturbance, resulting in poor concentration, irritability, and anxiety.
- Depression—caused by the direct effect of oestrogen deficiency on the central nervous system, or by the concept of the menopause, i.e. loss of fertility and fears of ageing.

Long-term complications of the menopause		
Symptoms/disease	**Cause**	**Consequence**
osteoporosis	oestrogen deficiency causes accelerated bone loss	increased risk of bone fractures, especially the femoral neck at the hip and crush fractures of the vertebrae
cardiovascular disease	oestrogens have a beneficial effect on the lipid profile in the blood and in doing so protect against cardiovascular disease	in the absence of oestrogens, there is an increased risk of coronary artery disease, myocardial infarction, and strokes
loss of collagen	oestrogen deficiency causes weakening in the pelvic ligaments, joints, and muscle, and loss of elasticity in the skin	predisposes to uterovaginal prolapse, immobility, muscle weakness and causes skin wrinkling

Fig. 16.3 Long-term complications of the menopause.

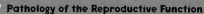

- Prolonged and irregular vaginal bleeding—caused by progesterone deficiency (progesterone is required to sustain the endometrium).
- Vaginal dryness, dyspareunia, and recurrent vaginal infections (due to loss of acidity)—caused by oestrogen deficiency.
- Urinary frequency and urgency —due to progressive atrophy of the lower urinary tract caused by oestrogen deficiency.

The diagnosis is usually evident from the patient's history—it is normally not necessary to measure hormone levels.

Hormone replacement therapy (HRT) is used to treat the menopausal symptoms and to prevent the long-term complications. HRT involves the continuous administration of natural oestrogens either by tablet or skin patch. Progestogens are included in the HRT for women who have not had a hysterectomy, these are taken for 12 days each month to prevent against endometrial carcinoma—but they do cause withdrawal bleeding and can cause pre-menstrual syndrome. HRT is contraindicated in patients with breast or endometrial cancer, or liver disease.

Men do not have an equivalent of the female menopause, although they may experience sexual dysfunction with age. They continue to produce testosterone and spermatozoa well into their eighties, although the amounts and quality produced decline. It is not understood what evolutionary pressure has caused females to lose their reproductive function with age and men to retain it; however, it is appropriate because the maternal and foetal outcome of pregnancy in elderly females is poor. Men, on the other hand, can father children at a greater age with no increased risks to themselves or to the foetus.

- **Outline the hormonal changes that occur at the time of the menopause.**
- **Discuss the effects caused by the menopause.**

INFERTILITY

Infertiliy is the inability to conceive after 1 year of unprotected intercourse. It is common—about 1 in 10 couples experience difficulty in conceiving. It may be caused by the male partner or the female partner, or both. Male infertility accounts for 30% of cases, 45% are caused by female infertility, and 25% of cases remain unexplained.

Abnormality in the sperm is the main cause of infertility in the male. Abnormalities include:

- Low sperrn counts (normal is >20 million/mL), called oligospermia, which may be due to or blockage in the epididymis (resulting from previous infective damage) or reduced spermatogenesis (resulting from infection or from genetic or endocrine disorders). Endocrine disorders include testosterone deficiency and hyperprolactinaemia.
- Decreased sperm quality due to asthenozoospermia, i.e. reduced motility (normal is >50% motile) or abnormal morphology. It may be caused by genetic disorders, raised scrotal temperature, genital-tract infections, varicocoele, or the presence of antisperm antibodies.

The main causes of infertility in the female are shown in Fig. 16.4. Other causes include sexual dysfunction or infrequency.

Treatment of infertility

Counselling and reassurance are important. Most couples complaining of infertility are not totally infertile and will benefit from education to maximize their chances of conception (e.g. maximizing their efforts during the fertile period by using the symptothermal family-planning method). Infertility is investigated by sperm microscopy, hormone investigations (e.g. FSH, LH, prolactin, progesterone, oestrogen, testosterone, thyroid hormone measurement), pelvic ultrasound and hysterosalpinography, if indicated (see Fig. 14.8). Determination and treatment of the specific cause is the most important method, but assisted-conception methods are available. These include:

- In-vitro fertilization (IVF)—oocytes harvested after hormone-induced superovulation are fertilized *in vitro*, and re-introduced into the uterus. This is the only effective method if the fallopian tubes are blocked.
- Gamete intrafallopian transfer (GIFT)—oocytes harvested after hormone-induced superovulation are

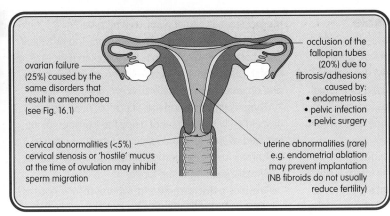

Fig. 16.4 Causes of infertility/subfertility in the female (showing their approximate frequencies in infertile couples).

ovarian failure (25%) caused by the same disorders that result in amenorrhoea (see Fig. 16.1)

occlusion of the fallopian tubes (20%) due to fibrosis/adhesions caused by:
• endometriosis
• pelvic infection
• pelvic surgery

cervical abnormalities (<5%) cervical stenosis or 'hostile' mucus at the time of ovulation may inhibit sperm migration

uterine abnormalities (rare) e.g. endometrial ablation may prevent implantation (NB fibroids do not usually reduce fertility)

re-introduced into the fallopian tubes along with sperm.

• Intrauterine insemination (IUI)—sperm is artificially delivered through the cervix.

dysfunction) and failure to ejaculate. Alcohol and drug treatment is the commonest cause, followed by psychological factors. The causes of erectile dysfunction are shown in Fig. 16.5.

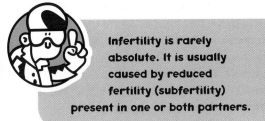

Infertility is rarely absolute. It is usually caused by reduced fertility (subfertility) present in one or both partners.

○ Discuss the causes of infertility.
○ How is infertility investigated and treated?

SEXUAL DYSFUNCTION

Sexual dysfunction in the male

This includes:

• Loss of libido—can be caused by systemic illness, stress, fatigue, depression, or an age-related decrease in testosterone levels.

• Impotence—describes the failure to maintain an erection suitable for vaginal penetration (erectile

The causes of erectile dysfunction in approximate order of frequency	
Cause	**Mechanism**
alcohol and drug treatment, e.g. narcotics, beta-blockers, antipsychotics, antidepressants	alcohol—acutely it reduces sensory nervous transmission from the penis to the brain and, chronically it damages the liver and testes which lowers the testosterone: oestrogen ratio (testosterone is required by nerves for them to transmit messages from the brain to stimulate reaction) beta-blockers reduce the blood flow to the penis antipsychotics antagonize neurotransmitters that mediate erection
psychological factors, e.g. anxiety and stress	stress reduces the sympathetic nervous stimulation of erection—this is often self-reinforcing as erectile dysfunction is a form of stress in itself
endocrine disorders, e.g. diabetes mellitus, hyperprolactinaemia	long term damage to the nerves and blood vessels of the penis caused by diabetes mellitus can result in erectile dysfunction
vascular disease, e.g. atherosclerosis of the iliac arteries	blood supply to the penis is insufficient to cause an erection
neuropathy, e.g multiple sclerosis	reduced sensation in the penis prevents erection

Fig. 16.5 Causes of erectile dysfunction, in approximate order of frequency.

Sexual dysfunction in the female

This includes:

- Loss of libido—often stems from psychological causes (e.g. confidence, trust, anxiety, depression, altered body image), but can be caused by vaginal infection, general illness, medications, and alcohol. It may mask other sexual problems or be attributed to relationship difficulties.
- Sexual arousal disorders—failure of vaginal lubrication and vasocongestion of the labia. A simple lubricant can be used and reassurance given.
- Vaginismus—pain on intercourse resulting from the involuntary contraction of the vagina upon penile penetration. It is a conditioned response to either previous dyspareunia or psychological factors (e.g. previous sexual anxiety or abuse). It can treated by vaginal dilators or by using behavioural therapy (e.g. sexual intercourse is banned for a time and other sexual behaviour encouraged until confidence is regained).
- Dyspareunia—pain on intercourse, which may be superficial or deep. Superficial dyspareunia is caused by lack of sexual arousal, vaginismus, cystitis, or vulval/vaginal infections. Deep dyspareunia can be caused by pelvic infections and endometriosis (see Chapter 17).
- Failure to reach orgasm (anorgasmia)—this is less often reported in females than in males because males are more likely to report failure of ejaculation whereas many females are able to feel sexually fulfilled without orgasm (depending on their feelings towards their partner).

Psychosexual counselling and education are used to treat sexual dysfunction that is non-organic and not related to drug treatments. Underlying psychological causes or complications must be recognized and explored. Both partners must involved in the therapy if possible.

DISORDERS OF THE PLACENTA AND PREGNANCY

Ectopic pregnancy

The fertilized ovum normally implants in the endometrium in the uterus. If it implants outside the uterine cavity the pregnancy is described as ectopic. This occurs in about 1 in 100 pregnancies in the UK but the incidence is higher in areas where pelvic inflammatory disease is more common. The prevalent site of ectopic implantation is the fallopian tube (97% of cases). Other sites include the ovary, broad ligament and omentum (these are extremely rare).

There is an increased risk of ectopic pregnancy associated with factors that delay the transport of the fertilized ovum along the fallopian tubes:

- Chronic pelvic inflammatory disease (PID)—causes fibrosis/scarring of the tubes.
- Previous pelvic surgery (e.g. laparoscopy)—causes adhesion formation that may distort the tubes.
- Use of intrauterine contraceptive devices—causes a low grade PID.
- Use of progesterone only pills—interferes with the transport of the ovum.

In tubal pregnancies the trophoblast erodes into the muscle of the fallopian tube and the embryo may receive an adequate blood supply during its early development. This allows the embryo to grow but the pregnancy usually terminates at 6–10 weeks gestation. This is because:

- The tubes are unable to distend to accommodate the growing embryo and the tubal muscles contract to expel it. This is referred to as tubal abortion. It causes intermittent, unilateral pelvic pain followed by mild to moderate bleeding per vagina.
- The trophoblast invades through blood vessels in the tubal wall, resulting in haemorrhage—either into the tube or rupturing through the wall into the peritoneal cavity. This is referred to as tubal rupture. It causes severe pelvic and abdominal pain, shock (due to intraperitoneal blood loss) and the patient may die.

Diagnosis of tubal pregnancies before they abort or rupture is difficult because a moderate amount of pelvic pain and irregular vaginal bleeding is not uncommon in normal pregnancies. In tubal pregnancies, the hCG pregnancy test is positive but ultrasound scanning will fail to demonstrate an intrauterine pregnancy. If no embryo is visualized, then a laparoscopy is performed to examine the tubes directly.

Treatment of tubal pregnancies is by:

- Surgical removal of the entire tube that contains the embryo (commonly performed following tubal rupture).
- Surgical removal of the embryo only, via an incision in the tube.

If an intrauterine pregnancy is discovered by ultrasound scan then the presence of an ectopic pregnancy can almost always be ruled out. Remember that a co-existing ectopic pregnancy may occur if there is more than one embryo (e.g. twin pregnancy).

A woman may miscarry before she even knows that she is pregnant (i.e. before she misses a period)—this is known as a 'silent abortion' and is indistinguishable from a period.

- Injection of methotrexate (cytotoxic drug) into the embryo under laparoscopic supervision. This kills the embryo and it is slowly reabsorbed by maternal tissues.

There is a 10% chance that subsequent pregnancies will be ectopic.

Miscarriage

Miscarriage (otherwise known as spontaneous abortion) is the expulsion of a foetus from the uterus before it is capable of extrauterine survival (i.e. any time between conception and 24 weeks gestation). It is common—1 in 7 diagnosed pregnancies miscarry in the first 3 months. In most cases there is no recurrent cause.

Possible causes include:
- Foetal abnormality (60%)—usually due to a chromosomal disorder.
- Placental abnormality (15%)—resulting from defective implantation.
- Maternal abnormality (25%)—e.g. systemic infection, diabetes, psychological stress, uterine abnormality/infection, cervical incompetence.

Symptoms include pelvic pain and bleeding as the products of conception are expelled from the uterus. Vaginal bleeding during pregnancy does not always indicate an inevitable miscarriage and the diagnosis is difficult because the pregnancy test remains positive for several days after foetal death. If products of conception are retained, they must be evacuated to prevent bleeding and infection.

Pre-eclampsia and eclampsia

Pre-eclampsia is a pregnancy-specific syndrome that affects 6% of pregnancies. It develops after 20 weeks gestation and is characterized by high blood pressure (>140/90 mmHg) and the presence of protein in the urine (proteinuria). It is often accompanied by fluid retention and oedema. The disorder originates in the placenta but it affects the whole body (see Fig. 16.6).

A patient with pre-eclampsia who becomes severely ill and has convulsions is said to have developed eclampsia. Eclampsia is very rare (1 in 2000 pregnancies) but it is a life-threatening condition—it causes cerebral haemorrhage and cardiac failure. The likelihood of disease progression is not predictable. Symptoms include headache, chest pain, epigastric pain, vomiting, and visual disturbances. (NB Pre-eclampsia is often asymptomatic and only rarely culminates in eclampsia.)

Pre-eclampsia is diagnosed by measuring the blood pressure and testing the urine for protein. The only way to cure pre-eclampsia is to terminate the pregnancy—it resolves within 10 days of delivery. If symptoms suddenly worsen and eclampsia is imminent then termination is crucial, whether or not the foetus is mature enough to survive. Asymptomatic pre-eclampsia is managed by:
- Regular measurement of blood pressure, proteinuria and foetal monitoring to monitor disease progression.
- Evaluation of renal and liver function tests, platelet counts and blood clotting factors.

Eclampsia is treated with:
- Anticonvulsant drugs to control the fits.
- Antihypertensive drugs to reduce the blood pressure.
- Caesarian section to deliver the foetus.

Neoplastic disorders of trophoblastic origin

Hydatidiform mole

A hydatidiform mole is a benign uterine tumour of trophoblastic tissue (i.e. formed from a fertilized ovum). It occurs in about 1 in 1000 pregnancies in the UK. The tumour may have completely or partially replaced the placenta—complete moles are entirely composed of hyperplastic chorionic villi, partial moles may still contain foetal tissue. They are caused by chromosomal abnormalities in the fertilized ovum. An affected woman will have exaggerated symptoms of pregnancy (e.g. severe morning sickness, early onset pre-eclampsia) and an abnormally large uterus.

Moles are diagnosed by:

- Foetal heart monitoring—no foetal heart is detectable.
- Ultrasound scanning—they have a 'snowstorm-like' appearance.
- Plasma human chorionic gonadotrophin (hCG) measurement—plasma hCG levels are extremely high because moles are derived from chorionic tissue that secretes hCG.

Treatment consists of:

- Suction evacuation of the uterus.
- Monitoring plasma hCG levels to ensure there is no recurrence (i.e. all the tumour cells were removed). This is important because 10% of moles develop into choriocarcinoma.

Choriocarcinoma

This is a highly malignant tumour that occurs in 1 in 20 000 pregnancies. Half these cases follow a benign mole, half follow abortion or childbirth. It is composed of trophoblastic tissue but no chorionic villi are formed. It secretes high levels of hCG, bleeds easily (resulting in bloody vaginal discharge) and its cells metastasise via the blood stream. It is diagnosed by histological examination of uterine curettings. Combination chemotherapy is extremely effective (almost 100%) and plasma hCG levels are monitored to evaluate the response to treatment.

Hypotensive drugs (e.g. methyldopa, hydralazine, β-blockers) only treat the symptoms of pre-eclampsia and have no effect on the underlying disease process. They may worsen placental perfusion and endanger the foetus. However, they are used to treat hypertension in severe pre-eclampsia (under close hospital supervision) if the foetus is still immature, but growing adequately, and the other tests are satisfactory.

- Discuss the causes and outcomes of ectopic pregnancy.
- List the causes of miscarriage.
- Outline the pathophysiology of pre-eclampsia and eclampsia and their treatment.
- Compare the types of trophoblastic tumours.

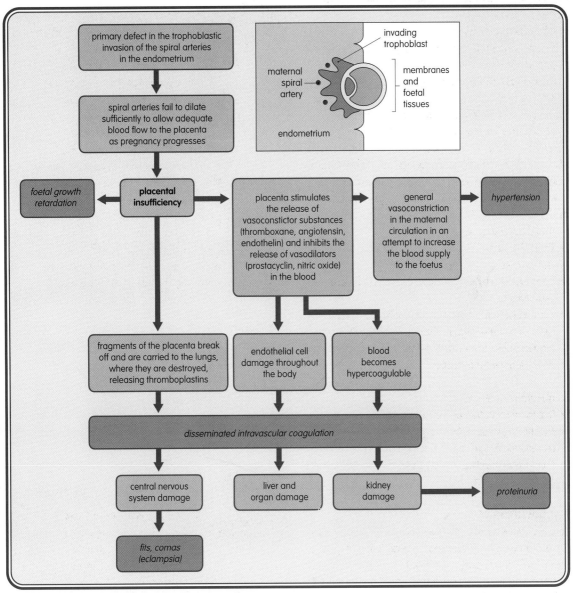

Fig. 16.6 Pathophysiology of pre-eclampsia and eclampsia. The primary defect is thought to be caused by an abnormality in the maternal immune response to the invading trophoblast. The pointers to that help to diagnose pre-eclampsia are shown in italic.

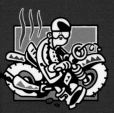

17. Pathology of the Female Reproductive System

Bartholin's cyst

This is the commonest disorder of the vulva and is caused by the obstruction of the duct of Bartholin's gland. (Fig. 17.1). The cyst almost always become infected, usually by staphylococci, gonococci, or coliform organisms, and may form an abscess. Cysts require surgical treatment and antibiotics to prevent infection.

Inflammation and infection

Genital herpes

This is a sexually transmitted disease caused by herpes simplex virus (usually HSV II).

It is highly infectious (80% of women in contact with male carriers become infected). The incubation period is short (3–7 days) and attacks recur every 3–4 weeks. Symptoms are usually severe and include:

- Burning, itching, hyperaesthesia and inflammation (oedema and erythema) of the infected area.
- Vaginal discharge.
- Dysuria and urinary retention (if the periurethral area is involved).
- Small indurated tender papules are found at the site of infection, these become vesicles and quickly break down to form shallow ulcers.
- Enlarged inguinal lymph nodes.
- General malaise, headache and neuralgia.

Genital warts

This is a sexually transmitted disease caused by human papilloma virus (HPV), of which there are 40 types. HPV infection causes wart formation and may also be associated with thickening of the vulval skin and mucosa. Possible sites of infection include the labia, perianal area, the perineum, the lower part of the vagina, and may even spread to the thighs.

Vulval dystrophy

Vulval dystrophy describes a spectrum of inflammatory disorders of the vulva. There are three main types:

- Primary atrophy—skin of the vulva degenerates, becomes dry, thin, shiny and contracts. It tends to

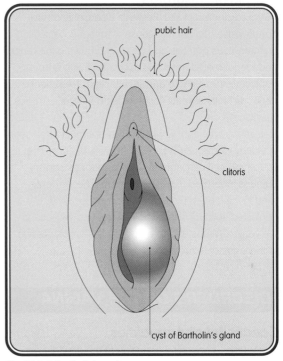

Fig. 17.1 A Bartholin's cyst.

occur in postmenopausal women and is usually associated with oestrogen deficiency (some cases are idiopathic). It causes vulval soreness and is treated using topical oestrogen creams.

- Lichen sclerosus—flat, pinkish-white patches appear on the vulva—these gradually coalesce and the vulva is moist and reddened. Vulval discomfort and severe pruritis accompany these patches. The tissues gradually become sclerotic (hardened and scarred), contract and scratching may induce lichenification (thickening of the epidermis). Lichen sclerosis can affect any area of skin of either sex, at any age, but is most commonly seen in the vulvoperineal skin of middle-aged women. Its cause is unknown. Treatment involves topical emollient creams, high dose hydrocortisone cream or local surgical excision (depending on its severity).

- Squamous hyperplasia—white plaques appear on the vulva, caused by increased production and growth of normal cells. It is associated with an increased risk of vulval carcinoma and plaques are excised.

Neoplastic disorders

Vulval carcinoma in situ (Bowen's disease) is a rare, non-invasive malignant disease. It presents as scaling, erythematous patches and histology shows a thickened and irregular epidermis. It is associated with human papillomavirus (HPV 16 and 18) infection. Treatment depends on its severity (local excision or total vulvectomy).

Invasive carcinomas of the vulva are most often seen in elderly women (>60 years), and 95% of cases are squamous cell carcinomas. They appear as solitary, painless indurated ulcers, and are most commonly sited in the labium majus. They spread locally if neglected, to involve the whole vulva, and will invade the vagina. Metastatic spread is via the lymph vessels to the inguinal lymph nodes.

DISORDERS OF THE VAGINA

Congenital abnormalities

Gynatresia—congenital occlusion of the genital tract—may be due to the complete absence of the vagina or to incomplete development.

Vaginal septae are quite common—the presence of a longitudinal septum produces a double vagina. This usually occurs in association with a double uterus. It is caused by the failure of the Mullerian ducts to fuse completely during development. Normal pregnancy and delivery are possible with a double vagina.

Inflammation and infection
Bacterial infections

Chlamydia trachomatis is a sexually transmitted disease that infects the vagina, and is also an important cause of chronic pelvic inflammatory disease (PID) and infertility. Initial symptoms are often mild. Vaginal discharge may be present, varying from watery to purulent, according to the severity of the infection.

Trichomonas vaginalis is another common cause of vaginitis in young women. It is sexually transmitted and causes the vaginal mucosa to become red and inflamed, with a frothy white discharge.

Fungal infection

Candida albicans is a fungal infection that causes thrush. The infection may be acquired through sexual contact or by endogenous infection (the organism is normally found in the rectum). The fungus can grow in the acid medium in the vagina and does not always cause symptoms. Symptomatic infection is most likely to arise when there are predisposing conditions, e.g.:
- Pregnancy.
- Immunosuppressive therapy.
- Antibiotic therapy.
- Glycosuria.
- Chronic anaemia.

Neoplastic disorders

Primary malignant tumours of the vagina are rare. Secondary tumours are more common and are especially extensive from cervical cancer. The patient complains of vaginal bleeding and discharge. If the bladder is involved, pain and dysuria will be experienced.

Approximately 85% of malignant vaginal tumours are squamous carcinomas, occurring in women over 60 years. The remainder include melanoma, sarcoma, adenocarcinoma, and clear-cell carcinoma, all of which tend to be associated with middle-aged or even young women.

In childhood, the vagina may be the site of development of a rhabdomyosarcoma, which is a polypoid, gelatinous mass that protrudes from the vagina.

Malignant tumours of the lower third of the vagina have a much poorer prognosis than those of the upper and middle thirds because spread to the inguinal lymph nodes is quicker and because of the danger to the bladder. Radical surgery is claimed to give good results.

DISORDERS OF THE CERVIX

Cervical ectropion

Cervical ectropion are common and often occur in response to high oestrogen levels during adolescence, pregnancy and in women who take the combined contraceptive pill. They appear as a red ring around the cervical os and are caused by an overgrowth of the columnar epithelium in this area. Ectropions secrete excess mucus and are prone to bleeding and infection.

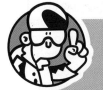

Inflammation and infection

Cervicitis (infection of the cervical epithelium) can be caused by *Chlamydia*, gonococci, and herpes. It is usually asymptomatic but can present with pelvic pain, vaginal discharge and dyspareunia.

Neoplastic disorders

Cervical Polyps

Cervical polyps are benign nodular or pedunculated growths arising from the endocervix. They are often associated with chronic cervicitis and are a common cause of irregular vaginal bleeding, especially after coitus. A polypoid fibroid of the uterus may present as a cervical polyp.

Cervical dysplasia and squamous cell carcinoma

Cervical dysplasia is the abnormal change in the epithelial cells present at the transformation zone of the cervix. The normal columnar epithelium is replaced by dysplastic squamous epithelium.

Dysplastic cells have the following features:

- Large nuclei, i.e. dysplastic cells have a high nuclear:cytoplasmic ratio.
- Irregular size and shape.
- Hyperchromatism, i.e. stain more deeply than normal cells.
- Loss regular structure.
- Increased number of mitotic figures.

Cervical dysplasia is regarded as the first of a series of changes that causes cervical intraepithelial neoplasia

At the transitional zone of the cervix, the columnar epithelium of the endocervix meets the squamous epithelium of the ectocervix. This region of the cervix is prone to dysplastic changes.

(CIN) and may subsequently lead to invasive carcinoma (Fig. 17.2). It takes approximately 10 years for the first signs of dysplasia to be converted into a carcinoma *in situ*.

Cytological examination of cervical smears (cells are scraped from the transitional zone) is used to screen for cervical cancer. If dysplastic or neoplastic cells are found then colposcopy is performed—i.e. the cervix is examined with a microscope, biopsies can be taken and electrodiathermy is used to destroy the abnormal cells. Treatment of pre-invasive carcinoma prevents the progression to carcinoma.

CIN is an important precursor of invasive squamous cell carcinoma. It is a pre-neoplastic proliferation and is usually associated with infections by human papilloma virus (HPV). HPV genotypes 16,18, and 33 of this virus are especially implicated in neoplastic cervical disease. Smoking and multiple sexual partners are also associated with an increased risk of cervical carcinoma.

Cervical carcinoma is a fungating, ulcerating or infiltrating tumour that spreads locally to the vagina,

Fig. 17.2 Stages of cervical dysplasia.

Stages of cervical dysplasia			
Stage	Histological grade	Description	Treatment
mild dysplasia	CIN I	basal layer of the cervical epithelium contains dysplastic cells	usually resolves spontaneously but smear test should be repeated in 4 months time and if CIN I still shows then colposcopy is performed
moderate dysplasia	CIN II	basal and middle layer of the cervical epithelium contains dysplastic cells	large loop diathermy excision of transitional zone (LLETZ) under colposcopy
servere dysplasia	CIN III	full thickness of cervical epithelium involved (equivalent to carcinoma *in situ*)	large loop diathermy excision of transitional zone (LLETZ) under colposcopy

pelvic wall, bladder and rectum, and via the blood and lymph vessels to other organs and lymph nodes. Patients with end stage disease usually die from uraemia as a result of the tumour blocking the urinary outflow tract.

Radical hysterectomy (removal of uterus, tubes, ovaries, upper third of the vagina, and pelvic lymph nodes) and radiotherapy are used to treat cervical carcinoma. The prognosis depends on the extent of the tumour growth—if confined to the cervix then the five year survival is 80%.

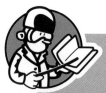

- Discuss vulvar dystrophy.
- Outline infections of the lower genital tract.
- Summarize the tumours of the vulva, vagina, and cervix.

DISORDERS OF THE ENDOMETRIUM AND MYOMETRIUM

Adenomyosis

This is an infiltration of the myometrium (muscular layer of the uterus) by ectopic deposits of immature endometrial cells. Macroscopically the uterus is enlarged. Commonly the enlargement is most marked on one aspect of the uterus (usually the posterior), giving rise to a tumour-like mass. The cut surface of the uterus shows typical small blood spots due to bleeding from the endometrial deposits. The uterus can become adherent to the rectum or adnexa.

The microscopic appearance of the uterus shows typical endometrial glands and stroma within the myometrium, although the stroma may be more prominent than the glands. Pain, menstrual upset and subfertility are the usual symptoms, caused by the cyclical bleeding from the ectopic endometrial deposits. For mild or no symptoms, no treatment is advised; for severe symptoms, a hysterectomy is advised.

Endometriosis

This is a very common gynaecological disorder, occuring in 12% of women (although not all have symptoms). It consists of ectopic deposits of endometrial cells in the lower part of the peritoneal cavity. Do not confuse this condition with adenomyosis!

The gross appearance shows ectopic deposits, varying in quantity from a few in one locality to a large number in another, distributed over the pelvic organs and peritoneum (Fig. 17.3). The ectopic deposits vary in size from pinpoint to 8 mm.

A typical lesion commonly appears as a round protruding vesicle that shows a succession of colours from blue to black to brown. The variation in colour is due to cyclical haemorrhage each month that corresponds with menstruation.

The main symptom is pelvic pain—this affects more than 80% of women with endometrial deposits. The pain tends begin premenstrually, reaching a peak during menstruation, and then subsides gradually. Chronic endometriosis may lead to scarring and the formation of adhesions as a result of cyclical haemorrhage. Adhesions may occlude the fallopian tubes and cause infertility.

Treatments aim to reduce pain and, if required, to restore fertility. Hormonal treatments suppress the disease symptoms by inhibiting ovarian function (e.g. danazol) and inhibiting cyclical endometrial development (e.g. continuous progestogens). Surgical treatment, using laparoscopy, involves the ablation of endometriotic deposits and removal of adhesions. Where fertility is not a problem, radical surgery to remove both ovaries is said to be a lasting cure for endometriosis since it removes the oestrogenic stimulus that promotes endometrial growth.

It is not known how endometriosis is caused but there are three theories:

- Retrograde spill of menstrual debris through the tubes—this has proven to take place in most women.
- Metaplasia of embryonic cells—these are derived from the primitive coelom and may remain in and around the pelvis and differentiate into ectopic endometrial tissue.
- Emboli of endometrial tissue may travel via blood and lymph vessels and become established in ectopic sites.

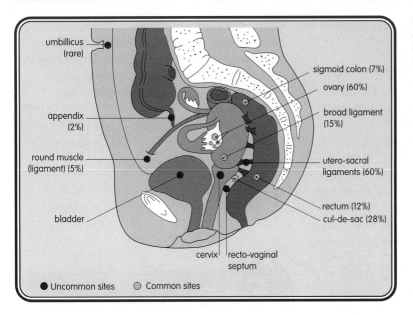

Fig. 17.3 Possible sites of extrauterine endometriosis (approximate frequencies are shown in brackets).

Labels in figure:
- umbillicus (rare)
- appendix (2%)
- round muscle (ligament) (5%)
- bladder
- cervix
- recto-vaginal septum
- sigmoid colon (7%)
- ovary (60%)
- broad ligament (15%)
- utero-sacral ligaments (60%)
- rectum (12%)
- cul-de-sac (28%)
- ● Uncommon sites ○ Common sites

Inflammation and infection

Acute endometritis (inflammation of the endometrium) may develop in response to infection following childbirth, abortion, and the insertion of an intrauterine contraceptive device; or be due to gonorrhoeal infection. This is a rare condition because the cervical mucus prevents the entry of infection into the uterus and because of the frequency with which the endometrium is shed. The diagnosis is histological and there are no specific signs or symptoms.

Endometrial hyperplasia

Endometrial hyperplasia tends to occur in women aged between 30–40 years. Patients present complaining of vaginal bleeding. There are three classifications of hyperplasia:

- Mild benign hyperplasia—the most common type. The endometrium has a characteristic 'Swiss cheese-like' appearance resulting from cystic glandular hyperplasia.
- Moderate hyperplasia—this demonstrates crowding of glands, stratified epithelium, and mitoses are relatively frequent.
- Severe hyperplasia—at this stage atypical premalignant cells are prominent and glands are distorted. It is also referred to as carcinoma *in situ*.

In young patients with mild hyperplasia who wish to remain fertile, conservative hormonal treatment may be sufficient. In severe cases, progestogens may be tried initially, but, if results are not satisfactory in 6–8 weeks, hysterectomy is recommended.

Neoplastic disorders
Endometrial polyps

Endometrial polyps are benign growths that are usually seen in the perimenopausal age range. They are thought to be caused by the overproliferation of glands in response to oestrogenic stimuli. The polyps vary in size from 1 to 3 cm, and appear as firm, smooth nodules within the endometrial cavity. They are clinically associated with menorrhagia, irregular menstrual bleeding and dysmenorrhoea. Polyps may ulcerate or undergo torsion.

Endometrial carcinoma

Endometrial carcinoma is one of the commonest malignant tumours of the female reproductive system. It is usually (75%) found in postmenopausal women between the ages of 55 and 65 years.

The usual complaint is of a blood-stained watery discharge, which, due to infection, often becomes foul smelling. Diagnosis is usually made by histological examination of endometrial curettings together with hysteroscopy.

The majority of tumours (60%) are adenocarcinomas. The tumour may be widespread or focal (e.g. in the form of a polyp) within the endometrial cavity. Invasion into the myometrium is slow and tumour cells are normally confined to the uterus at the time of diagnosis.

Treatment is with a combination of surgery (hysterectomy and bilateral salpingo-oophorectomy) and radiotherapy. The prognosis is generally good because the tumour tends to present early and tends to be confined to the uterus.

Myometrial tumours

Leiomyomas (fibroids) are benign tumours of the myometrium. They are the most common tumours in women (20% of women have fibroids). They are smooth, well-defined tumours of smooth muscle cells that bulge out of the uterine wall (see Fig. 17.4), and are usually multiple. Fibroids are oestrogen-dependent tumours which enlarge during pregnancy and atrophy after the menopause.

Most fibroids are asymptomatic. Symptoms depend on the size of the fibroids and their position in the uterus and include:

- Pelvic mass —fibroids can become very large.
- Urinary frequency and incontinence—caused by pressure on the bladder from a large fibroid.
- Painless menorrhagia—periods are heavy and prolonged due to distortion and enlargement of the uterine cavity.
- Infertility—fibroids may interfere with blastocyst implantation, however this is rare and most women with fibroids have no difficulty in conceiving.
- Pelvic pain—pedunculated submucous fibroids may undergo torsion and cause pain.

Symptomatic fibroids may be treated by hysterectomy or myomectomy (surgical removal of the fibroids). Gonadotrophin-releasing hormone (GnRH) analogues are usually administered for three months prior to myomectomy to help shrink the fibroids so the operation is easier.

Leiomyosarcomas are extremely rare malignant tumours of the myometrium that tend to occur in women aged 40–60 years.

- Compare adenomyosis with endometriosis.
- Why does endometritis rarely occur?
- Outline endometrial hyperplasia.
- What neoplastic disorders occur in the endometrium and myometrium?

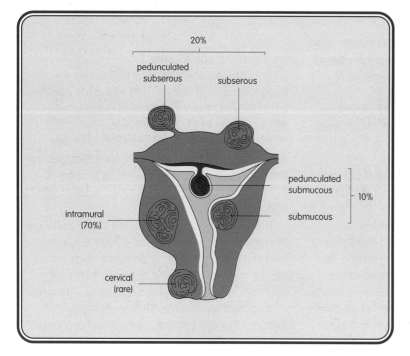

Fig. 17.4 Common sites for fibroids (benign tumours of the myometrium) in the uterus. The relative frequency for each type is shown.

DISORDERS OF THE OVARIES AND FALLOPIAN TUBES

Polycystic ovarian disease (Stein–Leventhal syndrome)

Polycystic ovarian disease occurs in 5% of women. The ovaries are enlarged and contain multiple benign follicular cysts—at least 15 in each ovary. The cysts do not mature normally and release excessive amounts of oestrogen and androgens (androstenedione and testosterone).

Patients maintain a persistent anovulatory (infertile) state, amenorrhoea, and often complain of hirsutism and obesity. It is associated with high plasma levels of LH, oestrogen, androgens, and low plasma levels of FSH. There is insulin resistance (which causes impaired glucose tolerance) and raised plasma insulin levels. Insulin suppresses the production of sex-hormone binding proteins in the liver so that the plasma levels of unbound (i.e. active) androgens is increased—this causes hirsutism and virilisation.

Treatment is directed towards four major problems:

- Amenorrhoea—a combined oral contraceptive is used to induce artificial menstruation and to suppress hypersecretion of ovarian androgens.
- Infertility—clomiphene can restore fertility. It is an anti-oestrogen that blocks oestrogen receptors in the hypothalamus, resulting in increased FSH release that stimulates normal follicular maturation.
- Obesity—a regimen of diet and exercise should be followed to improve the sensitivity to insulin.
- Hirsutism—in mild cases, shaving, depilatory creams, or electrolysis can be used. Severe cases can be treated with oestrogen and cyproterone acetate therapy. Oestrogens suppress ovarian androgen production and cyproterone acetate blocks androgen receptors.

Pelvic inflammatory disease (PID)

Infection of the fallopian tubes (salpingitis) usually involves the ovaries and peritoneum, and the combined infection is called pelvic inflammatory disease.

With acute PID, the history is often of a prolonged, painful menstrual period followed by the gradual onset of fever, pelvic pain, vaginal discharge and irregular vaginal bleeding. There is abdominal tenderness and extreme tenderness of the vaginal fornices. PID can be caused by:

- Ascending infection from the lower genital tract caused by sexually transmitted disease, e.g. *Chlamydia trachomatis, Neisseria gonorrhoea*. This is the most common cause.
- Direct infection from endogenous organisms in the vagina or gut, resulting from trauma due to childbirth, surgical abortion, or the insertion of a coil.
- Blood-borne infection, e.g. tuberculosis.
- Transperitoneal infection, e.g. from appendicitis.

Acute PID must be treated with antibiotics to avoid chronic infection. With chronic PID, the patient complains of pelvic pain made worse during menstrual periods, which are irregular and heavy. Dyspareunia is common. On vaginal examination, some swelling may be felt and the vaginal fornices are tender. All degrees of inflammation are met with, from salpingitis alone to a widespread inflammatory reaction involving all the pelvic tissue. The ascending infection first attacks the tubes, which are sealed off by oedema and adhesions. This causes infertility. Abscess formation may also occur within the ovary; and the uterus and fallopian tubes (normally mobile) become fixed by adhesions. Mild cases resolve spontaneously but may predispose to ectopic pregnancy. In advanced cases the only treatment is surgery to remove the uterus and fallopian tubes and maybe the ovaries.

Neoplastic disorders
Ovarian tumours

Benign and malignant ovarian tumours have no specific symptoms: menstrual function is seldom upset; pressure symptoms include increased frequency of micturition and dull pain in the lower abdomen. Consequently, malignant ovarian tumours often have a poor prognosis due to their late detection.

Small ovarian tumours remain in the pelvis and will only be detected on bimanual examination or by ultrasound. Large ovarian tumours fill the pelvis and usually lie between the uterus and sacrum.

Tumours of a moderate size may have a pedicle composed of the attenuated broad ligament and fallopian tube, which allows the tumour to be displaced from side to side.

Ovarian tumours may arise at any age, but are commonest between 30 and 60 years.

Their clinical significance is:

- They are particularly liable to be or to become malignant.
- In their early stages they are asymptomatic and painless.

- They grow to a large size and tend to undergo mechanical complications—torsion and perforation.

Ovarian tumours are classified according to their cellular origin. There are four broad categories of ovarian tumours which are shown in Fig. 17.5.

Epithelial tumours

There are four main types:

- Serous tumours are mainly benign cystic tumours (serous cystadenomas) that contain serous fluid. They can become very large (football size).
- Mucinous tumours are mainly benign cystic tumours (mucinous cystadenomas) that contain mucinous fluid.
- Endometrioid tumours are mainly malignant solid tumours (adenocarcinomas). They resemble endometrial carcinoma histologically and they cause similar symptoms.
- Brenner tumours are rare and are usually benign solid tumours.

Germ cell tumours

There are five main types:

- Dysgerminomas are solid, rare, and often malignant. They are undifferentiated tumours of the germinal epithelium that are equivalent to the male seminoma tumours that are found in the testes.
- Teratomas can have a cystic or solid form. The cystic

form is one of the commonest ovarian tumours. It may be found at any age, but normally occurs in women of childbearing age, and is often bilateral. It characteristically may contain numerous components including hair, sebaceous matter, teeth, and cartilage—this is because germ cells can differentiate into numerous cell types within the tumour and manufacture various materials. They are commonly benign but are particularly liable to undergo malignant change.

- Yolk sac tumours are rare, highly malignant tumours found in children and young adults. It produces α-foetoprotein (AFP)—blood levels can be used as a diagnostic test and as a means of monitoring the response to treatment.
- Choriocarcinoma of the ovary is very rare. It is derived from trophoblastic tissue (see Chapter 16) and hence produces human chorionic gonadotrophin (hCG).
- Gonadoblastoma is a rare mixed tumour composed of germ cell and sex-cord stromal cell types.

Sex-cord stromal tumours

These are rare and usually benign. The most common sex-cord stromal tumours are thecomas. Thecomas often produce oestrogens and can cause abnormal uterine bleeding and endometrial hyperplasia. The other sex-cord stromal tumours are listed in Fig. 17.5.

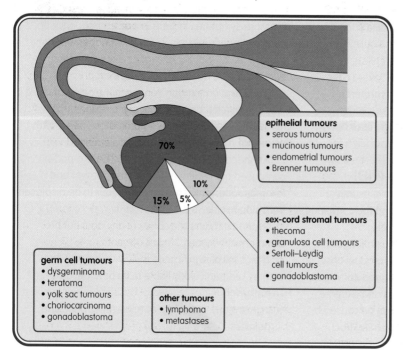

Fig. 17.5 Classification and relative incidence of the different types of ovarian tumours.

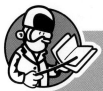

- **Discuss polycystic ovarian disease.**
- **Characterize PID.**
- **Describe the different types of ovarian tumours.**

Metastatic tumours

Various tumours metastasise to the ovary including endometrial, colon, stomach and breast adenocarcinoma.

Tumours of the fallopian tubes

The fallopian tubes are extremely resistant to malignant change; therefore tubal carcinomas are rare. The growth is usually an adenocarcinoma of the tubal epithelium which grows inwards and secretes a copious serosanguinous fluid that discharges into the vagina. The patient is usually in her 50s, and complains of pelvic pain and sometimes vaginal discharge.

DISORDERS OF THE BREAST

Congenital and anatomical anomalies

Supernumerary nipples (with or without breast tissue) occasionally occur along the 'milk line' which extends from the axilla to the groin. This is a minor congenital abnormality and the additional nipples are usually mistaken for moles or warts.

Congenital inversion of nipples occurs in many women. Nipple inversion normally corrects itself during pregnancy as the breast develops in preparation for lactation. NB breast carcinoma is suspected if nipple retraction occurs in a breast that was previous normal.

Inflammation and infection

Acute mastitis and breast abscess

Mastitis (breast infection) often occurs in the first week after delivery (a complication of lactation), or can be associated with a history of trauma. The portal of entry of the infective organism is cracks and fissures in the nipple and areola (*Staphylococcus aureus* is the commonest organism). Inflammation tends to be localized to one region, but can become widespread.

The initial infection may progress to abscess formation.

Symptoms include breast lump, breast pain, nipple discharge, high temperature, and malaise. These symptoms may present individually or together, and can be unilateral or bilateral. Cytological analysis of nipple discharge, fine-needle aspirate, or biopsy will show the presence of infection and inflammation. Antibiotics resolve most cases. Breast abscess may require surgical drainage.

Mammary duct ectasia

Duct ectasia (dilatation of ducts) is caused by inflammatory destruction of support tissues around the ducts. Its pathogenesis is uncertain. There is abnormal, progressive dilatation of the large mammary ducts, which accumulate retained secretory products and shed epithelium. It can be related to repeated pregnancy and lactation. It usually occurs in parous women in the perimenopausal age range.

Patients develop a firm, palpable breast lump. There is retraction of the nipple due to periductal fibrosis, and a blood-stained nipple discharge. Cytological examination of a fine-needle aspirate reveals inflammatory cells in the periductal region and significant fibrosis. Treatment is with antibiotics.

Fat necrosis

Breakdown of breast adipose tissue results in localised areas of inflammation. It occurs following episodes of trauma and is more frequent in obese and postmenopausal women. Necrotic fat appears yellow and haemorrhagic, and produces a hard, irregular breast lump, together with skin tethering and dimpling. A thorough examination is required to exclude a co-existing breast carcinoma. Cytological examination of a fine-needle aspirate reveals inflammatory cells and necrotic fat. Treatment is by excision combined with antibiotics to prevent secondary infection.

Fibrocystic disease

Fibrocystic disease is the most common disorder of the female breast (producing clinical symptoms in 10% of all women). It is a benign, non-neoplastic proliferative disease characterised by hyperplastic overgrowth of mammary lobules, ductules and stroma. It is caused by hormonal imbalance (excess of oestrogen or deficiency of progesterone) or a difference in responsiveness of breast tissue to oestrogen and progesterone. It most commonly occurs between the ages of 30 and 35 years

195

(there is a marked decrease in its incidence after the menopause because it is hormone dependent).
  Fibrocystic changes include:

- Mammary ducts dilate and cysts are formed—cysts may be large and produce a discrete breast lump, or may be small and multiple causing generalized 'lumpiness'.
- Fibrosis of the stroma—results in a hard lump that is often difficult to differentiate clinically from breast carcinoma.
- Epithelial hyperplasia—benign growth of normal epithelial cells that line the mammary ducts. Papillary processes may project into the duct lumen. This component of fibrocystic disease is associated with an increased risk of breast carcinoma (cysts alone do not predispose to breast carcinoma).
- Adenosis—benign proliferation, growth and fibrosis of the mammary lobules that contain the acini.

Diagnosis is made using fine-needle aspiration and mammography (see Fig. 14.10)—sclerosing lesions of the breast are most commonly seen in this way. Treatment and management consist of lumpectomy (if a discrete lump is present) and a diary of symptom occurrence and changes may be useful.

Neoplastic disorders
Benign tumours
The types of benign tumours are listed in Fig. 17.6. Diagnosis is made on the basis of:

- Presence of a breast lump.
- Mammography

Symptoms caused by inflammatory conditions of the breast and fibrocystic disease are often similar to those caused by breast carcinoma (i.e. breast lump, breast pain, nipple discharge). Breast disorders should be appropriately investigated to exclude the diagnosis of breast carcinoma.

- Cytological examination of a fine-needle aspirate from the lump.
- Histological examination of a tru-cut needle biopsy.

Treatment is by local excision of the lump (lumpectomy).

Malignant tumours (breast carcinoma)
Breast carcinoma is the commonest malignancy in women—it accounts for 20% of cancer deaths in women. Risk factors include:

- Age—peak incidence is 35–55 years of age, and it is rare below the age of 30.
- Family history of breast cancer—inheritable genetic mutations (e.g. in the tumour suppressor gene *p53*) have been linked to some families with a high incidence of breast cancer.
- Oestrogen imbalances/exposure—breast cancer is associated with increased exposure to:
  (A) high oestrogen levels, e.g. caused by ovarian tumours, obesity
  (B) oestrogen peaks that occur normally during the menstrual cycle, e.g. long length of reproductive life (early menarche, late menopause), nulliparity, late age of first child.
- Atypical epithelial hyperplasia in fibrocystic disease.

NB There is no proven increased risk with the oral contraceptive pill.

  There are numerous different types of breast carcinoma. They are classified depending on their invasiveness and their histological apppearance:

- Non-invasive (*in situ*) carcinoma—these tumours are confined to ducts (intraduct) or acini (intralobular).
- Invasive (infiltrating) carcinoma—there are a number of histologically distinct types, the most common one is infiltrating duct carcinoma (55% of cases). Paget's disease of the nipple is a specialized form of infiltrating duct carcinoma that spreads from its origin in the mammary ducts and invades the skin of the nipple.

In the UK, any woman has a 1 in 8 chance of developing breast cancer.

Types of benign tumours			
	Fibroadenoma	**Duct papilloma**	**Nipple adenoma**
incidence	most common benign tumour occurs in young women (often <30 years)	occurs in middle-aged women	rare
description	benign proliferation of fibrous and glandular breast tissue usually a well-circumscribed spherical nodule	benign papillary growth within a mammary duct	benign proliferation of epithelial cells beneath the nipple
effects	small, firm lump there is no increased risk of carcinoma	solitary lump bloody nipple discharge do not progress to carcinoma	mass beneath the nipple may ulcerate the skin 15% of tumours are associated with subsequent carcinoma

Fig.17.6 Types of benign tumours of the breast.

Infiltrating breast carcinoma spreads by:
- Local spread within the breast to involve the skin, nipple, pectoral muscles and the chest wall.
- Lymphatic spread to the axillary and internal thoracic lymph nodes.
- Blood-borne spread is especially to the lungs, liver, bone, and also to the ovaries, brain, and adrenal glands.

Patients often present with a solitary, painless lump in the breast and may have a retracted nipple, bloody nipple discharge, skin ulceration, and symptoms caused by secondary spread to the lungs, liver, and bone (e.g. backache, bone fractures, shortness of breath). Histological examination of a biopsy of the lump confirms the diagnosis. Investigations are required to deduce the extent of spread of the tumour, i.e. chest X-ray, bone scan, full blood count, liver function tests.

Treatment depends on the extent of spread (stage of the disease) and usually involves wide local surgical excision followed by radiotherapy, or radical mastectomy (removal of entire breast, pectoral muscles, and axillary lymph nodes). Chemotherapy combined with tamoxifen (oestrogen antagonist) may be given to prevent or treat metastases.

The prognosis depends on:
- The stage of the disease—the 5-year survival rate is 80% if no lymph nodes are involved, if skin and lymph nodes are involved it is 40%.
- The histological grade of the tumour cells—well differentiated tumours (i.e. still resemble cell of origin) have a better prognosis.

- Outline the congenital, inflammatory, and infective disorders of the breast.
- Discuss the changes that occur in fibrocystic breast disease.
- List the benign and malignant tumours of the breast.

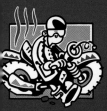

18. Pathology of the Male Reproductive System

DISORDERS OF THE PENIS

Congenital and anatomical abnormalities
Hypospadias

Hypospadias is the most common congenital abnormality of the penis, caused by the failure of the urogenital folds to fuse correctly over the urogenital sinus during development.

Normally, the urogenital folds fuse from the base of the penile shaft to the tip, resulting in the urethral meatus being sited at the tip of the glans.

If fusion is abnormal, the urethral meatus can be anywhere along the ventral surface of the penis—the commonest site is the inferior aspect of the glans (glandular hypospadias—see Fig. 18.1).

The meatus can also be anywhere along the line of the urethra on the penile shaft (penile hypospadias) or, very rarely, the meatus can be on the perineum, behind the scrotum, and the scrotum is bifid (perineal hypospadias).

Glandular hypospadias may be missed because it causes no symptoms and there is often a small pit where the external urethral meatus should be.

Penile hypospadias is often associated with a downward curvature of the penis (congenital chordee).

Hypospadias may interfere with potency and fertility, and is corrected surgically.

Epispadias

Epispadias is much rarer than hypospadias and is the same type of abnormality except that the urethra opens out onto the dorsal surface of the penis.

The commonest site for the meatus is at the base of the shaft, near the pubis.

Epispadias usually causes urinary incontinence and recurrent urinary infections, and is corrected surgically.

Phimosis

Phimosis is caused by the narrowing of the end of the foreskin (prepuce), resulting in failure of the foreskin to retract over the glans penis.

Congenital phimosis is very rare, but acquired phimosis results from scarring after trauma or infection.

Phimosis causes difficulty with micturition because the tight foreskin restricts the urinary flow. Paraphimosis is where micturition is normal but the prepuce is narrow enough to get stuck behind the glans penis after an erection, restricting venous blood flow and causing oedema.

Treatment is by circumcision.

Inflammation and infection
Genital herpes

This is a sexually transmitted disease caused by herpes simplex virus (usually HSV II).

Its incidence in the UK is increasing at present.

Genital herpes is a recurrent, acute skin infection that causes itching of the infected skin, followed by the appearance of itchy vesicles and painful skin erosions on the glans penis or the coronal sulcus. The inguinal lymph nodes are usually enlarged and painful.

Often, the primary infection is subclinical, and the virus then remains latent in the underlying skin or in the nerve ganglion that supplies that area of skin.

The latent virus can be reactivated (precipitated by fever, immunosuppression, stress, UV light) and causes recurrent attacks.

HSV infection is diagnosed clinically and by specific laboratory tests to identify the causative organism [tissue culture, electronmicroscopy, anti-HSV antibodies, polymerase chain reaction (PCR)].

Treatment with the antiviral drug acyclovir is appropriate for the initial episode and for asymptomatic recent sexual contacts, but for subsequent attacks treat

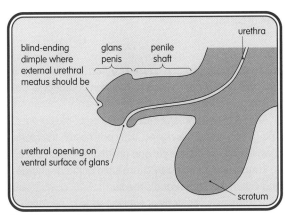

Fig. 18.1 Glandular hypospadias.

blind-ending dimple where external urethral meatus should be

glans penis

penile shaft

urethra

urethral opening on ventral surface of glans

scrotum

199

symptoms only (re-treat with acyclovir only if the patient is immunosuppressed).

The virus cannot be eliminated from the body, but treatment attempts to reduce its reactivation and to reduce symptoms.

Genital warts

This is a sexually transmitted disease caused by human papilloma virus (HPV subtypes 6, 11, 16, 18, 33).

Genital warts are benign, fleshy, hyperplastic skin lesions (condyloma acuminatum) that most commonly occur on the glans penis, the inner surface of the foreskin and in the external urethral meatus.

The incidence of genital warts is increasing in the UK at present.

HPV infection is diagnosed clinically (do not usually take samples to test for the presence of HPV).

Treatment comprises cryotherapy (spray the wart with liquid nitrogen to kill the infected cells) or podophyllin cream (apply weekly, leaving cream on for *only* 4 hours at a time, to burn the infected cells chemically).

Despite treatment, the warts often recur.

Syphilis

This is a sexually transmitted bacterial infection caused by *Treponema pallidum*.

Primary syphilis develops 9–90 days after inoculation, when a solitary, painless, ulcerated nodule (primary syphilitic chancre) appears at the infection site (usually on the glans penis, coronal sulcus, or the inner surface of the foreskin) and the inguinal lymph nodes are enlarged but not painful.

Secondary syphilis is a systemic disease but often involves the development of condylomata lata on the foreskin. Tertiary syphilis later affects the central nervous system.

Syphilis is diagnosed by dark-background

In all sexually transmitted diseases it is important to give advice on preventative measures (e.g. use of condoms) and to follow up sexual contacts in order to stop the spread of infection.

microscopy (of sample from primary chancre) and by serological tests (antibody tests using sample of patient's blood).

Treatment is with penicillin and probenecid (impedes renal excretion of penicillin to maintain concentrations); also treat recent sexual contacts.

Gonococcal urethritis (gonorrhoea)

This is a sexually transmitted bacterial infection caused by *Neisseria gonorrhoea*.

Symptoms include pain on urinating and a purulent urethral discharge.

Complications include periurethral abscesses, urethral stricture, proctitis, and epididymo-orchitis.

Its incidence is low in the UK.

Gonorrhoea is diagnosed by direct microscopy, and culture is used to determine the antibiotic sensitivity of the gonococcal stain (many are now resistant to penicillin).

Treatment is with penicillin or ceftriaxone (if penicillin resistant); also treat recent sexual contacts.

Non-gonococcal urethritis (NGU)

This is the most common sexually transmitted disease in the UK.

It is caused by *Chlamydia trachomatis*.

The symptoms and possible complications are the same as for gonorrhoea.

Tropical infections of *Chlamydia* serotypes L1–L3 can cause painless genital ulceration and persistent inguinal lymphadenopathy (lymphogranuloma venereum).

Chlamydial infection is suspected from the symptoms and the absence of *N. gonorrhoea* in direct microscopy, but is diagnosed by tissue culture (*Chlamydia* cannot be grown in normal culture), Giemsa stain, and antibody reaction tests.

Treatment is with oxytetracycline; also treat recent sexual contacts.

Thrush

This is a fungal infection caused by *Candida albicans*. It can be sexually transmitted but is often an endogenous infection.

Thrush causes balanitis (inflammation of the prepuce and glans penis) causing red, itchy patches on the glans, a white urethral discharge, and an irritant pale prepuce.

Thrush is diagnosed by Gram stain of the discharge and culture on Sabouraud's medium.

Treatment is with topical antifungals (e.g. nystatin); also treat recent sexual contacts.

Aseptic inflammation

This can be caused by:

- Dermatological disorders including psoriasis, dermatitis (irritant or allergic), lichenification (causes balanitis xerotica obliterans).
- Adverse drug reactions.
- Trauma (e.g. secondary to condom friction).

Neoplastic disorders

Benign tumours

Condylomata acuminata are small benign genital warts caused by HPV infection (see above); they do not have premalignant potential.

Treatment is with cryotherapy or podophyllin to destroy affected areas.

Malignant tumours

A carcinoma *in situ* (Bowen's disease) can occur anywhere on the skin, including the penis (where it is called erythroplasia of Queyrat)—it is a raised, red plaque that is a preinvasive squamous cell carcinoma (i.e. may progress to invasive squamous carcinoma).

Invasive squamous carcinoma of the penis (rare in the UK) occurs more commonly in elderly uncircumcised men and is associated with HPV infection—it is an ulcerating plaque, usually on the glans or inner surface of the foreskin, that invades surrounding structures and metastasizes to the inguinal lymph nodes.

Treatment is with radiotherapy, amputation, and lymph node dissection, depending on the extent of the tumour and its spread.

- Detail the developmental and neoplastic disorders of the penis.
- List the causes of infection and inflammation of the penis.

DISORDERS OF THE TESTES AND EPIDIDYMIS

Congenital and anatomical abnormalities

Cryptorchidism (undescended testes)

The testes develop *in utero* on the posterior abdominal wall and later descend to the scrotum (at birth, 80% have descended; at 1 year of age, 97% have descended).

Cryptorchidism can be unilateral or bilateral (1 in 5 are bilateral), are usually associated with congenital inguinal hernia, and the affected testis is normally small/underdeveloped (possible cause or effect of maldescent).

Undescended testes must be corrected surgically (before the age of 7 years) because intra-abdominal testes cannot produce spermatozoa (causes sterility if bilateral) and have a higher risk of malignant change.

Intra-abdominal testes can still produce testosterone, so there are no abnormal secondary sexual characteristics if it is retained into adulthood.

Retractile testes are testes that have descended normally but are still very mobile and can be drawn up to the external inguinal ring by the contraction of the cremasteric muscle—they should not be misdiagnosed as undescended testes.

Abnormalities of the tunica vaginalis (see Fig. 13.21)

Hydrocoele

A hydrocoele is a collection of fluid in the tunica vaginalis and is the commonest cause of an intrascrotal swelling.

Congenital hydrocoeles result from the retention of a patent processus vaginalis (the channel between the abdominal cavity and the scrotum that exists temporarily during development) and are sometimes associated with inguinal hernia—most disappear spontaneously; if they persist, they should be corrected surgically.

Secondary hydrocoeles may result from damage to the tunica vaginalis from infection, inflammation, or tumour growth. Treat the underlying condition that is causing the secondary hydrocoele (infection or neoplasm).

Haematocoele

A haematocoele is a haemorrhage into the tunica vaginalis.

It is usually caused by trauma to the scrotum or by a testicular tumour.

If the haemorrhage is not treated (i.e. drained and washed), the blood will clot and contract around the testis, causing it to become ischaemic and necrotic.

Hernia

An indirect inguinal hernia arises in the abdomen and can cause a scrotal mass. A hernial sac develops and passes through the inguinal ring into the scrotum, just as the spermatic cord does normally. The hernial sac can contain abdominal contents, e.g. bowel.

Indirect inguinal hernias can be congenital (caused by the retention of a patent processus vaginalis) or acquired (may occur at any age).

These hernias must be surgically corrected because they are liable to strangulate (due to a narrow hernial neck).

Testicular atrophy

Testicular atrophy may be caused by panhypopituitarism, where the anterior pituitary does not secrete sufficient levels of luteinizing hormone (LH) or follicle-stimulating hormone (FSH).

LH and FSH are gonadotrophic hormones that stimulate the testes to produce spermatozoa and to release testosterone. Lack of these hormones causes hypogonadism, reduced fertility, loss of secondary sexual characteristics, and loss of libido.

Treatment is by means of replacement therapy—if fertility is required, LH and FSH analogues are administered; if fertility is not required, testosterone needs to be replaced (to maintain 'maleness').

Other causes of testicular atrophy include excessive alcohol intake and illicit drug-taking.

Inflammation and Infection
Epididymitis and orchitis

Orchitis means inflammation of the testis, epididymitis means inflammation of the epididymis—both are usually caused by infection. Acute infections are usually caused by bacteria that tract up from the urethra following an untreated urinary tract infection. Causative organisms include:
- Coliform bacilli.
- *Chlamydia trachomatis.*
- *Neisseria gonorrhoea.*
- Mumps virus (which causes an orchitis in the absence of an epididymitis because they infect the testes via the bloodstream).

Symptoms include painful, swollen testis which may be accompanied by a secondary hydrocoele, general malaise, fever, and headache.

Complications may occur, e.g. testicular atrophy and

scarring, subfertility, epididymal cyst formation. They are usually diagnosed from the history of the episode, which can sometimes be confirmed by the presence of organisms and pus cells in the urine. Treatment is with appropriate antibiotics.

Chronic infections of the testes are painless and may be caused by tertiary syphilis (testicular gumma) or by tuberculosis, but both of these are now rare.

Granulomatous (autoimmune) orchitis

Granulomatous orchitis is a rare chronic inflammatory condition.

There is no infective agent and it may be caused by an autoimmune reaction—if the blood–testes barrier is breached, autoantibodies can destroy the developing spermatozoa in the seminiferous tubules and cause a chronic inflammatory reaction (the spermatozoa are normally protected from the body's immune system by the inability of the immune cells to pass through the blood–testes barrier).

The presenting signs are similar to those of a testicular tumour—the affected testis is firm and enlarged, and a secondary hydrocoele is sometimes found.

Trauma and vascular disturbances
Torsion of the testis

Torsion of the testis is where the testis (or, more commonly, the spermatic cord) becomes twisted and the blood supply is impaired or occluded—it is an acute surgical emergency.

Normal testes are fixed within the tunica vaginalis and therefore cannot twist—there must be an underlying congenital abnormality for torsion to occur (e.g. maldescended testis, abnormally long spermatic cord).

Torsion usually occurs spontaneously but can be precipitated by exertion.

The commonest age for torsion is 10–15 years.

The patient usually presents with severe pain in the testis and groin, and sometimes with lower abdominal pain (the nerve supply of the testes is from the T10 sympathetic pathway).

The twisted testis is extremely tender and swollen, and lies high in the scrotum.

If treatment is delayed, the testis will become ischaemic and infarcted owing to the compromised blood supply.

To treat, the testis is investigated surgically—if it is still viable, the cord is untwisted and the testis sutured to the tunica vaginalis to prevent a recurrence; if the testis has infarcted, it is removed.

During surgical repair of one testis, the other testis is also fixed to the tunica vaginalis to prevent it from twisting because the congenital abnormality predisposing to torsion is usually bilateral.

Varicocoele

A varicocoele is a bunch of dilated, varicose veins in the pampiniform plexus above the testes that feels like a 'bag of worms' and is reducible when the patient lies flat.

There is usually no obvious underlying cause but it is much more common on the left side than on the right.

Varicocoeles are usually harmless but very rarely they can be associated with an underlying renal carcinoma (the tumour grows down the renal vein and blocks the testicular vein, causing a varicocoele).

Patients with varicocoeles may have decreased spermatozoa production and hence be subfertile—this is because the intrascrotal temperature is raised owing to the increased amount of blood in the testicular vessels.

Management comprises reassurance and, if appropriate, treatment of the underlying cause.

Neoplastic disorders

Tumours of the testis are relatively uncommon (cause <1% of cancer deaths) but they are important to recognize because the peak incidence is in early adult life (they are the commonest form of malignancy in young adult males), they are often highly malignant, and many are curable.

Undescended testes are predisposed to neoplastic change (10-fold risk).

Patients often present with:
- A painless, enlarged, hard testis.
- Secondary hydrocoele.
- Lymph node enlargement in the retroperineum (NB the lymphatic drainage of the testes is to the para-aortic nodes and NOT via the inguinal lymph nodes).
- Metastases to the lungs or liver.
- Gynaecomastia (due to androgen or oestrogen secretion by Leydig cell tumours).

The tumour is diagnosed by scrotal ultrasound, and surgical examination (the testis is removed from the scrotum via an inguinal incision so that it can be inspected and biopsied if necessary—the spermatic cord must be clamped to prevent tumour cells being released into the circulation during this procedure). Chest X-ray, abdominal CT scan are used to look for metastases spread.

It is treated by orchiectomy (removal of testis) via an inguinal incision, followed by radiotherapy or chemotherapy, depending on the type of testicular tumour.

The prognosis depends on the type of tumour, but is generally very good (100% 5-year survival rate if lymph nodes are not involved, 95% if early lymph node involvement).

Testicular tumours may be derived from germ cells or from non-germ cells—see Fig. 18.2.

Germ cell testicular tumours

These comprise 90% of testicular tumours.

There are three types of tumour that are derived from germ cells:

Seminoma

This is an undifferentiated tumour of the germinal epithelium (may resemble spermatogonia cells).

The peak incidence is in 30–50-year-olds.

It presents as a painless swelling in the testis.

There is often early lymphatic spread to the para-aortic nodes and haematogenous spread to the lungs.

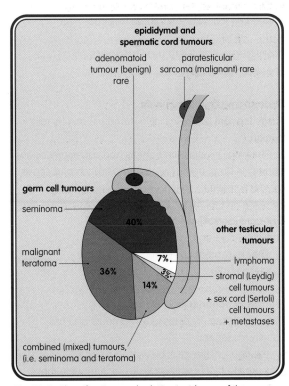

Fig. 18.2 Classification and relative incidence of the different types of testicular tumour.

Orchiectomy and radiotherapy cure most patients completely (seminomas are highly radiosensitive).

Teratoma

Teratomas are composed of various tissue types (endoderm, ectoderm, and mesoderm).

They are usually malignant (more so than seminomas).

The peak incidence is in those in their late 20s, but it may be seen in childhood.

Treatment comprises orchiectomy and combination chemotherapy to the affected lymph nodes.

The behaviour and prognosis of the tumour is related to the histological appearance of the tumour cells.

Yolk sac tumours and choriocarcinomas secrete α-foetoprotein (AFP) and/or β-human chorionic gonadotrophic (βhCG), which can be measured in the serum—these 'tumour markers' can be used to diagnose these rare tumours, to monitor treatment, and to detect metastases and recurrences from these tumours.

Combined tumours

These are mixed tumours composed of intermingled areas of seminoma and teratoma.

The behaviour and prognosis of the mixed tumours depend on the type of teratoma involved.

Non-germ-cell testicular tumours

These comprise 10% of testicular tumours.

Stromal (Leydig) cell tumours

These are rare (2% of testicular tumours) and usually benign.

They may produce androgens and cause precocious puberty in boys, or may produce oestrogen and cause gynaecomastia.

Sex-cord (Sertoli) cell tumours

These are rare and usually benign.

They may produce oestrogens and cause gynaecomastia.

Primary lymphoma (non-Hodgkin's)

These comprise 7% of testicular tumours and are usually malignant.

The peak incidence is between 60 and 80 years, and they are the most common testicular tumour in those aged over 65 years.

Metastatic tumours

These are usually only found incidentally at autopsy. Various tumours can metastasize to the testes, including bronchial and prostatic carcinoma and malignant melanoma.

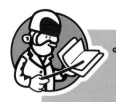

- **What are the congenital and anatomical disorders of the testes?**
- **List the infective, inflammatory and vascular disorders of the testes and epididymis.**
- **How does torsion of the testis occur?**
- **Name the different types of testicular tumours, their relative incidence, diagnosis, and treatment.**

DISORDERS OF THE PROSTATE GLAND

Inflammation and infection

Acute prostatitis

This is caused by infection with urethral organisms (e.g. coliform bacteria, *Neisseria gonorrhoea, Chlamydia trachomatis*) following urethritis or cystitis, or with faecal organisms (e.g. *Escherichia coli, Streptococcus faecalis*).

Patients may have symptoms of prostatism (urinary frequency), fever, and perineal pain; rarely, patients present with urinary retention (prostate becomes so inflamed and swollen that it obstructs the urethra, preventing the passing of urine).

The prostate gland is enlarged, soft, and tender on palpation.

Treatment is with antibiotics appropriate to the infective organism (a urine sample is tested as it will usually contain the causative organism).

Chronic prostatitis

This is caused by untreated or recurrent episodes of

acute infective prostatitis, or by tuberculosis infection (secondary to a tuberculous cystitis or epididymitis).

Granulomatous prostatitis

The aetiology of this is unknown (not caused by infection).

Inflammation causes the prostate to enlarge and sometimes obstruct the urethra.

Allergic prostatitis

This is usually associated with asthma.

The onset of symptoms is usually acute.

The inflammatory infiltrate contains a large number of eosinophils.

Benign prostatic hypertrophy

Prostatic hypertrophy commonly starts at the age of 50 years.

It is caused by hyperplasia (not neoplasia) of the lateral and periurethral areas of the prostate gland (see Fig. 18.3).

The increase in size of the prostate gland may cause urinary obstruction, not because it blocks the urethra directly, but because it disturbs the function of the internal urethral sphincter.

It occurs in 75% of elderly males, but only 5% have symptoms of 'prostatism' (i.e. difficulty in micturition involving urinary frequency, hesitancy, poor stream, and dribbling at the end of micturition).

If prostatic hypertrophy is severe and untreated, it can result in recurrent urinary tract infections (because of chronic retention of urine in the bladder and a poor urinary stream that fails to flush out pathogens), and eventually in impaired renal function.

Benign prostatic hypertrophy is not a premalignant lesion.

Treatment comprises **t**rans**u**rethral **r**esection of the hyperplastic **p**eriurethral zone (TURP)—the fragments carved off the prostate are examined histologically to exclude the possiblity of coexisting prostatic carcinoma.

Prostatic carcinoma

Prostatic carcinoma is an increasingly common form of cancer in the developed world (where it now accounts for 7% of cancer deaths).

The peak incidence is between 60 and 85 years.

It does not appear to be related to benign prostatic hyperplasia.

It is probably related to androgen hormones, e.g. testosterone (it is not seen in castrati).

It arises most commonly in the posterior and peripheral portion of the gland (cf. the distribution of benign hypertrophy, which surrounds the urethra and the lateral lobes).

Mode of spread

This comprises the following:

- Local spread within the gland leads to urinary obstruction and invasion into surrounding organs, e.g. bladder, urethra, seminal vesicles.
- Lymphatic spread is to the iliac and para-aortic lymph nodes.
- Retrograde venous flow sends metastases to the lumbar and sacral spine.
- Blood-borne spread is especially to the bones of the pelvis, spine, and skull, causing osteosclerotic lesions (this is unusual because metastases usually cause lytic lesions).

Clinical features

Symptoms are similar to those of benign prostatic enlargement, but they tend to progress more rapidly and often there are signs of metastatic disease present (e.g. back pain from bony metastases, general malaise, weight loss, anaemia).

Rectal examination reveals a hard nodule within the prostate gland; in a more advanced tumour, the median groove of the gland is obliterated (see Fig. 18.3).

Diagnosis

Prostatic carcinoma is diagnosed by:

- Measuring the level of prostate-specific antigen (PSA) and prostatic acid phosphatase (PAP) in the serum.
- Needle biopsy and histology.
- Plain X-rays to locate bone metastases.

Raised levels of PSA and PAP indicate the presence of prostatic carcinoma and their levels can be used to monitor the response to treatment.

Blood specimens for PSA and PAP measurement must be taken prior to rectal examination of the prostate to prevent error (examination cause excessive release of PSA and PAP).

Treatment

This comprises:

- Prostatectomy to remove the tumour.
- Radiotherapy to treat bone and lymph node metastases.

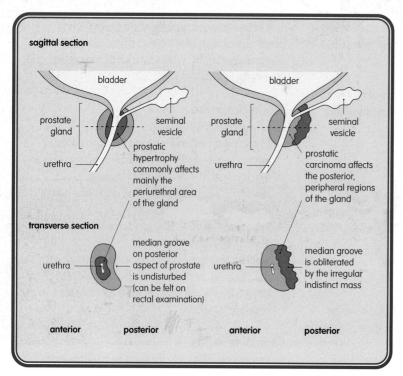

Fig. 18.3 Different regions of the prostate gland that are affected by benign hypertrophy and by malignant growth.

- Cyproterone acetate (a synthetic androgen antagonist) to block the effects of testosterone on the prostate.
- Gonadotrophin-releasing hormone (GnRH) analogues that when given continuously, block the release of LH from the anterior pituitary gland (and therefore cause the plasma testosterone levels to fall).

Prognosis

For a tumour confined to the gland (no metastases), the 5-year survival rate is 75%.

For a tumour involving the lymph nodes or bones, the 5-year survival rate is 35%.

THE MALE BREAST

Gynaecomastia

Gynaecomastia is a common cause of breast enlargement in men. It is caused by benign hyperplastic growth of the mammary ducts and connective tissues, resulting from an increase in the oestrogen–androgen ratio. Therefore, it occurs in syndromes where the plasma oestrogen levels are raised or the plasma testosterone levels are reduced (see Fig. 12.2). Its incidence is highest in adolescence and the majority of

cases are idiopathic. Treatment depends on the cause but surgical removal of breast tissue may be required if the breasts do not return to normal size.

Carcinoma of the male breast

Breast carcinoma in men is very rare compared to that in the female (male to female ratio is 1:100). Intraduct and infiltrating duct carcinoma are the prevalent types (see Chapter 17). It occurs in elderly men and they usually present with a lump or nipple discharge. The tumours are locally invasive and tend to have metastasized to the axillary lymph nodes and other organs (e.g. lungs, brain, bone, liver) by the time they are discovered. The prognosis is poor.

- Discuss the causes of prostatitis.
- What are the differences between prostatic hypertrophy and prostatic carcinoma?

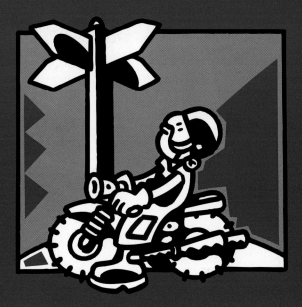

SELF-ASSESSMENT

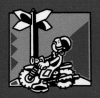

Multiple-choice Questions

Indicate whether each answer is true or false.

1. Causes of hypopituitarism include:
(a) Prolactinoma.
(b) Sheehan's syndrome.
(c) Severe head trauma.
(d) Sarcoidosis.
(e) Craniopharyngioma.

2. Regarding osteoporosis:
(a) Bone mass is abnormally reduced but mineralization is normal. T
(b) Afro-Caribbean women are more susceptible to it than Caucasian women. F
(c) It can be associated with acromegaly. F — Rickets + osteomalacia
(d) It can be caused by vitamin D deficiency. F
(e) Treatment with calcium supplements is not useful after the menopause. T

3. Concerning the contraceptive pill:
(a) To be effective, the combined pill needs to be taken continuously. F
(b) The combined pill contains synthetic oestrogen and progesterone and hence suppresses ovulation. T
(c) The combined pill causes fewer adverse side effects than the progesterone-only pill. F
(d) The progesterone-only pill is risk-free. F
(e) Using the combined pill as a means of contraception reduces the risk of developing ovarian cancer. T

4. Cortisol is a glucocorticoid hormone secreted by the adrenal cortex which:
(a) Promotes sodium reabsorption from the renal tubules. T
(b) Inhibits the pituitary secretion of ACTH. T
(c) Increases the total white-blood-cell count. T
(d) Suppresses the immune response. T
(e) Promotes protein catabolism. T

5. Regarding ectopic pregnancy:
(a) Implantation of the fertilized ovum outside the uterus is nearly always in the fallopian tubes. T
(b) It is commoner in females using the progesterone-only pill. T
(c) The human chorionic gonadotrophin (hCG) pregnancy test is negative in early pregnancy. F
(d) If no tubal pregnancy is visualised by ultrasound scan, then an ectopic can be ruled out. F
(e) Internal blood loss may occur. T

6. Pituitary adenomas:
(a) May affect visual acuity. F
(b) Are most commonly prolactinomas. T
(c) Usually upset the secretion of more than one pituitary hormone. F
(d) Must always be removed surgically. F
(e) Tend to grow rapidly and cause acute symptoms. F

7. Concerning types of hormones:
(a) Hormones derived from amino acids are stored in intracellular vesicles, ready for release. T
(b) Most hormones are steroid molecules. F
(c) Steroid hormones are synthesized in the mitochondria and smooth endoplasmic reticulum. T
(d) Peptide hormones are synthesized in the nucleus, rough endoplasmic reticulum, and Golgi apparatus. T
(e) Eicosanoid hormones also act as intracellular messengers. T

8. Regarding maternal adaptations to pregnancy:
(a) Nausea, breast tenderness, and urinary frequency are the only symptoms of pregnancy. F
(b) Blood pressure increases in early pregnancy. F
(c) Oestrogen stimulates respiration and causes the renal calyces to dilate. F
(d) All the organs involved in endocrine secretion are altered. T
(e) The myometrial cells hypertrophy. T

9. The insulin-induced hypoglycaemia stress test:
(a) Is used to test the ability of the anterior pituitary to increase its secretion of ACTH, GH, and prolactin. T
(b) Is stopped if the blood glucose falls below 2.2 mmol/L.
(c) Is contraindicated in patients with ischaemic heart disease and epilepsy.
(d) is use to diagnose diabetes insipidus.
(e) Is synonymous with the glucose tolerance test.

10. Parathyroid hormone:
(a) Is made in the parafollicular cells of the thyroid gland. F
(b) Is a steroid hormone. F
(c) Targets osteoclast cells (i.e. these cells have receptors for parathyroid hormone). F
(d) Stimulates calcium uptake from the gut directly. F
(e) Raises serum phosphate levels. F

11. Concerning the thyroid hormones, thyroxine (T_4), and tri-iodonine (T_3):
(a) T_4 and T_3 are stored extracellularly in the colloid as thyroglobulin. F
(b) T_4 is 5–10 times more potent in the tissues than T_3. F
(c) T_4 and T_3 are mainly transported in the blood bound to albumin. F 30% to albumin
(d) T_3 is converted into T_4 in the tissues. F
(e) T_4 and T_3 are secreted by the thyroid in equal quantities. F

12. A goitre can be caused by:
(a) Iodine deficiency. T
(b) Pregnancy. T
(c) De Quervain's thyroiditis.
(d) Hashimoto's thyroiditis. T
(e) Lithium.

13. Regarding development of the male and female reproductive systems:
(a) In the male, the mesonephric ducts develop into the vas deferens. T
(b) The scrotum in the male and the labia majora in the female are derived from the same embryological origin. T
(c) In the female, the primordial germ cells originate in the dorsal body wall. F
(d) In the female, oestrogen combined with the lack of testosterone causes the differentiation of the female external genitalia. T
(e) The testes and the ovaries both descend under the control of a gubernaculum. T

14. Concerning treatment of thyrotoxicosis:
(a) Propranolol can be given instead of surgery. F
(b) Carbamazepine is often used. F Carbimazole
(c) Persistently low levels of TSH is an indication for surgery. F
(d) Hypothyroidism may result after treatment. T
(e) Orbital decompression may be necessary because of thyroid eye disease. T

15. TSH secretion increases:
(a) After a partial thyroidectomy. T F
(b) When the basal metabolic rate falls. F
(c) During pregnancy. F
(d) When the diet is chronically iodine-deficient. T
(e) In Graves' disease. F

16. Regarding lactation:
(a) Oxytocin initiates the production of milk. F
(b) Development of the mammary glands occurs throughout pregnancy. T
(c) Suckling during breastfeeding stimulates prolactin secretion but inhibits oxytocin secretion. F
(d) Colostrum contains maternal antibodies. T
(e) Human milk has a higher fat content than colostrum. T

17. Regarding hypocalcaemia:
(a) Calcitonin deficiency can cause hypocalcaemia. F
(b) Pseudohypoparathyroidism (a possible cause of hypocalcaemia) is inheritable. T
↓ serum Ca++ (c) Hypocalcaemia is defined as a blood calcium level of less than 5.25 mmol/L. F
(d) Patients often present with numbness and paraesthesia in their hands and feet. T
(e) Chvostek's sign is positive. T

18. Concerning hormone receptors:
(a) Water-soluble hormones bind directly to G-protein molecules on the target cell surface. F
(b) Activated G-protein molecules activate adenyl cyclase or phospholipase C, which are located in the cell membrane.
(c) cAMP is the second messenger that binds to the endoplasmic reticulum and causes influx of calcium ions into the cell cytoplasm.
(d) Tyrosine kinase receptors have cAMP as their second messenger.
(e) Steroid hormones pass through the target cell membrane unaided and bind to intracellular receptors in the cytoplasm or in the nucleus.

19. Regarding the adrenal cortex:
(a) It is derived from ectodermal tissue. F
(b) It is composed of chromaffin cells. F — medulla
(c) The zona glomerulosa synthesizes mineralocorticoids. T
(d) The cells of the zona fasciculata are arranged in cords alongside blood sinusoids. T
(e) Blood flows from the outer layer inwards towards the adrenal medulla. T

20. The vagina:
(a) Has epithelium that undergoes cyclical changes during the menstrual cycle. T
(b) Has a pH of 5.6. T
(c) Has a rich sensory innervation. F
(d) Has a large number of glands. F
(e) Is lined by a simple columnal epithelium. F

21. Concerning Addison's disease:
(a) In the UK, it is most commonly caused by tuberculosis infection. F
(b) Hyperpigmentation is often present. T
(c) It is diagnosed using the dexamethasone test. F
(d) Patients commonly present with postural hypotension and hypoglycaemia. T
(e) There is often a family history of associated autoimmune diseases. T

22. Congenital adrenal hyperplasia:
(a) Is usually due to a deficiency of the enzyme 21-hydroxylase. T
(b) Causes a decrease in plasma cortisol and aldosterone concentrations. T
(c) Causes precocious puberty in males. T
(d) May present at birth with an acute addisonian crisis. T
(e) Has a poor prognosis even with treatment. F

23. Cushing's disease can cause:
(a) Hypokalaemia. T
(b) Hypertension. T
(c) Loss of body hair. F
(d) Low ACTH levels. F
(e) Cataracts.

24. Carcinomas of the vulva:
(a) Are usually noninvasive.
(b) Are most commonly found in the labium majorus.
(c) Spread locally if neglected.
(d) Are usually found in women under 60 years of age.
(e) Spread to inguinal lymph nodes.

25. The endocrine pancreas:
(a) Constitutes 20–25% of the wet weight of the pancreas.
(b) Develops from the midgut.
(c) Synthesizes insulin in the β cells of the islets of Langerhans.
(d) Secretes insulin and glucagon in equal amounts.
(e) Can be affected by haemochromatosis (congenital disorder of iron transport).

26. Concerning cyclical changes in the endometrium:
(a) The endometrium starts to proliferate after ovulation. F
(b) The uterine glands secrete a mucoid fluid that is rich in glycogen during the secretory phase of the menstrual cycle. T
(c) Approximately 30 mL of blood is lost each menstrual bleed. T
(d) The stratum functionale is shed during each cycle. T
(e) The myometrium contracts to expel the superficial endometrial tissue during menstruation. T

27. Regarding diabetes mellitus:
(a) The prevalence in the UK is approximately 1%. T
(b) It is diagnosed by testing for the presence of glucose in the urine. F
(c) Type 1 diabetes mellitus is inherited as an autosomal dominant trait. F
(d) Type 2 increases in prevalence in middle/old age. T
(e) Acute pancreatitis can cause diabetes mellitus. T

28. Metabolic effects of diabetes mellitus include:
(a) Loss of extracellular fluid. T
(b) Decreased glycogenolysis. F
(c) Decreased lipolysis. F
(d) Increased gluconeogenesis. T
(e) Intermittent periods of hypoglycaemia. F

29. Hypoglycaemia can be caused by:
(a) Insulinoma.
(b) Addison's disease.
(c) Liver failure.
(d) Alcohol.
(e) Anti-insulin-receptor antibodies.

30. Concerning the placenta:
(a) Immediately after fertilization the trophoblast develops finger-like projections called villi.
(b) The villi anchor the developing embryo.
(c) Maternal blood spaces within the decidua bathe the growing villi.
(d) It is expelled from the uterus during the second stage of labour.
(e) Its primary function is the synthesis of placental hormones.

31. Concerning puberty:
(a) The age when puberty occurs is genetically controlled.
(b) Breast development (thelarche) is the first change in females undergoing puberty.
(c) The time of onset of the pubertal growth spurt can affect the height achieved by the adult.
(d) Prepubertal boys and girls have an equal amount of body fat.
(e) Hypothalamic GnRH secretion is inhibited prior to puberty.

32. Concerning the ovaries:
(a) They are almond-shaped organs, each about 3 cm long. T
(b) They secrete mainly peptide hormones. F
(c) They contain ovarian follicles at various stages of development. T
(d) They contain about 1–2 million oocytes at birth. F
(e) They release approximately 400 oocytes during a woman's lifetime. T

33. Growth hormone secretion:
(a) Is controlled by the hypothalamus.
(b) Ceases after puberty. F
(c) Increases during fasting.
(d) Increases during sleep.
(e) Is regulated by the sex hormones.

34. Short stature in children can be caused by:
(a) Production of abnormal GH by the pituitary.
(b) Hypothyroidism.
(c) Rickets.
(d) Emotional deprivation.
(e) Cushing's syndrome.

35. Symptoms and signs of hypothyroidism include:
(a) Carpal tunnel syndrome.
(b) Heat intolerance.
(c) Amenorrhoea.
(d) Periorbital puffiness.
(e) Deafness.

36. Concerning the renin-angiotensin-aldosterone system:
(a) Renin is synthesized and stored in the juxtaglomerular granular cells.
(b) Renin is released into the blood in response to a rise in the renal blood pressure.
(c) Renin converts angiotensin I into angiotensin II.
(d) Aldosterone promotes sodium ion reabsorption from the kidney, colon, and stomach.
(e) Excess aldosterone secretion does not cause sodium retention.

37. Regarding testosterone:
(a) Production is stimulated by FSH.
(b) It is secreted by the Leydig cells.
(c) It stimulates spermatogenesis.
(d) The release of testosterone stimulates the pupils to dilate.
(e) Lack of testosterone causes loss of secondary sexual characteristics.

38. Insulin:
(a) Is a hormone composed of two peptide chains.
(b) Is secreted mainly in response to gut hormones.
(c) Circulates in the blood mostly bound to plasma proteins.
(d) Binds to a G-protein-coupled receptor on the target cell membrane.
(e) Inhibits lipolysis in adipose tissue.

39. Regarding secondary hyperparathyroidism:
(a) It results in hypercalcaemia.
(b) It can be caused by chronic renal failure.
(c) It can be caused by hypopituitarism.
(d) Parathyroid enlargement can usually be felt in the thyroid region.
(e) It may cause osteomalacia.

40. Galactorrhoea can be caused by:
(a) Metoclopramide.
(b) Prolactinoma.
(c) Bromocriptine.
(d) Hypothyroidism.
(e) Postpartum lactation.

41. Common causes of infertility include:
(a) Impotence.
(b) Hyperprolactinaemia.
(c) Fibroids.
(d) Hypothyroidism.
(e) Hydrocoele.

42. Regarding control of hormone secretion:
(a) Most hormones are secreted at a basal level but their secretion increases in response to nervous, endocrine, or biochemical stimuli.
(b) A high level of cortisol in the blood inhibits the secretion of corticotrophin-releasing hormone (CRH) from the hypothalamus.
(c) A high level of prolactin in the blood stimulates the secretion of prolactin-releasing hormone.
(d) GH stimulates glucagon secretion.
(e) The nervous system regulates hormone secretion.

43. Concerning hormonal changes during pregnancy:
(a) The presence of hPL (human placental lactogen) is diagnostic of pregnancy.
(b) Progesterone is the most important hormone in the maintenance of pregnancy.
(c) Oestrogens stimulate the production of oxytocin receptors in the myometrial cells.
(d) Maternal thyroid stimulating hormone (TSH) secretion increases.
(e) Maternal growth hormone secretion decreases.

44. Diabetes insipidus can be caused by:
(a) Idiopathic ADH deficiency.
(b) Head injury.
(c) Oat cell bronchial carcinoma.
(d) Hyperglycaemia.
(e) Polydipsia.

45. Herpes simplex II viral infections:
(a) Are sexually transmitted.
(b) Do not cause vaginal discharge.
(c) Are usually recurrent.
(d) Have a long incubation period.
(e) Are treated with penicillin.

46. Concerning treatment of diabetes mellitus:
(a) Insulin is administered by intramuscular injection.
(b) Insulin should not be given more than twice a day.
(c) During illnesses patients should reduce the number of insulin injections.
(d) Insulin is made using recombinant genetic techniques.
(e) Blood-insulin levels should be regularly monitored.

47. Swellings of the scrotum may be owing to:
(a) Inguinal hernia.
(b) Femoral hernia.
(c) Phimosis.
(d) Tertiary syphilis.
(e) Seminoma.

48. Concerning a phaeochromocytoma:
(a) It is a tumour of the adrenal medulla.
(b) It causes intermittent hypertension.
(c) 10% are bilateral.
(d) It may be familial and associated with other endocrine tumours.
(e) Propranolol and phenoxybenzamine are used in the long-term treatment.

49. Regarding ACTH:
(a) It is released by corticotrophic cells in the hypothalamus.
(b) It is a peptide hormone.
(c) Its secretion is high in the morning and low at night.
(d) The dexamethasone suppression test inhibits ACTH release.
(e) Excess release of ACTH causes Addison's disease.

50. Concerning hypothalamic-releasing hormones:
(a) Somatostatin stimulates GH release.
(b) TRH stimulates the release of both TSH and prolactin.
(c) Hypothalamic hormones only have to be secreted in small quantities to have an effect.
(d) Dopamine deficiency causes hyperprolactinaemia.
(e) Craniopharyngioma is a hypothalamic tumour that results in excessive secretion of hypothalamic-releasing hormones.

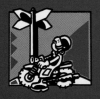

Short-answer Questions

1. Draw a labelled diagram to show how a hormone causes an intracellular response via the second messenger cyclic adenosine monophosphate (cAMP), and give three examples of hormone receptors that affect cAMP levels.

2. How is pelvic inflammatory disease (PID) caused and what are its symptoms and chronic complications?

3. Outline the development of the anterior pituitary gland.

4. How does the progesterone-only pill provide contraceptive protection, and list its advantages and disadvantages compared with the combined oral contraceptive pill.

5. Iodine deficiency can cause hypothyroidism. Explain why the thyroid gland requires iodine and give two examples of other disorders that can cause hypothyroidism.

6. Briefly describe the histology of the adrenal glands.

7. List the physiological effects of adrenaline.

8. What is the role of progesterone in pregnancy?

9. What are the causes of excess ADH (vasopressin) secretion and what are the expected symptoms and signs in a patient presenting with this disorder?

10. Explain how the body acquires 1,25-dihydroxycholecalciferol.

11. Draw and label a diagram of a mature spermatozoon.

12. Discuss the neuroendocrine control of lactation.

13. Describe the endometrial changes that occur in the normal (28 day) menstrual cycle if fertilisation does not occur.

14. Write short notes on insulin-like growth factors (IGF).

15. List reasons for prescribing hormone replacement therapy (HRT) to women during and after the menopause.

16. Where is cholecystokinin (CCK) secreted and what are its effects on the gastrointestinal system?

17. What emergency treatment is required for a patient with diabetic ketoacidosis? Why is it important to monitor the plasma potassium levels during this treatment?

18. What is secondary hyperparathyroidism and how is it caused?

19. List five pathologies that may present with a scrotal mass and how it is possible to differentiate between them on examination.

20. What is 'negative feedback inhibition' in respect of control of hormone secretion? Draw a flow diagram to show the negative feedback inhibition involved in cortisol release.

You know the tedious phrase—'always READ the question through carefully'—it's so obvious but it's so easy to misread a question, or to go off at a tangent, and write about the wrong subject.

Essay Questions

1. Discuss the management of thyroid disease.

2. Outline the embryological development of the reproductive tract in both males and females, paying particular attention to the hormones involved.

3. Describe the control of insulin and glucagon secretion.

4. Briefly describe the biosynthetic pathway of cortisol in the adrenal cortex. Which enzyme is deficient in patients with congenital adrenal hyperplasia and what are the consequences of this condition?

5. Draw a diagram to show the changes in blood levels of LH and FSH during the menstrual cycle. Discuss how pituitary secretion of LH and FSH is related to the circulating concentrations of oestrogen and progesterone. How are these hormonal relationships changed when a woman is taking a combined oral contraceptive pill (or is pregnant)?

6. Describe how the combined pituitary test is used to evaluate pituitary hormone secretion. Draw a graph (hormones measured in arbitrary units) showing the expected result if the patient has a prolactinoma.

7. List the functions of the placenta. In what ways is the placenta well-adapted for these purposes?

8. Why is calcium homoeostasis important and how are its plasma concentrations controlled?

9. Outline the sequence of events in the development of spermatogonia to spermatozoa, and its hormonal control.

10. Draw diagrams showing how peptide and steroid hormones (e.g. ACTH and cortisol) act on their target cells and list the differences between them.

Before you start scribbling, always jot down a PLAN of your essay—it may seem to be a waste of exam time, but it allows you to structure your thoughts and the resultant essay will be more ordered (which makes the examiner think that you actually understand it).

Always use annotated DIAGRAMS AND GRAPHS wherever possible when answering short answer and essay questions—it is a quick way of presenting a large amount of information in a limited time.

1. (a) T, (b) T, (c) T, (d) T, (e) T
2. (a) T, (b) F, (c) F, (d) F, (e) T
3. (a) F, (b) T, (c) F, (d) F, (e) T
4. (a) T, (b) T, (c) T, (d) T, (e) T
5. (a) T, (b) T, (c) F, (d) F, (e) T
6. (a) F, (b) T, (c) T, (d) F, (e) F
7. (a) T, (b) F, (c) T, (d) T, (e) T
8. (a) F, (b) F, (c) F, (d) T, (e) T
9. (a) T, (b) T, (c) T, (d) F, (e) F
10. (a) F, (b) F, (c) F, (d) F, (e) F
11. (a) T, (b) F, (c) F, (d) F, (e) F
12. (a) T, (b) T, (c) T, (d) T, (e) T
13. (a) T, (b) T, (c) F, (d) T, (e) T
14. (a) F, (b) F, (c) F, (d) T, (e) T
15. (a) T, (b) T, (c) F, (d) T, (e) F
16. (a) F, (b) T, (c) F, (d) T, (e) T
17. (a) F, (b) T, (c) F, (d) T, (e) T
18. (a) F, (b) T, (c) F, (d) F, (e) T
19. (a) F, (b) F, (c) T, (d) T, (e) T
20. (a) T, (b) T, (c) F, (d) F, (e) F
21. (a) F, (b) T, (c) F, (d) T, (e) T
22. (a) T, (b) T, (c) T, (d) T, (e) F
23. (a) T, (b) T, (c) F, (d) F, (e) T
24. (a) F, (b) T, (c) T, (d) F, (e) T
25. (a) F, (b) F, (c) T, (d) F, (e) T

26. (a) F, (b) T, (c) T, (d) T, (e) T
27. (a) T, (b) F, (c) F, (d) T, (e) T
28. (a) T, (b) F, (c) F, (d) T, (e) F
29. (a) T, (b) T, (c) T, (d) T, (e) T
30. (a) F, (b) T, (c) T, (d) F, (e) F
31. (a) T, (b) T, (c) T, (d) T, (e) T
32. (a) T, (b) F, (c) T, (d) F, (e) T
33. (a) T, (b) F, (c) T, (d) T, (e) T
34. (a) T, (b) T, (c) T, (d) T, (e) T
35. (a) T, (b) F, (c) T, (d) T, (e) T
36. (a) T, (b) F, (c) F, (d) T, (e) T
37. (a) F, (b) T, (c) T, (d) F, (e) T
38. (a) T, (b) F, (c) F, (d) F, (e) T
39. (a) F, (b) T, (c) F, (d) F, (e) F
40. (a) T, (b) T, (c) F, (d) T, (e) F
41. (a) T, (b) T, (c) F, (d) T, (e) F
42. (a) T, (b) T, (c) T, (d) F, (e) T
43. (a) F, (b) T, (c) T, (d) F, (e) T
44. (a) T, (b) T, (c) F, (d) F, (e) F
45. (a) T, (b) F, (c) T, (d) F, (e) F
46. (a) F, (b) F, (c) F, (d) T, (e) F
47. (a) T, (b) F, (c) F, (d) T, (e) T
48. (a) T, (b) T, (c) F, (d) T, (e) F
49. (a) F, (b) T, (c) T, (d) T, (e) F
50. (a) F, (b) T, (c) T, (d) T, (e) F

1. Draw fully and label Fig. 1.7

   Hormone receptors that increase cAMP levels intracellularly include: receptors for GRH, CRH, dopamine, LH, FSH, TSH, hCG, ACTH, PTH, glucagon, VIP, vasopressin, prostalandins, adrenaline (α_2 receptor), somatostatin, and angiotensin II.

2. Pelvic inflammatory disease (PID) is infection of the fallopian tubes, ovaries, and pelvic peritoneum. It can be caused by:
   • Ascending infection from the genital tract caused by sexually transmitted disease, e.g. *Chlamydia trachomatis* or *Neisseria gonorrhoea.*
   • Direct infection from endogenous organisms in the vagina or gut, caused by trauma due to childbirth, surgical abortion, or insertion of a coil.
   • Blood-borne infection, e.g. tuberculosis.
   • Transperitoneal infection, e.g. from appendicitis.

   Symptoms include fever, pelvic pain, menorrhagia, dysmenorrhoea, vaginal discharge, and deep dyspareunia. If acute PID is unrecognised or inadequately treated it may become chronic. This may result in abscess formation, peritonitis, and septicaemia. Chronic inflammation causes fibrosis—adhesions develop between the pelvic organs and at the end of the fallopian tubes, resulting in tubal blockage. Complications include infertility and ectopic pregnancy.

3. Draw and annotate Fig. 2.5 (parts 1–4)

   1. The anterior pituitary gland develops from the ectoderm of the primitive oral cavity.
   2. An outgrowth, called Rathke's pouch, extends upwards until it meets the infundibulum (the outgrowth of the diencephalon that forms the posterior pituitary gland).
   3. The stalk of Rathke's pouch then regresses and the connection with the roof of the pharynx is lost. Occasionally nests of squamous cells are retained in this area and these can give rise to cysts or tumours that may secrete hormones.
   4. The regression of Rathke's stalk means that the anterior pituitary loses the blood and nerve supply from the oral cavity. It develops a very rich blood supply—pituitary arteries from the internal carotid artery, and portal veins from the hypothalamus grow down into it. It does not develop a direct neural link with the hypothalamus.

4. The progesterone-only pill does nto reliably suppress ovulation—it provides contraceptive protection by:
   • Inhibiting the changes in the cervical mucous that normally occur around ovulation so that the migration of sperm is reduced.
   • Increasing the rate of ovum transport so it reaches the endometrium before implantation can take place.
   • Inhibiting endometrial proliferation so that implantation does not occur.

Progestogen-only pill compared to combined pill	
Advantages	**Disadvantages**
• Contains no oestrogen, so there is no increased risk of thromboembolic disease, dyslipidaemia, hypertension • Can be taken during breastfeeding • Can be recommended to older women who smoke	• Less effective (especially in younger women) • Only a 3 hr leeway in which to take the pill • May cause irregular bleeding, breast discomfort, and symptoms of premenstrual tension • Increased risk of ectopic pregnancy

Fig. SAQ 4

5. The thyroid gland requires iodine to synthesize its hormones (thyroxine and tri-iodothyronine). Both these hormones are iodinated tyrosine derivatives—thyroxine contains four iodine molecules, tri-iodothyronine contains three. Iodine is actively pumped into the thyroid gland to supply it with sufficient quantities for hormone production.

   Hypothyroidism can be caused by autoimmune disease (Hashimoto's thyroiditis) or can result from previous treatment for thyrotoxicosis (iatrogenic hypothyroidism)—e.g. too much thyroid removed/damaged by surgery or antithyroid drugs.

6. The adrenal gland is divided into two developmentally distinct regions—the adrenal cortex and the adrenal medulla. The adrenal cortex is further divided into three layers—zona glomerulosa, zona fasciculata, zona reticularis.

   Draw and annotate Fig. 5.3 (no need to draw the individual cells but sketch the zones and make it obvious that some cells are arranged in clumps, others in cords, etc.)

7. Adrenaline is the hormone of 'fight or flight'. It prepares the body for increased mental and physical exertion. It has the following effects:
   1. Increases the blood supply to specific organs via its actions on the:
      - Heart—increases the heart rate and force of contractions.
      - Blood vessels—causes generalised vasoconstriction but vasodilates the arterioles to the muscles, lungs, and heart.
      - Kidney—increases renin release.
   2. Increases oxygen uptake in the lungs by stimulating ventilation and dilating the bronchioles.
   3. Increases plasma levels of substrates required for energy production via its actions in:
      - Liver—increases glycogenolysis.
      - Adipose tissue—increases lipolysis.
      - Pancreas—increases glucagon secretion, reduces insulin secretion.
   4. Increases the efficiency of skeletal muscle contractions.
   5. Increases heat loss (by stimulating sweating in the skin).
   6. Dilates the pupils.
   7. Stimulates the brain, causing increased alertness, agitation, and sensation of fear.

8. Progesterone induces secretory changes in the endometrium to prepare it for implantation. Progesterone secretion increases continually as pregnancy proceeds and is essential for its maintenance. During pregnancy progesterone has numerous important effects, including:
   - The prevention of miscarriage or premature labour—it inhibits prostaglandin secretion in the myometrium so that the uterine muscles do not contract and expel the foetus.
   - Metabolic changes that are required during pregnancy in order to supply the mother and the foetus with adequate nutrition—it stimulates appetite and promotes the storage of body fat.
   - The stimulation of respiration of so that the increased demand for oxygen and the removal of carbon dioxide are met. It sensitises the respiratory centre to carbon dioxide.

9. The syndrome of inappropriate ADH secretion (SIADH) is the name given to excessive vasopressin (ADH) secretion. SIADH can be caused by:
   - Ectopic secretion of ADH, e.g. bronchial carcinomas may secrete large amounts of ADH.
   - Excessive secretion of ADH from the pituitary due to drugs, trauma, infections, and other endocrine disorders (e.g. adrenal insufficiency).

   Clinical features range from asymptomatic to severe. Symptoms include nausea, vomiting, headache, apathy, and muscle weakness. If severe, SIADH may result in convulsions, coma, and death.
   Signs include hypertension, low plasma osmolality, hyponatraemia, but it does NOT cause oedema.

10. 1,25-dihydroxycholecalciferol is the active form of vitamin D. The inactive form (cholecalciferol) is acquired by the body from two sources:
    - 90% is synthesized by photo-isomerization in the skin under the influence of ultraviolet light. The isomer produced is vitamin D_3.
    - The remaining 10% is acquired from the diet. The main sources of dietary vitamin D are fish and eggs. The absorbed form is vitamin D_2.

    Vitamin D_2 and vitamin D_3 are activated into 1,25-dihydroxycholecalciferol. This occurs in the liver and kidney by the enzymes 25 hydroxylase and 1∝-hydroxylase. Parathyroid hormone stimulates the synthesis of 1∝-hydroxylase in the kidney.
    Draw and annotate Fig. 8.5.

11. Draw and label Fig. 10.18

12. Draw and annotate Fig. 11.12.
    The 'suckling reflex' ensures adequate milk production during lactation. The nipples are stimulated during suckling, and this stimulus is conveyed to the hypothalamus via neural pathways and alters the secretion of prolactin and oxytocin. Prolactin initiates the production of milk in the alveolar cells once the plasma oestrogen levels decline after pregnancy. Oxytoxin is secreted by the posterior pituitary gland, and stimulates milk ejection. Suckling stimulates further prolactin and oxytocin secretion, resulting in more milk secretion. Hence lactation is maintained by frequent suckling via a positive feedback loop mechanism.

13. Draw the changes that occur to endometrium during the menstrual cycle from Fig 10.14 and explain that there are three phases to the endometrial cycle:
    1. Menstrual phase (days 1–4)—the surface epithelium and the stratum functionale become necrotic and are shed via the vagina. Clotting is inhibited and torn veins continue to seep blood for approximately 5 days.
    2. Proliferative phase (days 4–13)—stromal and epithelial cells proliferate in the stratum basale to replenish the stratum functionale (under the influence of oestrogens) and spiral arteries extend into it. Glandular epithelium migrates to cover the surface of the endometrium.
    3. Secretory phase (days 14–28)—endometrial glands enlarge (under the influence of progesterone), become corkscrew shaped and secrete a mucoid fluid that is rich in glycogen. The endometrium thickens and becomes oedematous. The spiral arteries lengthen.

    Towards the end of the secretory phase, the spiral arteries contract periodically. This restricts the blood flow to the surface epithelium and stratum functionale and they become ischaemic.

14. IGFs are peptide hormones that stimulate the growth of soft tissues and bones. They are called insulin-like growth factors because they have a similar structure to pro-insulin and can bind to insulin receptors as well as their own receptors. They are synthesized by many different cell types, but mainly in the liver and fibroblasts.

They exist as two forms, IGF-1 and IGF-2. Their secretion is stimulated by growth hormone (GH) from the pituitary gland. IGF mediate the action of GH (IGF are also called somatomedins because they mediate the effect of GH). Plasma levels of IGF are constant in the adult but during development the levels are higher (peak levels are at 12–17 years of age).

Both forms of IGF act on the G1 phase of the cell cycle. They promote growth and differentiation in bone, muscle, and adipose cells. They stimulate chondrocyte proliferation in bone, protein synthesis in muscle, and lipolysis in adipose tissue. IGF-1 induces cell division in cells that have already differentiated (clonal expansion), but the function of IGF-2 is unknown. IGF-1 plasma levels correlate with increases in body size, IGF-2 plasma levels correlate with height velocity.

15. HRT preparations are prescribed during and after the menopause to:
- Treat acute menopausal symptoms (e.g. hot flushes, sweating).
- Protect against the long-term complications of menopause (e.g. osteoporosis and cardiovascular disease).
- Treat dyspareunia, vaginal discomfort/dryness, and recurrent vaginal infections.
- Treat menopause-related depression.
- Treat prolonged and irregular vaginal bleeding (if no other cause is found).
- Reduce urinary symptoms (e.g. frequency, urgency) caused by atrophy of the lower urinary tract.
- Protect against loss of collagen which weakens the pelvic ligaments, joint ligaments, muscles, and skin elasticity—i.e. it helps prevent uterovaginal prolapse, immobility, muscle weakness, and wrinkling.

16. CCK is secreted by I-cells in the lining of the duodenum. It has four main actions on the gastrointestinal system:
- It stimulates pancreatic enzyme secretion.
- It causes the gall bladder to contract.
- It enhances the effects of the hormone secretion.
- It may contribute to saiety (via its effect in the hypothalamus).

17. First assess the patient—he or she will be dehydrated and hyperglycaemic. Dehydration is more life-threatening than hyperglycaemia and should be corrected as a priority. Intravenous isotonic saline is given to rehydrate the patient. Low dose insulin is administered intravenously to correct the hyperglycaemia.

It is important to monitor plasma potassium levels because insulin treatment causes the cells to take up glucose, and as they do so potassium enters along with it. Hence the danger is hypokalaemia which may cause cardiac arrhythmias. If hypokalaemia develops it may be necessary to administer intravenous potassium.

18. Secondary hyperparathyroidism is a disorder where parathyroid hormone secretion is elevated because the calcium levels in the blood are persistently low.

Persistent hypocalcaemia (and hence secondary hyperparathyroidism) can be caused by:
- Calcium malabsorption (e.g. due to vitamin D deficiency, or to coeliac disease).
- Renal failure (due to failure of vitamin D activation in the kidney). This disorder is otherwise known as renal osteodystrophy because the bones become painful and susceptible to fractures.

19. Inguinoscrotal hernia, testicular tumour, hydrocoele, varicocoele, epididymal cyst.
- A mass caused by an inguinoscrotal hernia arises in the abdomen so you cannot feel above the mass in the scrotum, and it may be reducible or tender.
- A mass that is solid and feels to be part of the testis is likely to be a testicular tumour.
- A mass caused by a hydrocoele is cystic (i.e. translucent when a light is shined through it) and surrounds the testis (i.e. is not part of the testis).
- A mass caused by a variocoele lies above the testis, feels like a 'bag of worms' and often reduces when the patient lies flat.
- A mass caused by an epididymal cyst is small, firm, cystic, and lies within the epididymis (i.e. it feels separate from the testis).

20. Negative feedback inhibition is where the presence or effects of a hormone in the circulation act back on the cells that secrete the hormone to prevent further secretion.

Draw and fully label Fig. 5.7. Annotate the diagram to show that the negative feedback is:
- Mainly at the hypothalamus and the higher centres of the brain (not much at the pituitary gland).
- More effective in the evening (which causes plasma cortisol levels to be lower in the evening and higher in the morning).

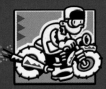

Index

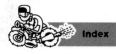

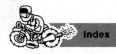